Medical Imaging: A Case-Based Approach

Medical Imaging: A Case-Based Approach

Editor: Gracie McKinley

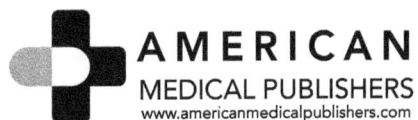

AMERICAN
MEDICAL PUBLISHERS
www.americanmedicalpublishers.com

AMERICAN
MEDICAL PUBLISHERS
www.americanmedicalpublishers.com

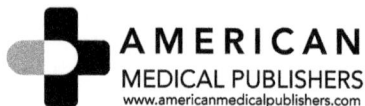

Cataloging-in-Publication Data

Medical imaging : a case-based approach / edited by Gracie McKinley.
    p. cm.
Includes bibliographical references and index.
ISBN 978-1-63927-075-0
1. Diagnostic imaging. 2. Imaging systems in medicine. 3. Radiography, Medical. I. McKinley, Gracie.
RC78.7.D53 M43 2022
616.075 4--dc23

American Medical Publishers,
41 Flatbush Avenue,
1st Floor, New York,
NY 11217, USA

ISBN 978-1-63927-075-0 (Hardback)

Contents

Preface

I am honored to present to you this unique book which encompasses the most up-to-date data in the field. I was extremely pleased to get this opportunity of editing the work of experts from across the globe. I have also written papers in this field and researched the various aspects revolving around the progress of the discipline. I have tried to unify my knowledge along with that of stalwarts from every corner of the world, to produce a text which not only benefits the readers but also facilitates the growth of the field.

Medical imaging is a technique used to create the visual pictures of the interior of a body. It is used for clinical analysis, medical intervention and also involves a visual representation of the function of some organs and tissues. Medical imaging establishes a database of normal anatomy and physiology to make it possible to identify abnormalities and helps in diagnosing and treating a disease. As it is a part of biological imaging, it includes radiology which uses the imaging technologies of X-ray radiography, tactile imaging, thermography, ultrasonography, endoscopy, elastography, magnetic resonance imaging, etc. Medical imaging is primarily used in clinical trials as a tool to enable rapid diagnosis with visualization and quantitative assessment. This book aims to shed light on some of the unexplored aspects of medical imaging and the recent researches in this field. It presents researches and studies performed by experts across the globe. The extensive content of this book provides the readers with a thorough understanding of the subject.

Finally, I would like to thank all the contributing authors for their valuable time and contributions. This book would not have been possible without their efforts. I would also like to thank my friends and family for their constant support.

Editor

Small average differences in attenuation corrected images between men and women in myocardial perfusion scintigraphy

Elin Trägårdh[1*], Karl Sjöstrand[2], David Jakobsson[1] and Lars Edenbrandt[1]

Abstract

Background: The American Society of Nuclear Cardiology and the Society of Nuclear Medicine state that incorporation of attenuation-corrected (AC) images in myocardial perfusion scintigraphy (MPS) will improve image quality, interpretive certainty, and diagnostic accuracy. However, commonly used software packages for MPS usually include normal stress databases for non-attenuation corrected (NC) images but not for attenuation-corrected (AC) images. The aim of the study was to develop and compare different normal stress databases for MPS in relation to NC vs. AC images, male vs. female gender, and presence vs. absence of obesity. The principal hypothesis was that differences in mean count values between men and women would be smaller with AC than NC images, thereby allowing for construction and use of gender-independent AC stress database.

Methods: Normal stress perfusion databases were developed with data from 126 male and 205 female patients with normal MPS. The following comparisons were performed for all patients and separately for normal weight vs. obese patients: men vs. women for AC; men vs. women for NC; AC vs. NC for men; and AC vs. NC for women.

Results: When comparing AC for men vs. women, only minor differences in mean count values were observed, and there were no differences for normal weight vs. obese patients. For all other analyses major differences were found, particularly for the inferior wall.

Conclusions: The results support the hypothesis that it is possible to use not only gender independent but also weight independent AC stress databases.

Background

Stress myocardial perfusion scintigraphy (MPS) is widely regarded as a clinically useful noninvasive imaging modality for diagnosing patients with suspected coronary artery disease [1-3]. However, Compton scatter and depth-dependent reduction of spatial resolution degrade MPS image quality and decrease test accuracy. In addition, localized soft-tissue attenuation by the breasts, lateral chest wall, and abdomen may create artefacts that mimic true perfusion abnormalities and decrease test specificity [4,5].

Several studies have reported an increase in the diagnostic accuracy (through higher specificity) for the detection of coronary artery disease when MPS is attenuation corrected (AC) [6-12]. The American Society of Nuclear Cardiology and the Society of Nuclear Medicine conclude in their joint position statement from 2004 [6] that incorporation of AC in addition to ECG gating with MPS images will improve image quality, interpretive certainty, and diagnostic accuracy. These combined results are anticipated to have a substantial impact on improving the effectiveness of care and lowering health care costs. However, commonly used software packages for MPS usually only include a normal stress database for non-attenuation corrected (NC) images.

* Correspondence: elin.tragardh@med.lu.se
[1]Clinical Physiology and Nuclear Medicine Unit, Skåne University Hospital, Lund University, Malmö, Sweden
Full list of author information is available at the end of the article

The three most commonly used software packages for viewing and quantifying MPS are Emory Cardiac Toolbox (Emory University), 4D-MSPECT (Invia Medical Imaging Solutions) and Quantitative Perfusion SPECT (Cedars Sinai). The Emory Cardiac Toolbox uses 3 populations for generating a normal database [13]: (1) a normal group of 30 patients with a low likelihood of coronary artery disease; (2) a criteria group of 60 patients with different perfusion abnormalities; and (3) a prospective validation group of 60 patients. This is done for both male and female patients. A second step is used to calibrate regionally how many standard deviations below the mean best separate normal from hypoperfused segments. The 4D-MSPECT uses a normal database comprising patients with a low pretest likelihood of coronary artery disease [14]. The database has more than 40 patient studies. The Quantitative Perfusion SPECT software also creates normal limits by use of low likelihood patients [15].

The aim of the present study was to develop and compare different normal stress databases for MPS with respect to both NC and AC images and with respect to both gender and the presence vs. absence of obesity. The principal hypothesis was that AC images show smaller differences between men and women compared with NC images, thus allowing for a gender independent AC normal stress database. Previous studies with the same aim [16-18] have all used a different technique than the one described herein for selecting the patients for the normal stress database. Our approach is most applicable to hospitals desiring to create normal stress databases for MPS that are optimized to their own patient populations.

Methods
Study population
Patients who underwent 99mTc MPS at Skåne University Hospital in Malmö, Sweden, in 2008, for suspected coronary artery disease or for the management of known coronary artery disease, were considered for inclusion. The study was approved (# 647/2008) by the ethics committee on human research at Lund University, Sweden, and complies with the Declaration of Helsinki. The normal population was found using the following steps:

1) Patients were included if they had a normal test result, meaning neither fixed nor reversible perfusion defects, normal ejection fraction ($\geq$ 60% for women, $\geq$ 55% for men) and normal end diastolic volume ($\leq$ 132 ml for women, $\leq$ 181 ml for men) [19] based on the final report according to clinical routine. Both NC and AC images were used for interpretation. The physicians who interpreted the images had

access to all patient history and exercise protocol, but were not aware that the patients might be included in a study. The EXINI heart™ (EXINI Diagnostics AB, Lund, Sweden) software package was used for interpretation [20]. This software displays MPS images, quantifies perfusion defects and cardiac function, and gives diagnostic advice based on artificial neural networks.

2) From the group with normal findings in step 1, patients with documented diabetes, coronary artery disease, previous myocardial infarction, previous revascularization, electrocardiographic signs of myocardial infarction (based on computer interpretation), presence of pre-excitation, paced rhythms and left bundle branch block were excluded. After this, 131 men and 213 women were included.
3) Bull's eye plots for these patients were created, and obvious 'non-normal' patients were excluded (5 men and 8 women). Finally, 126 men and 205 women were included in the study group. These patients were further divided into one group of normal weight and one group of obese (body mass index (BMI) > 30 kg/m^2) patients.

MPS
The MPS studies were performed using a 2-day gated stress/non-gated rest Tc-99m-tetrofosmin protocol, starting with injection of 600 MBq Tc-99m-tetrofosmin at stress. Patients were stressed using either maximal exercise on an ergometer or pharmacological test with adenosine. The exercise was continued for at least 1 min after the injection of the tracer and the adenosine infusion at least 2 min after the injection of the tracer. Normal findings at stress were not followed by a rest study. Not definitely normal stress studies were followed by a rest study with injection of 600 MBq Tc-99m-tetrofosmin.

Stress and rest acquisition began about 60 min after the end of the injection of Tc-99m-tetrofosmin. Images were obtained according to established clinical protocols, using SPECT over 180° elliptical, autocontour rotations from the 45° right anterior oblique position, with a dual-head gamma camera, e.cam (Siemens AG Medical Solutions, Erlangen, Germany). Patients were imaged in the supine position. Low energy high-resolution collimator and a zoom factor of 1.0 were used with 64 (32 views per camera) projections in a 128 × 128 matrix and an acquisition time of 25 s per projection. Stress images were gated to the electrocardiogram using 8 frames per cardiac cycle. No automatic motion-correction program was applied; instead the acquisition was repeated if motion was detected. This was decided by the physician in charge of the study, based on qualitative criteria. Tomographic reconstruction and calculation of short and long axis slice images were performed using e. soft (Siemens AG Medical Solutions, Erlangen, Germany). NC images were reconstructed with filtered back-projection. A 2D Butterworth pre-reconstruction filter was used with clinical frequency of 0.45, order 5. AC images were reconstructed with an iterative algorithm, 6 iterations [21] where a ramp filter was applied on the error projection prior to backprojection. A Butterworth filter with a clinical frequency of 0.40, order 5, was applied for regularization. Attenuation maps were generated from simultaneous transmission measurement using a Gd-153 multiple-line source (Siemens AG Medical Solutions, Erlangen, Germany) [22]. The cut-off frequencies of the filters were selected so that the noise level in the AC images was similar to that in the NC images.

Image processing
Normal stress perfusion databases were developed as follows: Each normal stress map was scaled such that its median value, in the region or regions including the 10% pixels with highest count values was made equal. This normalization makes the stress data equal in a region that is likely to show the most normal perfusion.

Statistical analysis
The comparison method consisted both of a pixel-by-pixel analysis and a segmental analysis. The following tests were carried out for all patients, for patients with normal weight, and for obese patients: NC men vs. NC women; AC men vs. AC women; NC men vs. AC men; and NC women vs. AC women. For all patients, also NC normal weight vs. NC obese; and AC normal weight vs. AC obese were carried out. For all women and all men, the following tests were carried out: NC normal weight vs. NC obsese; and AC normal weight vs. AC obese. Groups where compared using two-sample t-tests for men vs. women comparisons, and paired t-tests for AC vs. NC comparisons. The level of statistical significance was set at $\alpha = 0.001$. The database images are of size 65-by-65 pixels yielding a total of 4225 tests for each comparison. Due to random components in the images such as noise, many of these tests may be rejected also when the null hypothesis (no difference) is true everywhere. To adjust for this effect a non-parametric permutation scheme outlined in [23] was employed. The method proceeds by computing pixelwise differences between groups when the group assignment for the images is perturbed. For such datasets, one does not expect significant differences, and we record the maximal absolute t-value as a measure of the most extreme outcome given no differences. This procedure is repeated many times (here, 500), yielding an empirical distribution of maximal t-values. The original (unperturbed) t-value image is then thresholded at the t-value corresponding to the $100*(1 - \alpha)$th percentile of the maximal t-value distribution. This procedure provably maintains strong control over type-I errors, meaning that the probability of declaring a difference at any pixel when in fact there is none is at most α. Furthermore, the probability of falsely declaring a difference at a specific pixel, regardless of any true difference elsewhere, is at most α.

The area for the different segments was created in the following way: The apical segment was delineated from apex to 30% of the distance to the base. The rest of the area was divided into four equally sized areas: lateral, inferior, septal and anterior, without overlap. The most basal 10% were not included into the segmental analysis in order to avoid differences in perfusion pattern due to differences in the basal delineation of the left ventricle.

Results
Description of patients
For the 205 women, mean age was 59 years (ranging from 29 to 87 years). For the 126 men, mean age was 56 years (ranging from 27 to 86 years). Forty (40) women were regarded as obese (mean BMI 34.0 kg/m^2) and 165 women had normal body weight (mean BMI 24.6 kg/m^2). For men, 24 were obese (mean BMI 33.1 kg/m^2) and 102 had normal weight (mean BMI 25.5 kg/m^2).

All patients
Figure 1 shows the normal stress data base for AC men, AC women, NC men and NC women, respectively. Included also are the areas with a significant difference (green or yellow) in mean counts. In the AC databases, when comparing men and women, only very small areas of the bull's eye plot show a statistically significant difference, whereas there were large areas of significant differences within the other groups tested. When comparing women within the NC and AC databases, the largest difference in mean counts was found in the inferior wall (lower in the NC group). The same result was found in men. For men and women in the NC group, men showed lower mean counts in the inferior wall. When comparing men and women in the AC group, the largest differences were found in small areas in the apex and lateral wall. Table 1 shows differences in mean count values (± 2 standard deviations), from a scale ranging from -100 to 100 (0 meaning no difference), in different groups for different segments.

Patients divided into groups based on BMI
Figure 2 shows the normal stress databases and the statistically significant differences between them, when

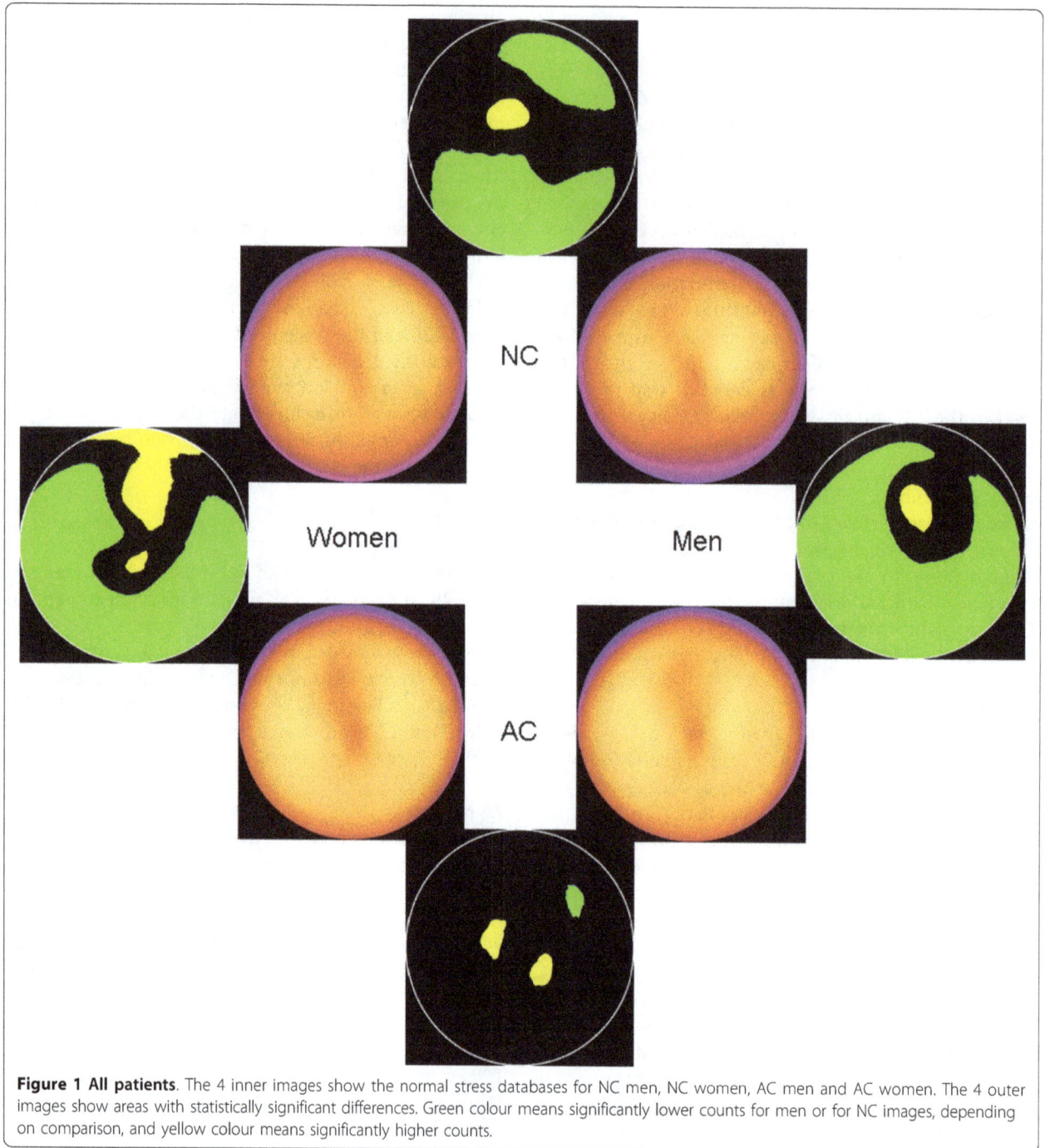

Figure 1 All patients. The 4 inner images show the normal stress databases for NC men, NC women, AC men and AC women. The 4 outer images show areas with statistically significant differences. Green colour means significantly lower counts for men or for NC images, depending on comparison, and yellow colour means significantly higher counts.

only including patients with BMI < 30 kg/m². In the AC database, when comparing men and women, no statistically significant differences were found. When comparing NC women with AC women, mean counts were lower in the NC women in the basal inferolateral wall. For the other groups (NC women vs. NC men and NC men vs. AC men) differences were found in the inferior wall.

Figure 3 shows the normal stress databases and the significant differences between them, for patients with BMI > 30 kg/m². Also for these patients, no statistically significant differences were found when comparing mean counts between AC women and AC men. For all other analyses (NC women vs. AC women, NC men vs. AC women, NC women vs. NC men), there were significant differences in the inferior wall.

Table 1 Differences in mean count values (± 2 standard deviations), from a scale ranging from -100 to 100 (0 meaning no difference), in different groups for different segments

	Women (NC/AC)	Men (NC/AC)	NC (Women/Men)	AC (Women/Men)
Apical	1.5 (± 3.9)	1.0 (± 6.2)	2.1 (± 6.6)	2.1 (± 2.4)
Lateral	-3.9 (± 8.5)	-4.1 (± 9.6)	-1.6 (± 4.0)	-2.1 (± 3.3)
Inferior	-7.4 (± 8.4)	-14.0 (± 7.5)	-6.6 (± 4.4)	-0.6 (± 3.5)
Septal	-5.9 (± 5.0)	-7.6 (± 7.5)	-0.7 (± 6.4)	0.5 (± 3.2)
Anterior	2.4 (± 6.0)	0.4 (± 7.1)	-1.6 (± 6.3)	-0.2 (± 4.0)

When comparing NC normal weight men with NC obese men, no statistically significant differences was found. This was also true when comparing AC normal weight men with AC obese men, and AC normal weight women with AC obese women. When comparing NC normal weight women with NC obese women, 0.1% of the total area (inferoseptal, midventricular wall) had statistically different mean count values between the groups (data not shown). When instead dividing all patients into groups of NC normal weight, NC obese, AC normal weight and AC obese (no gender separation) we found significant differences between NC normal weight and NC obese individuals, but no differences between AC normal weight and AC obese individuals (Figure 4).

Discussion

We compared NC and AC normal stress databases for men and women and demonstrated that there were significant differences in mean counts in large areas of the left ventricle when comparing NC men and NC women, as well as when comparing NC men and AC men, and NC women and AC women. The differences were much smaller when comparing AC men and AC women. No significant differences were found when comparing AC normal weight and AC obese individuals, whereas there were significant differences when comparing NC normal weight and NC obese individuals. Thus, we have demonstrated that AC eliminates the differences between gender and body weight, which supports the hypothesis that it is possible to use a gender independent and body weight independent AC stress database. Use of such a database would be favourable because only one stress database therefore becomes necessary and nuclear cardiologists need not learn to distinguish between different possible attenuation artefacts.

The reason for the small areas of statistical difference between AC men and AC women (all patients), compared to no statistical difference when comparing AC men and AC women (normal weight patients and obese patients) was probably due to the first comparison being

less susceptible to type-II statistical error given the larger number of individuals involved.

A previous study by Grossman et al [16] investigated the accuracy of an AC database quantification program for the detection and localization of coronary artery disease and evaluated its application to a heavy patient population as compared with standard uncorrected methods. They found no statistically significant differences when comparing AC perfusion distributions of normal men and women, whereas significant differences were found in the same NC studies. They also found that AC improved quantitative analysis, yielding a significantly higher normalcy rate and specificity without a significant loss in sensitivity, even in an obese patient population. In their study, only 26 men and 22 women were included in the normal group (compared to 126 men and 205 women in our study). They also did not perform any studies on the differences between overweight patients and patients with normal weight for the normal stress database. Previous studies by Ficaro et al [17] and Slomka et al [18] also included a lower number of patients in the normal stress database (20 men and 20 women; 50 men and 50 women, respectively). Ficaro et al [17] found no significant differences between the male and female AC distributions, whereas Slomka et al [18] noted some gender differences for the AC normal database. Slomka et al [18] also investigated body mass index-specific normal limits, and found no significant differences between normal studies of low-BMI and high-BMI patients for either the AC or NC data set. None of these previous studies have used a pixel-by-pixel analysis, but instead only examined segmental differences in the 17-segment model.

The pre-installed databases of normal values in commercial software programs are generally based on the results obtained in a U.S. population, and may not be optimal for assessing a population form another country. It has previously been shown that there are major differences between US and Japanese normal databases in nuclear cardiology [24], particularly in the apex and in the anterior wall in females and in the inferior wall in males. Similar results have been found in a Chinese [25] as well as a Spanish population [26]. We believe that in an ideal situation, every clinic should create its own normal stress database, instead of using the ones offered by the company providing the imaging evaluation software. Different cameras with different techniques used (for example filtered backward projection or iterative reconstruction) produce images that may not be directly comparable to the normal stress database included in the software nor to the distribution of body habitus in the population. Creating normal databases, however, consumes time and resources. Properly implemented AC methods should remove differences in the normal

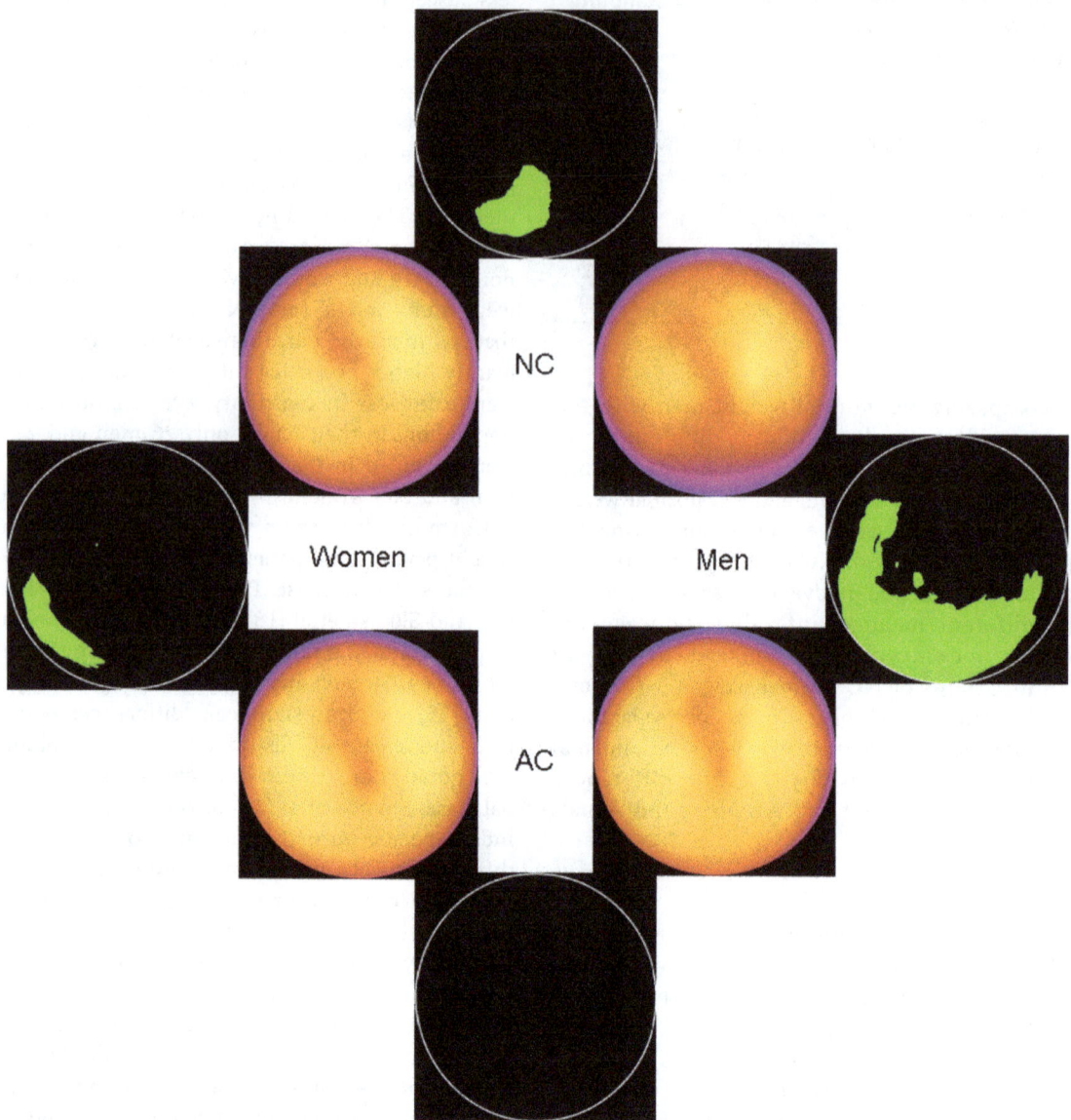

Figure 2 **Patients with normal weight**. The 4 inner images show the normal stress databases for NC men, NC women, AC men and AC women. The 4 outer images show areas with statistically significant differences. Green colour means significantly lower counts for men or for NC images, depending on comparison, and yellow colour means significantly higher counts. There are no significant differences between AC men and AC women (bottom black circle).

perfusion distribution that are due to variations in body habitus including gender, as shown in the present paper. For clinics using AC methods, a gender independent and body-weight independent stress database is easier to create than to produce separate databases for male and female subjects with different weights.

In this study a Gd-153 transmission source was used for attenuation correction. In the computed tomography - single photon emission computed tomography hybrid devices, computed tomography-based correction may perform differently than a radionuclide-source correction. We believe that methods for attenuation correction other than

Gd-153 also will also reduce the influence on gender and body habitus on MPS images, as indicated by other studies [13-15], but when a different technique is used, it is probably necessary to create a new normal stress database.

Further studies are needed to evaluate the accuracy of the image interpretation when using a gender- and body weight independent normal stress database such as the one described herein.

Study limitations
One study limitation is that the included individuals were not a random sample from the healthy population, but

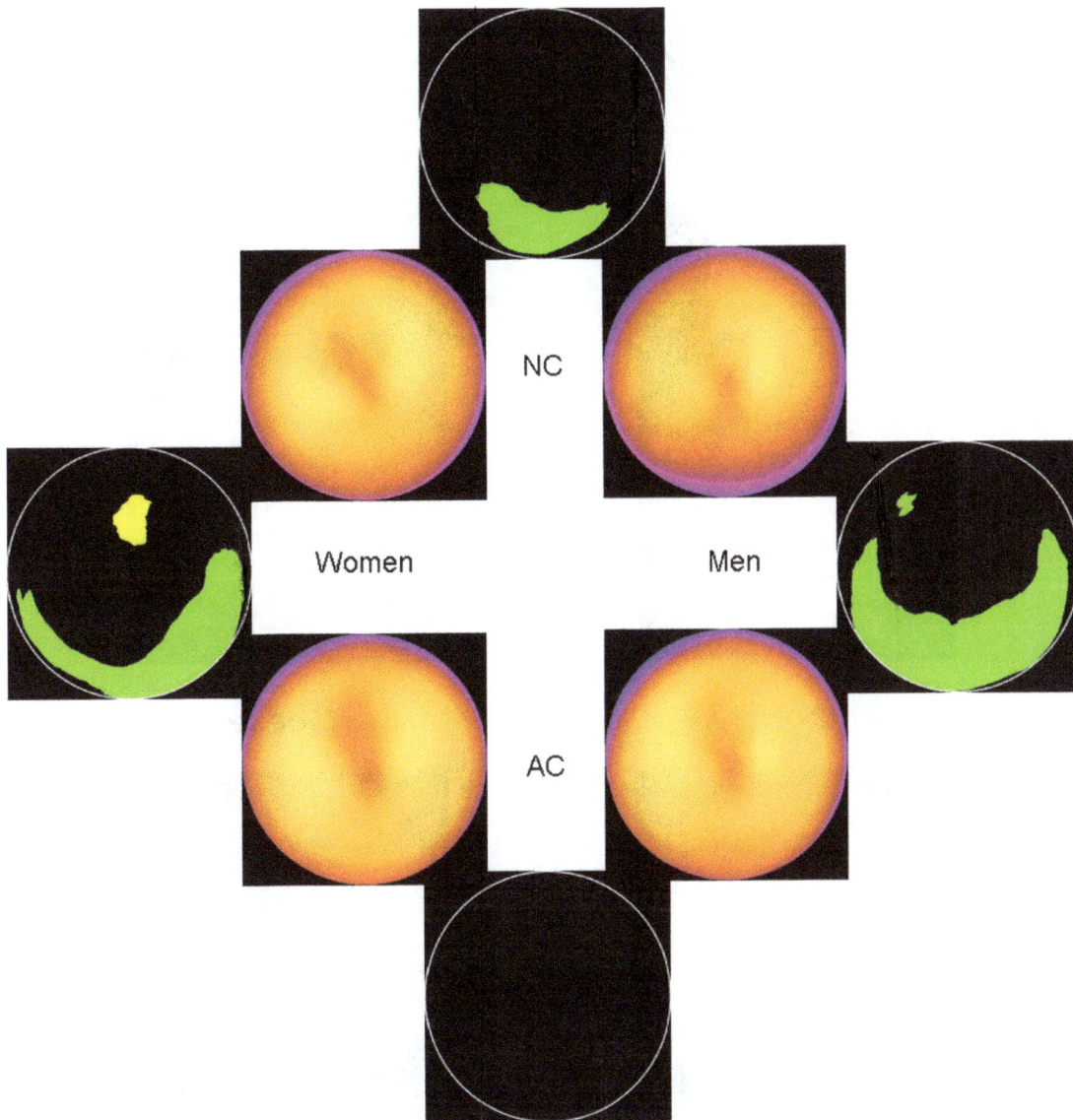

Figure 3 Obese patients. The 4 inner images show the normal stress databases for NC men, NC women, AC men and AC women. The 4 outer images show areas with statistically significant differences. Green colour means significantly lower counts for men or for NC images, depending on comparison, and yellow colour means significantly higher counts. There are no significant differences between AC men and AC women (bottom black circle).

instead "healthy patients". Another limitation is that the number of obese patients was low compared to patients with normal weight. For the selection of the normal population, only MPS was used and not any other imaging modality. If coronary angiography was used to select normal patients, patients with a "non-normal" MPS, but a normal coronary angiography, could have been included in the normal database. It might be that "pseudo-pathological" MPS are excluded from our study, which ought to be included. However, if we had required a normal coronary angiogram for inclusion, patients with microvascular disease might have been included in the normal MPS stress database, which would have been equally problematic.

Conclusion

In conclusion, differences in mean counts when comparing men and women in the AC group were much smaller than when comparing the other groups; no differences were found in this group when dividing patients according to body weight. The results support the hypothesis that it is possible to use gender independent and body weight independent AC stress databases. Use of such databases would be favourable because only

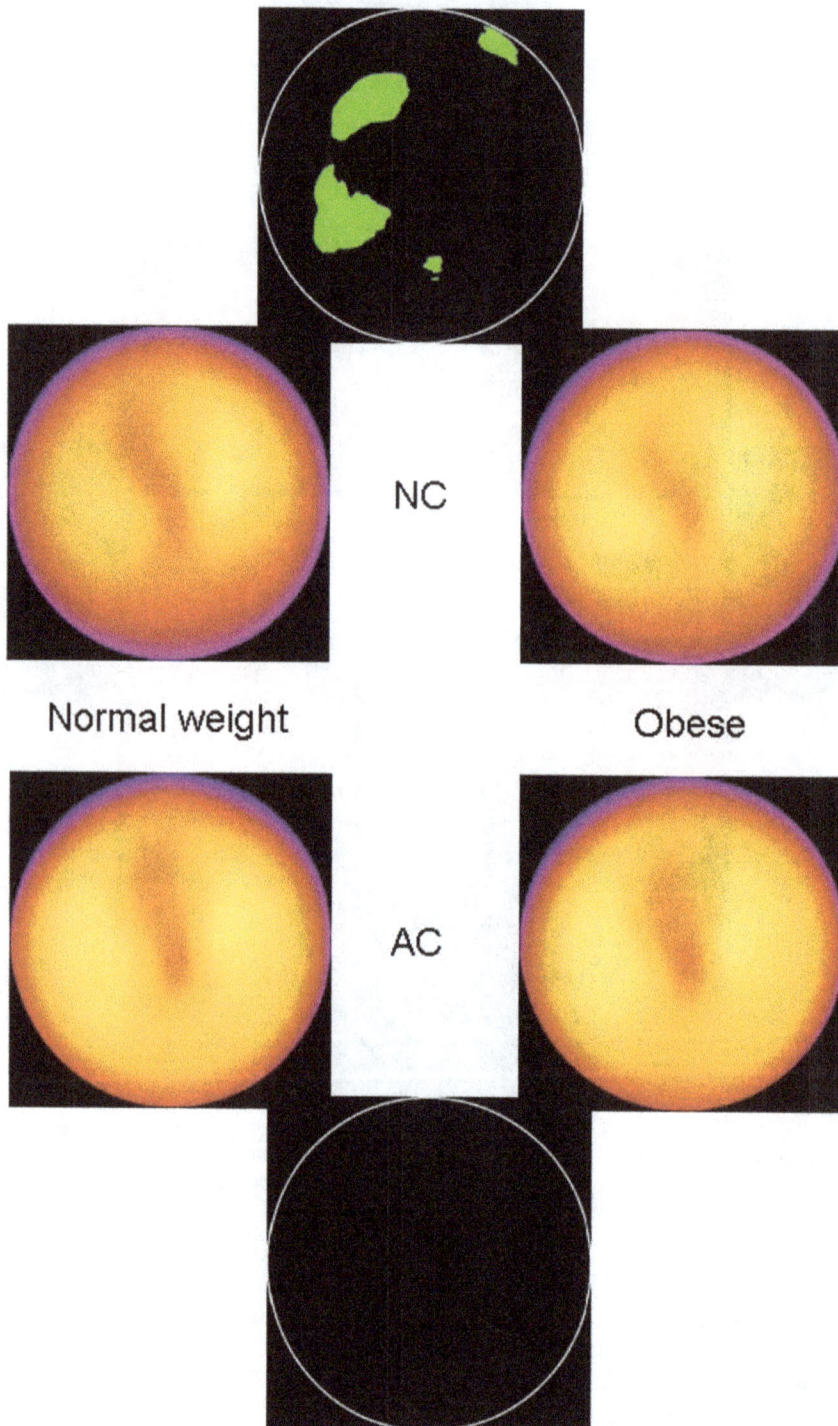

Figure 4 All patients. The 4 inner images show the normal stress databases for NC normal weight individuals, NC overweight individuals, AC normal weight individuals and AC overweight individuals. The 2 outer images show areas with statistically significant differences. There are no significant differences between AC normal weight and AC overweight individuals (bottom black circle).

one database therefore becomes necessary and nuclear cardiologists need not learn to distinguish between different possible attenuation artefacts.

List of Abbreviations Used

AC: attenuation-corrected; BMI: body mass index; MPS: myocardial perfusion scintigraphy; NC: non-attenuation-corrected

Acknowledgements

This study was supported by the Medical Faculty at Lund University.

Author details

[1]Clinical Physiology and Nuclear Medicine Unit, Skåne University Hospital, Lund University, Malmö, Sweden. [2]Informatics and Mathematical Modeling, Technical University of Denmark, Copenhagen, Denmark.

Authors' contributions

ET participated in the design of the study, the selection of patients and drafted the manuscript. KS and DJ performed the statistical analyses, image processing and helped in drafting the manuscript. LE participated in the design of the study and helped in drafting the manuscript. All authors read and approved the final manuscript.

Declaration of Competing interests

LE, KS and DJ are employed by and stockholders of EXINI Diagnostics, Lund, Sweden.

References

1. Hachamovitch R, Berman DS, Kiat H, Cohen I, Cabico JA, Friedman J, Diamond GA: Exercise myocardial perfusion SPECT in patients without known coronary artery disease. *Circulation* 1996, 93:905-914.
2. Hachamovitch R, Berman DS, Shaw LJ, Kiat H, Cohen I, Cabico JA, Friedman J, Diamond GA: Incremental prognostic value of myocardial perfusion single photon emission computed tomography for the prediction of cardiac death. *Circulation* 1998, 97:535-543.
3. Iskander S, Iskandrian AE: Risk assessment using single photon emission computed tomography technetium-99m-sestamibi imaging. *J Am Coll Cardiol* 1998, 32:57-62.
4. DePuey EG, Garcia EV: Optimal specificity of thallium-201 SPECT through recognition of imaging artefacts. *J Nucl Med* 1989, 30:441-449.
5. Corbett JR, Ficaro EP: Clinical review of attenuation-corrected cardiac SPECT. *J Nucl Cardiol* 1999, 6:54-68.
6. Heller GV, Links J, Bateman TM, Ziffer JA, Ficaro E, Cohen MC, Hendel RC: American Society of Nuclear Cardiology and Society of Nuclear Medicine joint position statement: attenuation correction of myocardial perfusion SPECT scintigraphy. *J Nucl Cardiol* 2004, 11:229-230.
7. Gallowitsch HJ, Sykora J, Mikosch P, Kresnik E, Unterweger O, Molnar M, Grimm G, Lind P: Attenuation-corrected thallium-201 single-photon emission tomography using a gadolinium-153 moving line source: clinical value and the impact of attenuation correction on the extent and severity of perfusion abnormalities. *Eur J Nucl Med* 1998, 25:220-228.
8. Hendel RC, Merman DS, Cullom SJ, Follansbee W, Heller GV, Kiat H, Groch MW, Mahmarian JJ: Multicenter clinical trial to evaluate the efficacy of correction for photon attenuation and scatter in SPECT myocardial perfusion imaging. *Circulation* 1999, 99:2742-2749.
9. Links JM, Becker LC, Rigo P, Taillefer R, Hanelin L, Anstett F, Burckhardt D, Mixon L: Combined corrections for attenuation, depth-dependent blur, and motion in cardiac SPECT: a multicenter trial. *J Nucl Cardiol* 2000, 7:414-425.
10. Links JM, DePueyo EG, Taillefer R, Becker LC: Attenuation correction and gating synergistically improve the diagnostic accuracy of myocardial perfusion SPECT. *J Nucl Cardiol* 2002, 9:183-187.
11. Thompson RC, Heller GV, Johnson LL, Case JA, Cullom SJ, Garcia EV, Jones PG, Moutray KL, Bateman TM: Value of attenuation correction on ECG-gated SPECT myocardial perfusion imaging related to body mass index. *J Nucl Cardiol* 2005, 12:195-202.
12. Masood Y, Liu YH, Depuey G, Taillefer R, Araujo LI, Allen S, Delbeke D, Anstett F, Peretz A, Zito MJ, Tsatkin V, Wackers FJ: Clinical validation of SPECT attenuation correction using x-ray computed tomography-derived attenuation maps: multi-center clinical trial with angiographic correlation. *J Nucl Cardiol* 2005, 12:676-686.
13. Garcia EV, Faber TL, Cooke CD, Folks RD, Chen J, Santana C: The increasing role of quantification in clinical nuclear cardiology: The Emory approach. *J Nucl Cardiol* 2007, 14:420-432.
14. Ficaro EP, Lee BC, Kritzman JN, Corbett JR: Corridor4DM: The Michigan method for quantitative nuclear cardiology. *J Nucl Cardiol* 2007, 14:455-465.
15. Germano G, Kavanagh PB, Slomka PJ, Van Kriekinge SD, Pollard G, Berman DS: Quantititation in gated perfusion SPECT imaging: The Cedars-Sinai approach. *J Nucl Cardiol* 2007, 14:433-454.
16. Grossman GB, Garcia EV, Bateman TM, Heller GV, Johnson LL, Folks RD, Cullom SJ, Galt JR, Case JA, Santana CA, Halkar RK: Quantitative Tc-99m sestamibi attenuation-corrected SPECT: Development and multicenter trial validation of myocardial perfusion stress gender-independent normal database in an obese population. *J Nucl Cardiol* 2004, 11:263-272.
17. Ficaro EP, Fessler JA, Shreve PD, Kritzman JN, Rose PA, Corbett JR: Simultaneous transmission/emission myocardial perfusion tomography. Diagnostic accuracy of attenuation-corrected 99mTc-sestamibi Single-Photon Emission Computed Tomography. *Circulation* 1996, 93:463-473.
18. Slomka PJ, Fish MB, Lorenzo S, Nishina H, Gerlach J, Berman DS, Germano G: Simplified normal limits and automated quantitative assessment for attenuation-corrected myocardial perfusion SPECT. *J Nucl Cardiol* 2006, 13:642-651.
19. Lomsky M, Johansson L, Gjertsson P, Björk J, Edenbrandt L: Normal limits for left ventricular ejection fraction and volumes determined by gated single photon emission computed tomography - a comparison between two quantification methods. *Clin Physiol Funct Imaging* 2008, 28:169-173.
20. Lomsky M, Gjertsson P, Johansson L, Richter J, Ohlsson M, Tout D, van Aswegen A, Underwood SR, Edenbrandt L: Evaluation of a decision support system for interpretation of myocardial perfusion gated SPECT. *Eur J Nucl Med Mol Imaging* 2008, 35:1523-1529.
21. Wallis JW, Miller TR: Rapidly converging iterative reconstruction algorithms in single-photon emission computed tomography. *J Nucl Med* 1993, 34:1793-1800.
22. Hawman EG, Ray M, Xu R, Vija AH: An attenuation correction system for a dedicated small FOV, dual head, fixed-90°, cardiac gamma camera using arrays of Gd-153 line sources. *IEEE Nucl Science Symposium Conference Record* 2006, 3:1806-1810.
23. Nichols TE, Holmes AP: Nonparametric permutation tests for functional neuroimaging: A primer with examples. *Human Brain Mapping* 2002, 15:1-25.
24. Nakajima K, Okuda K, Kawano M, Matsuo S, Slomka P, Germano G, Kinuya S: The importance of population-specific normal database for quantification of myocardial ischemia: comparison between Japanese 360 and 180-degree databases and a US database. *J Nucl Cardiol* 2009, 16:422-430.
25. Li D, Li D, Feng J, Yuan D, Cao K, Chen I: Quantification of myocardial perfusion SPECT studies in Chinese population with Western normal databases. *J Nucl Cardiol* 2010, 17:486-493.
26. Cuberas-Borrós G, Aquadé-Bruix S, Boronat-de Ferrater M, Muxí-Pradas MA, Romero-Farina G, Castell-Conesa J, Aliaga V, García-Dorado D, Candell-Riera J: Normal myocardial perfusion SPECT database for the Spanish population. *Rev Esp Cardiol* 2010, 63:934-942.

2

Bronchus sign on thin-section computed tomography is a powerful predictive factor for successful transbronchial biopsy using endobronchial ultrasound with a guide sheath for small peripheral lung lesions

Tomoyuki Minezawa[1], Takuya Okamura[1], Hiroshi Yatsuya[2], Naoki Yamamoto[3], Sayako Morikawa[1], Teppei Yamaguchi[1], Mariko Morishita[4], Yoshikazu Niwa[1], Tomoko Takeyama[1], Yuki Mieno[1], Tami Hoshino[1], Sakurako Uozu[1], Yasuhiro Goto[1], Masamichi Hayashi[1], Sumito Isogai[1], Masaki Matsuo[5], Toru Nakanishi[1], Naozumi Hashimoto[4], Mitsushi Okazawa[6] and Kazuyoshi Imaizumi[1*]

Abstract

Background: Recent advances in bronchoscopy, such as transbronchial biopsy (TBB) using endobronchial ultrasonography with a guide sheath (EBUS-GS), have improved the diagnostic yield of small-sized peripheral lung lesions. In some cases, however, it is difficult to obtain adequate biopsy samples for pathological diagnosis. Adequate prediction of the diagnostic accuracy of TBB with EBUS-GS is important before deciding whether bronchoscopy should be performed.

Methods: We retrospectively reviewed 149 consecutive patients who underwent TBB with EBUS-GS for small-sized peripheral lung lesions (≤30 mm in diameter) from April 2012 to March 2013. We conducted an exploratory analysis to identify clinical factors that can predict an accurate diagnosis by TBB with EBUS-GS. All patients underwent thin-section chest computed tomography (CT) scans (0.5-mm slices), and the CT bronchus sign was evaluated before bronchoscopy in a group discussion. The final diagnoses were pathologically or clinically confirmed in all studied patients (malignant lesions, 110 patients; benign lesions, 39 patients).

Results: The total diagnostic yield in this study was 72.5 % (95 % confidence interval: 64.8–79.0 %). Lesion size, lesion visibility on chest X-ray, and classification of the CT bronchus sign were factors significantly associated with the definitive biopsy result in the univariate analysis. In the multivariate analysis, only the CT bronchus sign remained as a significant predictive factor for successful bronchoscopic diagnosis. The CT bronchus sign was also significantly associated with the EBUS findings of the lesions.

Conclusion: Our results suggest that the CT bronchus sign is a powerful predictive factor for successful TBB with EBUS-GS.

Keywords: EBUS-GS, CT bronchus sign, Diagnostic yield, Thin-section CT, Peripheral lung lesion

* Correspondence: jeanluc@fujita-hu.ac.jp
[1]Division of Respiratory Medicine and Clinical Allergy, Department of Internal Medicine, Fujita Health University, 1-98 Dengakugakubo, Kutsukake-cho, Toyoake, Aichi 470-1192, Japan
Full list of author information is available at the end of the article

Background

Recent studies of lung cancer screening by low-dose computed tomography (CT) have demonstrated a definite advantage for detecting early-stage lung cancer [1–3]. Both chronic obstructive pulmonary disease and pulmonary fibrosis, rapidly growing health problems especially in the older population, are frequently associated with lung cancer [4, 5]. In patients with such diseases, a chest CT scan is essential for disease evaluation or monitoring. An increasing number of small-sized peripheral lung lesions are being found incidentally during the follow-up of these diseases [6]. Accordingly, there is an urgent need for the development of strategies to confirm the pathological diagnosis of small-sized lung lesions. Bronchoscopy has been the mainstay diagnostic method for pulmonary lesions. Recent advances in newer bronchoscopic techniques, such as endobronchial ultrasound (EBUS) or the use of virtual navigation systems, have enabled us to approach small peripheral lung lesions that are invisible on fluoroscopy [7]. However, recent studies have shown that a final diagnosis cannot be reached by bronchoscopy even with the most advanced techniques available today in a certain percentage of patients [8].

Recent developments in molecular targeted therapy for lung cancer have increased the need to obtain bronchoscopic biopsy specimens sufficient for molecular analysis [9]. Various diagnostic procedures other than bronchoscopy, such as CT-guided percutaneous needle aspiration biopsy (CTNAB) and surgical biopsy, are also available. Physicians must choose the most suitable procedure with which to establish a diagnosis in patients who present with lung lesions. It is very important to predict the possibility of obtaining an adequate bronchoscopic tissue specimen for pathological and molecular diagnosis. Based on the present analysis, CT bronchus sign on thin-section CT (TSCT) at the initial evaluation seems to be the most reliable predictive factor for successful biopsy by bronchoscopy. The results of this study provide both patients and doctors with useful information that will allow for informed consent in the selection of a diagnostic procedure.

Methods

Patients

The medical records of consecutive patients who underwent bronchoscopy in Fujita Health University Hospital from April 2012 to March 2013 were retrospectively reviewed. The institutional review committee (Fujita Health University Institutional Review Board) approved this study protocol, which was conducted in accordance with the tenets of the Declaration of Helsinki (approval number Fujita 14-152). All patients provided written informed consent before undergoing bronchoscopy.

Evaluation before bronchoscopy

All patients underwent chest TSCT (0.5 mm slice) within 1 month before bronchoscopy. TSCT images were generated using a nonenhanced multidetector CT system (Aquilion One Vision Edition; Toshiba Medical Systems, Tokyo, Japan). The CT scan parameters were as follows: tube current, automatic exposure control SD7; tube voltage, 120 kV; rotation speed, 0.5 s/rot; table speed, BP 1.39; reconstruction filter, FC51 AIDR 3D WEAK; window width, 1600; and window level, −600. We used automatic exposure control, the volume helical scan mode, and multi-planar reconstruction images.

We did not use a virtual bronchoscopic navigation system. Each bronchoscopist studied the patient's chest X-ray and TSCT images before the procedures and identified the size and location of the lesions and the respective bronchus. In every case, we confirmed these findings and identified the target bronchus to approach by group discussion. We investigated the bronchus sign on CT, which was identified as the presence of a bronchus directly leading to the target lesion (CT bronchus sign) [10]. In each case, we categorized the relationship between the target lesion and the nearest bronchus into three types of CT bronchus signs (A to C). In type A, the responsible bronchus clearly reached the inside of the target lesion. In type C, no bronchus could be detected in relation to the lesion. When the CT findings could be categorized into neither type A nor C, the CT bronchus sign was categorized as type B (Fig. 1). Two bronchoscopists (T.M. and K.I.) independently assessed each TSCT scan and determined the type of each CT bronchus sign (A, B, or C). When the two bronchoscopists recommended different types, the final type was determined by discussion.

Bronchoscopic procedures

After administration of local pharyngeal anesthesia, all patients were lightly sedated with individually calculated dose of intravenous midazolam as reported elsewhere [11]. Transbronchial biopsy (TBB) using EBUS with a guide sheath (EBUS-GS) was performed according to the standard Kurimoto method [12]. A 20-MHz radial type ultrasound probe with an external diameter of 1.4 mm (UM-S20-17S; Olympus Medical Systems, Tokyo, Japan) connected to an endoscopic ultrasonography system (EU-M30S; Olympus Medical Systems) was used in all cases. We mainly used a bronchoscope with a 2.0-mm-diameter working channel (BF-P260F; Olympus Medical Systems) for a guide sheath with an external diameter of 1.9 mm (K-201 kit equipped with a biopsy forceps and cytological brush; Olympus Medical Systems). According to the size or location of the lesion, the operator could use a 1T260 bronchoscope with a 2.6-mm-diameter working channel with the guide sheath

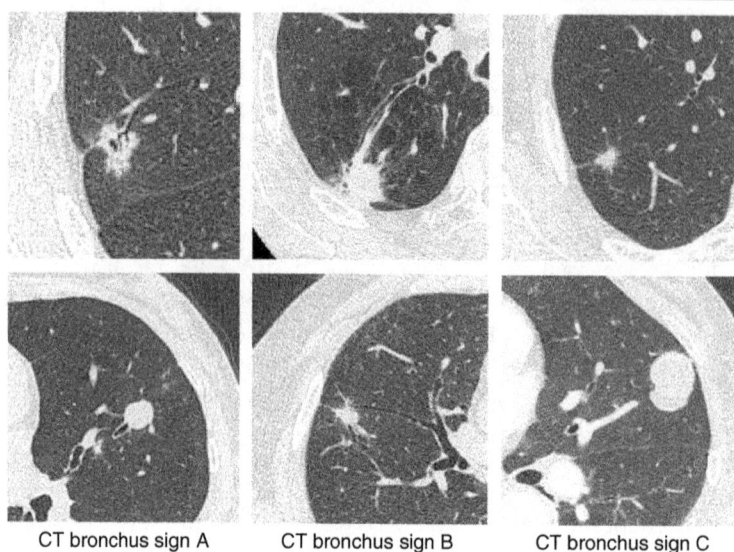

CT bronchus sign A   CT bronchus sign B   CT bronchus sign C

Fig. 1 CT bronchus sign. According to TSCT (0.5-mm reconstruction), we categorized the CT bronchus sign in each case into three types **a** to **c** according to the relationship between the nearest bronchus and the target lesion. In type *A*, the responsible bronchus clearly reached the inside of the target lesion. In type *C*, no bronchus could be detected in relation to the lesion. When the CT findings could be categorized into neither type *A* nor *C*, the CT bronchus sign was categorized as type *B*

kit K203 (external diameter of the guide sheath: 2.55 mm) (Olympus Medical Systems). We took 12 biopsy samples when using the K201 kit and nine samples using the K203 kit. Nine bronchoscopists performed the procedures in this study. Five of them had less than 7 years of experience as a bronchoscopist (range: 2–6 years), whereas four had more experience (range: 7–21 years).

Diagnostic evaluation of TBB results (positive diagnostic criteria by bronchoscopy)

In this study, we evaluated the bronchoscopic diagnostic yield in both malignant and non-malignant diseases (including inflammatory disease). Thus, we determined the evaluation criteria for judgment of successful (diagnostic) bronchoscopy according to previous reports [8, 13]. Lesions with evident malignant findings on histological examination or class IV/V findings on cytological examination were defined as malignant. For benign lesions, when bronchoscopy demonstrated a distinct histologic pattern (such as epithelioid granuloma or intra-alveolar organization) or the presence of bacteria accompanied by reasonable radiologic and clinical findings, we determined that the bronchoscopy was successful. All benign lesions were followed for more than 12 months to confirm that the lesions had remained stable or improved by appropriate therapy.

Statistical methods

Statistical analyses were carried out using JMP software (ver. 8.0; SAS Institute, Inc., Cary, NC). A binomial proportion confidence interval (CI) was calculated for diagnostic yield. Differences in proportions were evaluated with the χ^2 test. Spearman rank correlation was used to identify the association between two ordinal variables. Multivariate logistic regression analysis was used to identify factors associated with diagnostic yield independent of other variables. We entered all variables that were significantly ($p < 0.05$) associated with diagnostic yield in the univariate analyses into the multivariate analysis. The final model was determined by a backward variable selection method, and odds ratios and the 95 % CIs are presented. A p-value of <0.05 was considered to indicate statistical significance. All analyses were two-sided.

Results

Patient characteristics and details of lesions

We retrospectively reviewed 149 consecutive patients who underwent TBB with EBUS-GS. Table 1 shows the characteristics of the studied patients and targeted lesions. The median age of the patients was 70 years (range: 32–86 years). There was no sex difference. The size of the lesions ranged from 7.5 to 29.7 mm, and the median size was 19.6 mm. Five patients (3.4 %) had lesions smaller than 10 mm in diameter. Seventy-seven lesions (51.7 %) were located in the upper lobe and 17 (11.3 %) were located in superior segment of the lower lobe. Twenty-one cases (14.1 %) exhibited ground glass opacity (GGO), including 17 cases with pure GGO lesions. The number of bronchial branches that reached the target lesion from the trachea ranged from 3–8 (median: 5). Chest X-ray and TSCT were assessed as

Table 1 Characteristics of Patients and Targeted Lesions (*n* = 149)

Variable (patients)	
Age	
yrs. median (range)	70 (32–86)
Gender	
Male, number (%)	86 (57.7 %)
Female, number (%)	63 (42.3 %)
Variable (lesions)	
Size of the lesion (diameter)	
mm, median (range)	19.6 (7.5–29.7)
Location of the lesions	
Upper lobe	77 (51.7 %)
Lingular lobe or middle lobe	19 (12.8 %)
Superior segment of the lower lobe	17 (11.3 %)
Lower lobe (except for superior segment)	36 (24.2 %)
Chest X-ray findings of the lesions	
Clearly visible	77 (51.7 %)
Vague or invisible	72 (48.3 %)
Thin slice CT features	
GGO	21 (14.1 %)
Solid	128 (85.9 %)
Number of the branch reach to the lesion	
mean	5.03
3	12 (7.9 %)
4	32 (21.5 %)
5	55 (36.9 %)
6	35 (23.6 %)
7	12 (8.1 %)
8	3 (2.0 %)
CT bronchus sign [a]	
A	86 (57.8 %)
B	49 (32.9 %)
C	14 (9.3 %)

GGO ground glass opacity, [a]CT bronchus sign: see Methods

radiological findings evaluable before the decision regarding whether to perform bronchoscopy. On the initial chest X-rays, the targeted lesions were clearly visible in 77 patients (51.7 %) and vague or invisible in 72 patients (48.3 %). After careful assessment of chest TSCT by two bronchoscopists, we determined the type of CT bronchus sign of each lesion: A (86 lesions, 57.8 %), B (49 lesions, 32.9 %), and C (14 lesions, 9.3 %) (Table 1, Fig. 1). The median bronchoscopic examination time was 55 min (range: 43–71 min). The mean total dose of lidocaine used was 345 mg (range: 240–550 mg). Ten patients (6.7 %) had complications including five with pneumothorax requiring pleural

drainage, four with pneumonia and one with a transient delirium. No severe complications occurred during this study. Final diagnosis of targeted lesions are shown in Table 2.

Factors associated with bronchoscopic diagnosis

In total, 72.5 % (95 % CI: 64.8–79.0) cases could be diagnosed with TBB using EBUS-GS. The diagnostic yield of malignant diseases and non-malignant diseases was 78.2 % and 56.4 %, respectively (Table 3). The diagnostic yield was significantly higher in malignant than in non-malignant diseases (*p* = 0.0089). We examined clinical factors that can be obtained at the outpatient clinic for their potential ability to predict the bronchoscopic diagnostic yield. Lesion diameter, lesion visibility on chest X-ray, and the CT bronchus sign were significantly associated with the diagnostic yield in the univariate analyses (Table 4). In the logistic regression analysis, the CT bronchus sign was the only significant factor associated with successful achievement of a bronchoscopic diagnosis. The diagnostic success rate for lesions with a CT bronchus sign type A was 11.1 times higher than that for lesions with a CT bronchus sign type C (Table 5). More than 90 % of malignant lesions with a CT bronchus sign type A could be diagnosed successfully. Conversely, the bronchoscopic diagnostic yield was extremely low in lesion with a CT bronchus sign type C

Table 2 Final diagnosis of targeted lesions (*n* = 149)

Malignancy (*n* = 110)	
Lung cancer	
Adenocarcinoma	72
Squamous cell carcinoma	14
Large cell carcinoma	2
NSCLC	4
Adenosquamous	1
Small cell carcinoma	4
Metastatic cancer	12
Lymphoma	1
Non-malignancy (*n* = 39)	
NTM	10
Organizing pneumonia	10
Non-specific inflammation	6
Fungal infection	3
Benign tumor	2
Bacterial pneumonia	2
Sarcoidosis	2
Tuberculosis	2
Others	2

NSCLC non-small cell lung cancer, not otherwise specified, *NTM* non-tuberculosis mycobacteriosis. Others include pulmonary infarction and asbestos-related fibrosis

Table 3 Diagnostic yield (all cases)

Diagnostic yield		
All cases	72.5 % (108/149)	
Malignancy	78.2 % (86/110)	
Non-malignancy	56.4 % (22/39)	$p = 0.0089$*

*Significant difference between malignancy and benign lesions

(36.4 % and 0.0 % in malignant and non-malignant lesions, respectively) (Fig. 2).

Diagnostic yield according to the combination of CT bronchus sign with chest X-ray findings and lesion size

In the daily clinical setting, we must decide whether a patient should undergo bronchoscopy at the initial evaluation in the outpatient clinic. Informed consent for bronchoscopy should include the probability of establishing a pathological diagnosis. We evaluated the diagnostic yield of bronchoscopy according to the combination of a CT bronchus sign, lesion visibility on the initial chest X-ray, and lesion size (Table 6). When target lesions with a CT bronchus sign type A were clearly visible on chest X-ray, the diagnostic yield for the lesions was high (88.0 % for all lesions and 98.6 % for malignant lesions). The diagnostic yield for malignant lesions with both a CT bronchus sign type A and clear visibility on chest X ray was extremely high (100.0 % for lesions 20–30 mm in diameter and 94.6 % for those <20 mm diameter). When the target lesions showed a CT bronchus sign type B accompanied by vague or invisible chest X-ray findings, the diagnostic yield was around 60 %. In five patients with lesions of <10 mm in diameter (range: 7.5–9.9 mm) (type A in two patients

Table 5 Logistic regression analysis of factors on diagnostic yield of TBB using EBUS-GS

Variables		HR	(95%CI)	p value
Visibility on Chest X-ray	Clearly visible	2.03	0.90–4.59	$P = 0.087$
	Vague or invisible	Ref.		
CT bronchus sign[a]	A	11.1	2.99–41.2	$P < 0.001$*
	B	4.62	1.24–17.2	$P = 0.023$*
	C	Ref.		

* significant difference, [a] See Methods. *Ref.* reference

and B in three patients), a bronchoscopic diagnosis could be obtained in both patients with the type A sign. In 17 patients with pure GGO lesions, the CT bronchus signs were A in 10 lesions, B in 5 lesions and C in two lesions. The diagnostic yield was 80 % in type A, 60 % in B, and 0 % in C.

Relationship between CT bronchus sign and EBUS findings

Previous reports have emphasized the role of the EBUS findings of the target lesion for successful bronchoscopic diagnosis [12, 14]. When an EBUS probe is located in the center of ("within") the target lesion, the probability of successful diagnosis would be higher than when the probe is located next to ("adjacent to") or outside ("invisible") the target lesion. Thus, we evaluated the relationship between the CT bronchus sign and EBUS findings in each case. As shown in Fig. 3, the CT bronchus sign and EBUS findings were well correlated with each other (Spearman rank correlation coefficient $r = 0.556$, $p < 0.001$). Nearly 70 % of lesions with a CT

Table 4 Contribution of clinical factors available before bronchoscopy to diagnostic yield (all cases)

Variables		Diagnostic yield	p value
Lesion diameter	<20 mm	51/80 (63.8 %)	0.01*
	≥20 mm	57/69 (82.6 %)	
Lesion location	Upper lobe or sup segment of lower lobe	40/56 (71.4 %)	0.82
	Middle or lower lobe [a]	68/93 (73.1 %)	
Feature of the lesion	GGO	12/18 (66.7 %)	0.24
	Solid	96/131 (73.2 %)	
Visibility of the lesion on Chest X-ray	Clearly visible	59/72 (81.9 %)	0.01*
	Vague or invisible	49/77 (63.6 %)	
Number of bronchial branch to reach the lesion	≥5	35/50 (70.0 %)	0.63
	≤4	73/99 (73.7 %)	
Operator's experience (years)	≥7	34/52 (65.4 %)	0.16
	≤6	74/97 (76.3 %)	
CT bronchus sign[b]	A	72/86 (83.7 %)	0.001*
	B	32/49 (65.3 %)	
	C	4/14 (28.6 %)	

* significant difference, [a] except for superior segment of the lower lobe, [b] See Methods

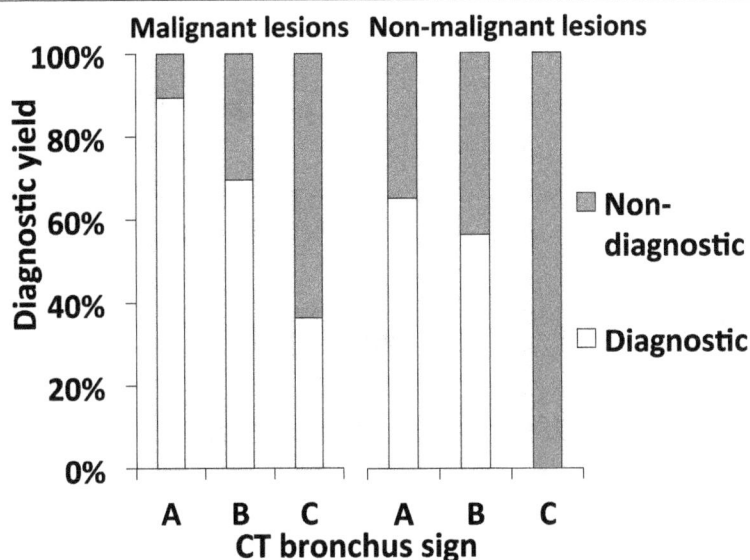

Fig. 2 CT bronchus sign and bronchoscopic diagnostic yield. The CT bronchus sign was a significant factor associated with a positive bronchoscopic diagnosis. In particular more than 90 % of malignant lesions with a CT bronchus sign type A could be diagnosed successfully. Conversely, in benign lesions, the bronchoscopic diagnostic yield was 0 % in lesions with a CT bronchus sign type C

bronchus sign type A showed a "within" finding on EBUS.

Discussion

It is clinically important to determine which diagnostic modality would be the most reliable and safest for patients with unknown peripheral lesions in the outpatient clinic. Although recent advances in bronchoscopic technologies, including EBUS-GS, have improved the diagnostic yield of bronchoscopy, other modalities such as CTNAB or surgical biopsy might be preferable for some patients. However, these procedures may also be associated with specific complications. Notably, CTNAB is often complicated by pneumothorax and occasionally more serious complications such as air embolism or

tumor dissemination along the biopsy route [15]. Thus, it is sometimes difficult to recommend the most suitable diagnostic method to a patient at the initial evaluation. Our study shows that the CT bronchus sign as evaluated by TSCT is the most powerful predictive factor for successful bronchoscopic diagnosis of small peripheral lesions. The physician should encourage the patient to undergo bronchoscopy if the target lesion exhibits a CT bronchus sign type A. On the contrary, if the patient's lung lesion shows a CT bronchus sign type C, the patient should be offered an alternative diagnostic procedure, such as CTNAB or surgical biopsy.

In this study, we assessed all patients' TSCT images as their radiological findings at their initial evaluation. However, because it may be difficult to perform TSCT

Table 6 Diagnostic yield according to the CT bronchus sign, Chest X-ray findings and lesion size

CT bronchus sign	Visibility on Chest X-ray	Lesion size	Diagnostic yield % (total/malignancy)
A	Clearly visible	All size	88.0/98.6
		≥20 mm	91.9/100
		<20 mm	76.9/94.6
	Vague or invisible	All size	77.8/82.8
		≥20 mm	83.3/83.3
		<20 mm	75.0/82.4
B	Clearly visible	All size	68.8/90.9
		≥20 mm	87.5/83.3
		<20 mm	60.0/100
	Vague or invisible	All size	63.6/59.1
		≥20 mm	50.0/50.0
		<20 mm	65.2/64.3

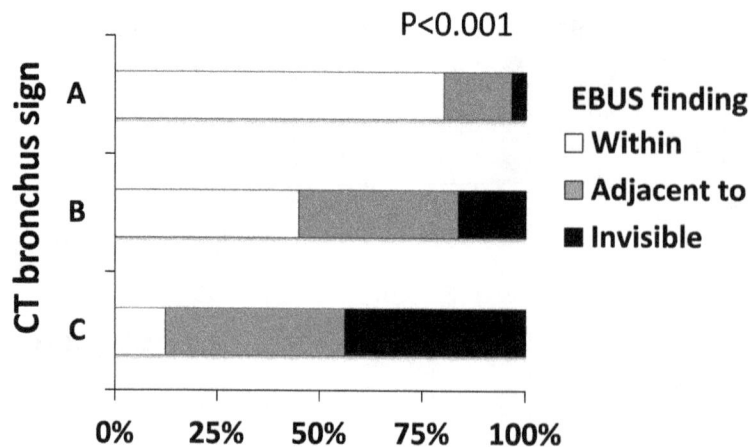

Fig. 3 Relationship between CT bronchus sign and EBUS findings. The CT bronchus sign was highly correlated with the EBUS findings Spearman rank correlation coefficient $r = 0.556$, $p < 0.001$. Nearly 70 % of lesions with a CT bronchus sign type A showed a "within" finding on EBUS

for every patient at some institution, our results might only be valid for bronchoscopy performed at medical centers or educational hospitals in which TSCT is readily available. Future studies are warranted to assess whether conventional CT findings can also be used to predict the results of bronchoscopic biopsy. Our retrospective analysis may also indicate that the differential bronchoscopic diagnostic yield can be determined according to the combination of the CT bronchus sign and chest X-ray findings. This would be useful information that could be offered to patients as a standard method by which to estimate the diagnostic yield of TBB with EBUS-GS. However, these issues must be confirmed in a future prospective study.

Other reports have emphasized that EBUS findings are the most important factor for obtaining pathological results in bronchoscopy with EGUS-GS [12, 14]. These reports have shown that an EBUS finding of "within," which means that an EBUS probe can be introduced inside the lesion, is strongly related to a high diagnostic yield. In the present study, we demonstrated that a CT bronchus sign type A was significantly related to a "within" EBUS finding. These results might indicate that we can predict EBUS findings from the CT bronchus sign on TSCT at the initial evaluation. Most recently, Evison et al. [16] reported that the presence of a bronchus sign on CT was the only independent predictor of all predefined outcomes, including lesion identification with radial EBUS, positioning of the probe within the center of the lesion, and accurate pathological diagnosis. However, they evaluated larger lesions (nearly 70 % of lesions were >30 mm in diameter) than those in the present study (all lesions were <30 mm in diameter). Our study cohort included five patients with lesions of <10 mm in diameter and 17 with pure GGO lesions. Although the

diagnostic yields in these cases were lower than in other cases, a CT bronchus sign type A was still well correlated with a higher diagnostic yield. Taken together, our results clearly indicate that a CT bronchus sign is a powerful predictor of successful bronchoscopy, even in smaller lung lesions.

Our study has some limitations. First, this was a retrospective analysis in a single institution. Because the diagnostic yield may vary among institutions, the usefulness of the CT bronchus sign should be confirmed in a multicenter prospective study. Notably, in the present study, young bronchoscopists with less than 7 years of experience performed about two-thirds of all procedures, and the experience level of the examiner was not related to the diagnostic yield. We speculated that the usefulness of the CT bronchus sign may be universal and independent of differences among institutions or bronchoscopists. Second, it has been reported that the ability to obtain a fluoroscopic view of the lesion significantly influences the success of a bronchoscopic diagnosis. However, a fluoroscopic view of the target lesion is usually difficult to obtain at the patient's first visit to an outpatient clinic. Therefore, we assessed the chest X-ray findings of the target lesions at the initial evaluation in this study. Third, we did not use a virtual navigation system or rapid on-site examination of the cytological findings. Both of these methods are well known to improve the bronchoscopic diagnostic yield even when using the EBUS-GS system [17–19]. However, we also showed a higher diagnostic yield than those reported in previous studies that used a virtual navigation system and/or rapid on-site examination. Based on the findings of this study, we can say that the CT bronchus sign is an important and useful predictive marker with or without the use of virtual technology or on-site cytological evaluation.

Conclusions

In summary, the CT bronchus sign associated with target lesions on TSCT is a useful predictive marker for successful bronchoscopic diagnosis of small peripheral lung lesions. Physicians should perform TSCT and evaluate the CT bronchus sign associated with the target lesion before deciding whether bronchoscopy is suitable for the patient.

Abbreviations

CT: Computed tomography; EBUS-GS: Endobronchial ultrasonography with a guide sheath; TBB: Transbronchial biopsy; CTNAB: Computed tomography guided needle aspiration biopsy; TSCT: Thin-section computed tomography; GGO: Ground glass opacity; CI: Confidence interval.

Competing interests

The authors declare that they have no competing interests.

Authors' contributions

TM participated in the design of the study, evaluation of the CT images, and drafting the manuscript. TO participated in the evaluation of the CT images. HY performed the statistical analysis. NY helped to draft the manuscript. SM participated in the design of the study. TY participated in the evaluation of the CT images and performed the statistical analysis. MM revised the manuscript. YN participated in the evaluation of the CT images. TT participated in the evaluation of the CT images. YM participated in the design of the study and the evaluation of the CT images. TH revised the manuscript. SU helped to draft the manuscript. YG participated in the design of the study. MH revised the manuscript. SI participated in the evaluation of the CT images. MM helped to draft the manuscript. TN participated in the evaluation of the CT images. NH revised the manuscript. MO revised the manuscript. KI participated in the design of the study, evaluation of the CT images, and drafting the manuscript. All authors read and approved the final manuscript.

Acknowledgements

The authors thank Mrs. Naomi Maeda for her excellent secretarial help. They also thank Mrs. Chikako Hibiya and Ms. Noriko Hiramatsu for their generous technical assistance.

Author details

[1]Division of Respiratory Medicine and Clinical Allergy, Department of Internal Medicine, Fujita Health University, 1-98 Dengakugakubo, Kutsukake-cho, Toyoake, Aichi 470-1192, Japan. [2]Department of Public Health, Fujita Health University, Toyoake, Aichi, Japan. [3]Laboratory of Molecular Biology & Histochemistry, Fujita Health University, Toyoake, Aichi, Japan. [4]Department of Respiratory Medicine, Nagoya University Graduate School of Medicine, Nagoya, Japan. [5]Department of Respiratory Medicine, Chubu Rosai Hospital, Nagoya, Japan. [6]Department of Respiratory Medicine, Daiyu-kai Hospital, Ichinomiya, Aichi, Japan.

References

1. Aberle DR, Adams AM, Berg CD, Black WC, Clapp JD, Fagerstrom RM, et al. Reduced lung-cancer mortality with low-dose computed tomographic screening. N Engl J Med. 2011;365(5):395–409.
2. Kovalchik SA, Tammemagi M, Berg CD, Caporaso NE, Riley TL, Korch M, et al. Targeting of low-dose CT screening according to the risk of lung-cancer death. N Engl J Med. 2013;369(3):245–54.
3. de Koning HJ, Meza R, Plevritis SK, ten Haaf K, Munshi VN, Jeon J, et al. Benefits and harms of computed tomography lung cancer screening strategies: a comparative modeling study for the U.S. Preventive Services Task Force. Ann Intern Med. 2014;160(5):311–20.
4. Hashimoto N, Matsuzaki A, Okada Y, Imai N, Iwano S, Wakai K, et al. Clinical impact of prevalence and severity of COPD on the decision-making process for therapeutic management of lung cancer patients. BMC Pulm Med. 2014;14:14.
5. Tomassetti S, Gurioli C, Ryu J, Decker P, Ravaglia C, Tantalocco P, et al. The impact of lung cancer on survival of Idiopathic Pulmonary Fibrosis. Chest. 2014 in press.
6. de-Torres JP, Casanova C, Marin JM, Zagaceta J, Alcaide AB, Seijo LM, et al. Exploring the impact of screening with low-dose CT on lung cancer mortality in mild to moderate COPD patients: a pilot study. Respir Med. 2013;107(5):702–7.
7. Steinfort DP, Vincent J, Heinze S, Antippa P, Irving LB. Comparative effectiveness of radial probe endobronchial ultrasound versus CT-guided needle biopsy for evaluation of peripheral pulmonary lesions: a randomized pragmatic trial. Respir Med. 2011;105(11):1704–11.
8. Tamiya M, Okamoto N, Sasada S, Shiroyama T, Morishita N, Suzuki H, et al. Diagnostic yield of combined bronchoscopy and endobronchial ultrasonography, under LungPoint guidance for small peripheral pulmonary lesions. Respirology. 2013;18(5):834–9.
9. Kim L, Tsao MS. Tumour tissue sampling for lung cancer management in the era of personalised therapy: what is good enough for molecular testing? Eur Respir J. 2014 in press.
10. Gaeta M, Pandolfo I, Volta S, Russi EG, Bartiromo G, Girone G, et al. Bronchus sign on CT in peripheral carcinoma of the lung: value in predicting results of transbronchial biopsy. AJR Am J Roentgenol. 1991;157(6):1181–5.
11. Ogawa T, Imaizumi K, Hashimoto I, Shindo Y, Imai N, Uozu S, et al. Prospective analysis of efficacy and safety of an individualized-midazolam-dosing protocol for sedation during prolonged bronchoscopy. Respir Investig. 2014;52(3):153–9.
12. Kurimoto N, Miyazawa T, Okimasa S, Maeda A, Oiwa H, Miyazu Y, et al. Endobronchial ultrasonography using a guide sheath increases the ability to diagnose peripheral pulmonary lesions endoscopically. Chest. 2004;126(3):959–65.
13. Shinagawa N, Nakano K, Asahina H, Kikuchi E, Ito T, Matsuno Y, et al. Endobronchial ultrasonography with a guide sheath in the diagnosis of benign peripheral diseases. Ann Thorac Surg. 2012;93(3):951–7.
14. Kurimoto N, Inoue T, Miyazawa T, Morita K, Matsuoka S, Nakamura H. The usefulness of endobronchial ultrasonography-guided transbronchial needle aspiration at the lobar, segmental, or subsegmental bronchus smaller than a convex-type bronchoscope. J Bronchology Interv Pulmonol. 2014;21(1):6–13.
15. Tomiyama N, Yasuhara Y, Nakajima Y, Adachi S, Arai Y, Kusumoto M, et al. CT-guided needle biopsy of lung lesions: a survey of severe complication based on 9783 biopsies in Japan. Eur J Radiol. 2006;59(1):60–4.
16. Evison M, Crosbie PA, Morris J, Martin J, Barber PV, Booton R. Can computed tomography characteristics predict outcomes in patients undergoing radial endobronchial ultrasound-guided biopsy of peripheral lung lesions? J Thorac Oncol. 2014;9(9):1393–7.
17. Oki M, Saka H, Kitagawa C, Kogure Y, Murata N, Adachi T, et al. Rapid on-site cytologic evaluation during endobronchial ultrasound-guided transbronchial needle aspiration for diagnosing lung cancer: a randomized study. Respiration. 2013;85(6):486–92.
18. Asano F, Matsuno Y, Tsuzuku A, Anzai M, Shinagawa N, Yamazaki K, et al. Diagnosis of peripheral pulmonary lesions using a bronchoscope insertion guidance system combined with endobronchial ultrasonography with a guide sheath. Lung Cancer. 2008;60(3):366–73.
19. Iwano S, Imaizumi K, Okada T, Hasegawa Y, Naganawa S. Virtual bronchoscopy-guided transbronchial biopsy for aiding the diagnosis of peripheral lung cancer. Eur J Radiol. 2011;79(1):155–9.

3

Diagnostic accuracy of left ventricular longitudinal function by speckle tracking echocardiography to predict significant coronary artery stenosis

Ingvild Billehaug Norum[1,2*], Vidar Ruddox[1,2†], Thor Edvardsen[2,3†] and Jan Erik Otterstad[1]

Abstract

Background: Patients evaluated for acute and chronic chest pain comprise a large, heterogeneous group that often provides diagnostic challenges. Although speckle tracking echocardiography (STE) has proved to have diagnostic value in acute coronary syndrome it is not commonly incorporated in everyday practice.
The purpose of the present systematic review was to assess the diagnostic accuracy of left ventricular (LV) longitudinal function by STE to predict significant coronary artery stenosis (CAD+) or not (CAD-) verified by coronary angiography in patients with chest pain suspected to be of cardiac ischemic origin.

Methods: 4 electronic databases; Embase, Medline, Cochrane and PubMed ahead-of print were searched for per 19.05.14. Only full-sized articles including > 40 patients were selected.

Results: A total of 166 citations were identified, 16 full-size articles were assessed of which 6 were found eligible for this review. Of 781 patients included 397 (60 %) had CAD+. The overall weighted mean global longitudinal strain (GLS) was −17.2 % (SD = 2.6) among CAD+ vs. -19.2 % (SD = 2.8) in CAD- patients. Mean area under curve in 4 studies for predicting CAD+ ranged from 0.68 to 0.80. The study cut-off levels for prediction of CAD+ in the ROC analysis varied between −17.4 % and −19.7 % with sensitivity from 51 % to 81 % and specificity between 58 % and 81 %. In 1 study GLS obtained during dobutamine stress echocardiography (DSE) had the best accuracy. Regional strain measurements were not uniform, but may have potential in detecting CAD.

Conclusions: GLS measurements at rest only have modest diagnostic accuracy in predicting CAD+ among patients presenting with acute or chronic chest pain. The results from regional strain, layer specific strain and DSE need to be verified in larger studies.

Keywords: Coronary artery disease, Speckle tracking, Strain imaging, Left ventricular function, Chest pain

Background

In recent years it has become increasingly apparent that a large number of patients classified as low risk for acute coronary syndrome (ACS) and without diagnostic cardiac biomarkers represent the most prevalent group of patients admitted to hospital with chest pain [1–3]. In addition, we see numbers in our outpatient clinic referred for evaluation of stable chest pain. Up to 1/3 of patients with chest pain who are referred to coronary angiography have no significant coronary artery stenosis [4]. Though this investigation is generally safe, it has well known risk of complications and is also costly. Exercise testing is widely used for selecting patients for coronary angiography, but has its clear limitations as emphasized in the European guidelines for stable coronary artery disease [5]. In stable coronary artery disease, coronary computed tomography angiography (CTA) is a non-invasive alternative to assess coronary anatomy, but according to expert consensus only selected patients should be considered for CTA [5]. In guidelines concerning

* Correspondence: ingvild.billehaug.norum@siv.no
†Equal contributors
[1]Department of Cardiology, Vestfold Hospital Trust, Pb 2168, 3103 Tønsberg, Norway
[2]University of Oslo, Faculty of Medicine, Pb 1078 Blindern, 0316 Oslo, Norway
Full list of author information is available at the end of the article

ACS [6] CTA is said to be useful to exclude ACS or other causes of chest pain, but due to limited availability and also the concern of radiation it is to our knowledge not commonly used in this setting worldwide. Thus we are in need of a simple, non-invasive method to improve the selection of patients who are referred to coronary angiography.

For several years measurements of left ventricular deformation, hereunder strain by speckle tracking echocardiography (STE), has been studied to evaluate global and regional left ventricular systolic function. Strain imaging has proven useful in several clinical settings i.e. evaluation of cardiotoxicity, ventricular function in heart transplant recipients and in acute coronary syndrome [7–11]. As pointed out by Feigenbaum [12], in spite of its feasibility and potential clinical value, yet only a few academic centers have incorporated it into everyday practice of echocardiography, and even then on a limited basis. Arguments being that STE is time consuming and provides results that are difficult to interpret. He advocates a simplified method incorporating solely measurements of longitudinal strain (LS) that might overcome some of these issues and make it easier to include STE in common clinical evaluation.

The purpose of this review is to evaluate the diagnostic accuracy of global (G) and regional (R) longitudinal strain to predict the presence or absence of significant CAD. A prerequisite for including studies was that all patients had undergone LS measurements and a subsequent coronary angiogram preferably < 2 months apart, subdividing them into significant coronary artery disease (CAD+) and no CAD (CAD-). The main objective was to assess the diagnostic accuracy of LS to predict CAD+ in these studies.

Methods

We searched for studies that included patients who had been evaluated for significant CAD being related to chest pain, either in the acute setting such as suspected ACS, or electively with a question of stable angina pectoris. Previously known CAD may influence the strain-measurements and thereby represent a bias. Therefore, studies defining exclusion criteria for established CAD on presentation, such as a history of myocardial infarction (MI), previous percutaneous coronary intervention (PCI), open heart surgery or severe wall motion abnormalities were preferably included. We made some compromises leaving the possibility to include studies where a minority of patients had obvious CAD. Included studies should in principal also have excluded patients with overt heart failure, LV systolic dysfunction, atrial fibrillation or frequent ventricular premature complexes, also due to the possibility of influencing strain measurements.

In case of discrepancies in the assessment of inclusion or exclusion criteria, the problem was solved through consensus. We searched the following 4 electronic databases: Embase (1980 to 2014 week 20), Ovid MEDLINE (1946 to May 19.2014), Cochrane library and PubMed ahead-of-print as per May 19. 2014. The search strategy combined text words and subject headings identifying reports related to speckle tracking and angiography. The search strategy is presented in Additional file 1. In case of lacking data or questions of the methodology applied, the first authors were contacted for additional information. Only full text articles in the English language were accepted. Abstracts, reviews, letters to the editor, current opinions etc. were excluded from this review.

Consecutive series of > 40 patients who had been evaluated for significant CAD by left ventricular GLS and, eventually regional LS (RLS) measurements with a subsequent coronary angiography were included. CAD+ should have been defined as a minimum of at least one stenosis > 50 % or ≥70 % reduction of the arterial luminal area. Studies of LS at rest and, eventually during a stress test could be included. There should be a clear definition of how GLS and RLS were assessed. Provided LS measurements had been performed, studies with additional circumferential strain measurements were also included.

Selected studies should preferably present receiver operating characteristic (ROC) analysis for diagnostic accuracy including area under curve (AUC) values with an optimal cutoff and sensitivity and specificity of the strain method applied to predict CAD+. In principle, the LS values were compared between those with CAD+ vs. CAD-. The mean differences of the respective mean LS values in patients with CAD + vs. CAD- were calculated by simple subtraction for each study. For summary measures a plot depicting the mean values and SDs for GLS in both the CAD+ and the CAD- group from each study was constructed. A similar plot was constructed for the 4 studies that provided RLS data. We used STATA (version 12.0) and combined data from the different studies to make two virtual combined samples, CAD+ ($n = 397$) and CAD- ($n = 381$) respectively. We did not have access to raw data, but the mean and variance of the combined samples could be calculated from the reported values in the original studies. The mean GLS of the combined CAD+ sample, for instance, was calculated by taking the weighted mean of the reported GLS means of CAD+ patients from each study, the weights being each study's relative size in the combined sample. The variances, and corresponding standard deviations, were found using standard formulas for pooled variance. A crucial implicit assumption in this process is that all studies we included used random samples from the same two populations (chest pain or other anginal equivalent and CAD- or CAD+) with no selection bias nor measurement bias being present in any of the studies (see "Discussion" for an elaboration on this point). We then assumed that LS values for CAD- and CAD+ are both normally distributed.

Results

After database screening a total of 166 unique titles and abstracts were identified. A flow diagram of the studies selected is shown in Fig. 1 including principal reasons for excluding 10 full text articles [13–22]. A more detailed description explaining the arguments for exclusion of these studies (published between 2007 and 2014) is provided in Additional file 2. The six studies included [23–28] on basis of our predefined criteria were published between 2011 and 2014. No additional studies outside the search could be retrieved from screening reference lists in various reviews and full text articles.

Description of individual studies
One study based upon the use of an Artida (Toshiba) system

In the study of Sarvari et al. [23] 77 patients were prospectively referred to a single tertiary coronary care center with suspected non-ST-elevation acute coronary syndrome (NSTE-ACS) for coronary angiogram. Exclusion criteria were preexisting CAD, defined by a history of previous MI, PCI and open chest surgery. Echocardiography was performed 1–2 h prior to the invasive procedure and within 48 h after the last episode of chest pain. LV strain was measured from a parasternal short-axis view of the LV at the level of the papillary muscle for circumferential strain and 3 apical views for LS. The Artida system allows analysis of the 2D images for endocardial, mid-myocardial and epicardial strains.

Peak negative systolic strains from the 3 layers in 16 longitudinal LV segments were averaged from each myocardial layer to calculate GLS. Layer-specific strain measurements were also used for RLS. RLS was calculated based on the perfusion territories of the 3 major coronary arteries in a 16 segment model, modified according to

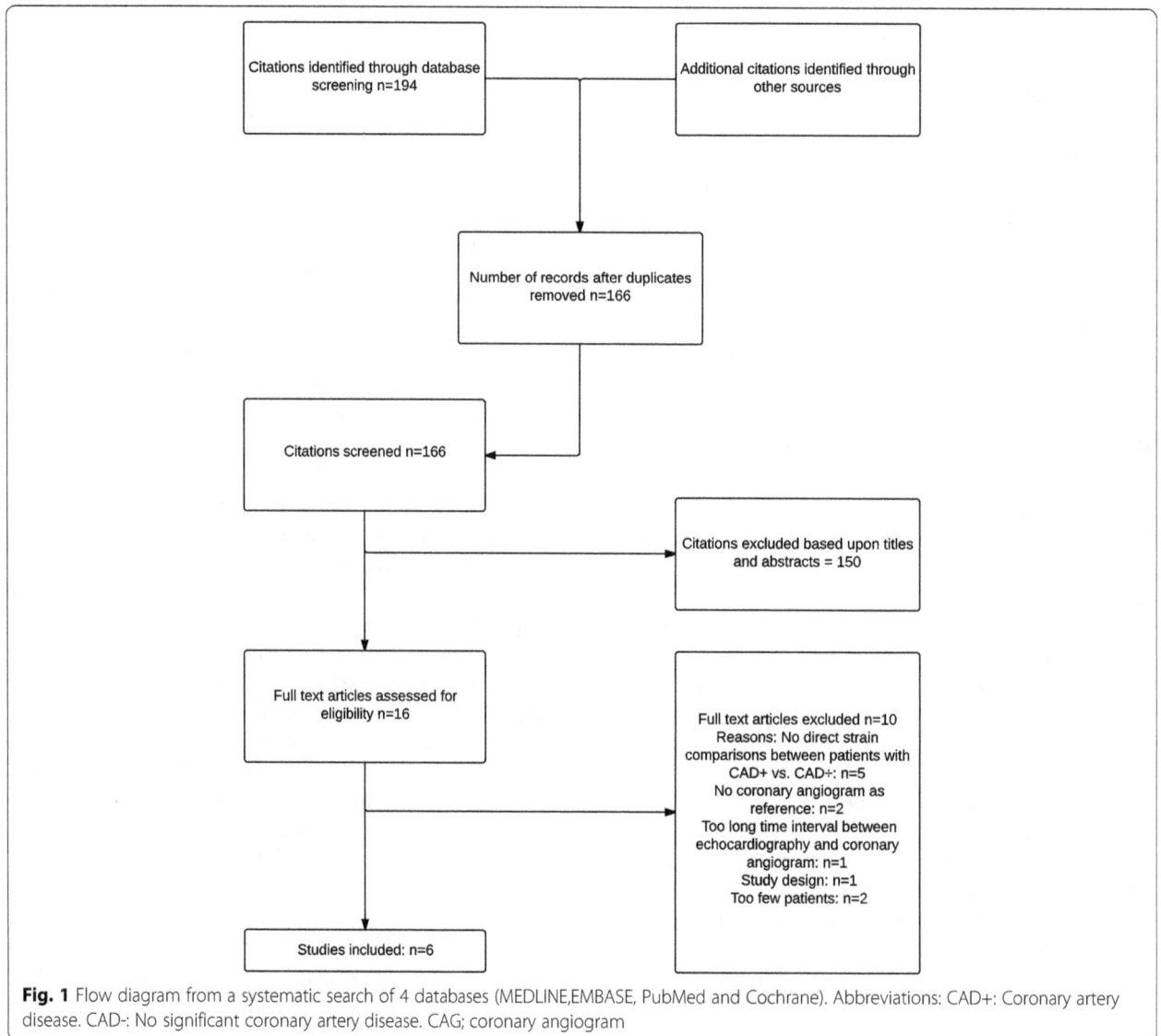

Fig. 1 Flow diagram from a systematic search of 4 databases (MEDLINE,EMBASE, PubMed and Cochrane). Abbreviations: CAD+: Coronary artery disease. CAD-: No significant coronary artery disease. CAG; coronary angiogram

Cerquieira et al. [29], by averaging all segmental peak systolic strain values within each territory and termed territorial longitudinal strain (TLS) in the article.

Global circumferential strain (GCS) was measured for each myocardial layer from one parasternal short axis view (papillary muscle level) in 6 circumferential LV segments. Wall motion was visually assessed and a 16 segment model and wall motion score index was calculated for each patient as the average of the segmental values. Data for endocardial strain values only is presented in Table 1.

Patients with CAD+ had worse function in all 3 myocardial layers assessed by GLS and GCS compared with CAD- patients. The average differences between CAD+ and CAD- patients from the endocardial layer were 3.9 % for GLS; 5.2 % for RLS, and 5.0 % for GCS. The absolute differences between endocardial and epicardial strain values were significantly lower in patients with CAD+ than in those with CAD- (Table 1). ROC analysis revealed high AUC values for endocardial and mid-myocardial RLS and GCS compared to those obtained from the epicardial layers ($p < 0.05$), from wall motion score index ($p < 0.01$) and LVEF ($p < 0.001$). The optimal cut-off value for identifying patients with CAD + was −16.4 % for endocardial RLS with a sensitivity/specificity/positive (PPV) and/negative (NPV) predictive value of 89 %/81 %/73 %/93 % respectively. No such detailed data is presented for GLS in the publication. With multivariate regression analyses, including parameters influencing myocardial function, endocardial RLS (per1% change) was the only predictor of the presence of CAD+ (OR 2.10, 95 % CI 1.5 – 3.1, $p < 0.001$).

In conclusion, assessment of layer-specific strain by 2D STE might identify NSTE-ACS patents with CAD. Endocardial function was found to be more affected in CAD+ compared with epicardial function and LVEF, with endocardial and mid-myocardial RLS having the best diagnostic accuracy.

4 studies based upon GE equipment at rest

Elective diagnostic coronary angiography Montgomery et al. [24] retrospectively studied 2D STE characteristics in 123 consecutive patients who underwent stress echocardiography, and subsequently coronary angiography within 10 days. In this study 23 patients had been excluded due to obvious CAD, LVEF < 40 % or severe wall motion abnormalities. However a total of 9 subjects (7 %) included had prior revascularization procedures (five CABG).

The diagnostic power of GLS at rest was compared with the wall motion score index during stress for detecting CAD+. STE was performed on all 3 apical views at rest and mean GLS was calculated. For RLS peak LAD segmental strain measurements were compared, and the RLS values presented in Table 2 express LAD segmental peak

systolic strain as well as the ROC analysis for GLS and RLS. The mean differences in GLS and RLS between CAD+ and CAD- patients were 2.3 % and 2.7 % respectively. In the ROC analysis the sensitivity/specificity of the strain cut-off points listed in Table 2 were comparable to a cut-off point for wall motion score index ≥ 1.13 (68 %/ 70 %) measured during stress. In conclusion GLS measurements at rest did not differ from wall motion score index during stress for identification of patients with CAD+. The study did not incorporate strain measurements during stress.

Smedsrud et al. [25] included 86 patients and investigated whether the duration of LV early systolic lengthening could accurately identify patients with CAD+. Since LS measurements also were performed, the study was included in the present review. Consecutive patients were referred to elective coronary angiography because of stable chest pain. Echocardiography was performed immediately before coronary angiography. Exclusion criteria were ACS, a history of MI and/or any evidence of scar by late enhancement on contrast-enhanced MRI or previous heart surgery. GLS was measured from the 3 apical views model and was based upon the peak negative systolic strain value. RLS was calculated as the average of the segments belonging to each perfusion territory of the 3 major coronary arteries [29]. The average difference between patients with CAD+ and CAD- was 1.8 % and 2.2 % for GLS and RLS respectively, In the ROC analysis GLS showed poor sensitivity for predicting CAD+ (Table 2), with a PPV of 0.73 (95 % CI 0.57-0.86) and NPV of 0.63 (95 % CI 0.54-0.69). In contrast to the modest diagnostic accuracy of GLS and RLS the prolonged duration of systolic lengthening showed a far better accuracy with an AUC of 0.83 (95 % CI 0.75-0.92) for predicting CAD+.

In a large study Biering- Soerensen et al. [26] enrolled 296 consecutive patients with suspected stable angina pectoris. 3 patients were excluded due to poor quality of the echocardiographic images. The remaining 293 participants were all examined with echocardiography, including 2DSE and exercise test followed by coronary angiography (median 25 days with interquartile range 14– 45 days (T. Beiering-Soerensen, personal communication). Exclusion criteria were known ischemic heart disease, congestive heart failure, heart valve disease, LVEF < 50 %, intraventricular conduction disturbances, pathological Q-waves and arrhythmias. This is the only study where CAD+ was defined as stenosis with ≥ 70 % reduction of the arterial lumen, which corresponds to 50 % reduction in arterial diameter. GLS was calculated from the average of 18 segments (GLS[18]) as well as from 12 segments (GLS[12]), derived from 6 basal and 6 midventricular segments, thereby excluding the 6 apical segments. RLS was termed regional peak systolic strain and measured in 18 segments from all views. Multiple regression models were

Table 1 Layer-specific left ventrcular strain measurements at rest using CAG as reference for CAD

Study	Indication	CAG	Strain values (%)			Differences endo-epic. strain			AUC for CAD+, TLS/GCS (%)
			CAD+	CAD-	p-value	CAD+	CAD-	p-value	
Sarvari [23]	Suspected NSTE-ACS n = 77	CAD+ n = 49	TLS: −14.0 ± 3.3	−19.2 ± 2.2	<0.001	Δ2.4 ± 3.6	Δ5.3 ± 2.1	<0.001	Endocardial: 0.91/0.85
		CAD- n = 28	GCS: −19.3 ± 4.0	− 24.3 ± 3.4	<0.001	Δ2.4 ± 3.7	Δ10.4 ± 3.0	<0.001	Mid-myocardial: 0.91/0.87
			GLS: −15.3 ± 2.2	−19.2 ± 2.2	<0.001	Δ2.4 ± 3.8	Δ5.3 ± 2.1	<0.001	Epicardial: 0.79/0.68

Strain values and differences between andocardial and epicardial strain are presented as mean ± SD

NSTE-ACS Non-ST elevation acute coronary syndrome, CAG Coronary angiography, CAD+ Coronary artery disease, defined as coronary artery stenosis ≥ 50 %, TLS Territorial longitudinal strain, GCS Global circumferential strain, endo endocardial, epic epicardial, AUC Area under the curve for ROC analysis of prediction of CAD being present or not

Table 2 4 studies on measurements of left ventricular strain at rest to predict CAD+ using coronary angiogram as reference

Study	n	CAG	GLS (%)	p CAD+ vs CAD-	TLS (%)	pCAD+ vs CAD-	AUC for CAD+ (95 % CI)	Cut-off	Sensitivity	Specificity
Montgomery [24]	123	CAD+ n = 56[a]	−16.8 ± 3,2				GLS 0.72 (0.63-0.82)	− 17.8 %	66 %	76 %
		CAD- n = 67	−19.1 ± 3.4	0.0002			TLS 0.73 (0.62 - 0.83)	− 18.3 %	69 %	70 %
	109	LAD+ n = 35[c]	−19 ± 2.8		−18.68 ± 3.3					
		LAD- n = 74	−17.5 ± 2.7	0.0001	−21.14 ± 3.3					
Smedsrud [25]	86	CAD+ n = 43[a]	−17.7 ± 3.0		−17.9 ± 3.5		GLS 0.68 (0.56-0.79)	−17.4 %	51 %	81 %
		CAD- n = 43	−19.5- ± 2.6	0.003	−20.1 ± 2.9	0.015	TLS 0.67 (0.52-0.82)	n.a.	n.a.	n.a.
Biering-Sørensen [26]	293	CAD+ n = 107[b]	−17.1 ± 2.5[b]				GLS 0.68 (0.62-0.74)[d]	− 18.4 %	74 %	58 %
		CAD- n = 186	− 18.8 ± 2.6	<0.001						
Shimoni [27]	97	CAD+ n = 69[a]	−17.3 ± 2.4		−9.1 ± 3.2		GLS 0.80	−19.7 %	81 %	67 %
		CAD- n = 28	−20.8 ± 2.3	<0.001	−12.9 ± 2.3	<0.001	TLS 0.75	−12.6 %	77 %	68 %

Abbreviations and definitions: CAD+ was defined as ≥ 50 % stenosis [a] in one or more coronary arteries and as ≥ 70 % luminal area reduction[b]
LAD: Left anterior desending [c]subset of 109 patients where TLS in the LAD territory was performed. [d] GLS from 12 segments. TLS = territorial longitudinal strain, defined specifically in the text from each study

constructed and significant stenosis in the LAD, RCA and LCX were tested as independent predictors of RLS in each of the 18 segments. The typical disitribution of these three arteries were adopted from Lang et al. [30], incorporating that some segments have variable coronary perfusion. RLS values are not reported directly in the article.

GLS[12] data is presented in Table 2, since this was the only independent predictor of CAD+ remaining after multivariate adjustment. The mean difference in GLS[12] between patients with CAD+ vs. CAD- was 1,7 %. As presented in Fig 1 in the Data Supplement of the article, RLS was significantly lower in segments supplied by stenotic coronary arteries compared with nonstenotic arteries in a pattern closely mimicking the anatomic perfusion area. When the data from GLS[12] and the exercise test was combined in ROC analysis, the AUC was significantly higher than that for the exercise test alone (0.84 versus 0.78, p = 0,007.). In conclusion GLS[12] peak systolic strain at rest was found to be an independent predictor of CAD+ and significantly improved the diagnostic performance of exercise testing.

Patients hospitalized with acute chest pain The study of Shimoni et al. [27] included 97 consecutive patients, hospitalized with chest pain and suspected CAD, who had LVEF > 50 % and normal regional LV systolic function. Patients with ST-elevation MI at presentation or a history of myocardial infarction were excluded. This study was included by consensus among the authors, since 21 patients (22 %) had previous revascularization. A control group of 51 patients referred to stress echocardiography for evaluation of atypical chest pain was not evaluated in our review, because they had no coronary angiography. GLS was measured from the apical views. RLS was computed as that segment with the least negative strain value during systole using the segmental division of the three major coronary arteries introduced by Cerquira et al. [29]. Although this study incorporated a histogram with different variation in strain measurements, the data included in Table 2 is based upon peak systolic strain values obtained from 16-segment model. The mean difference between patients with CAD+ vs-CAD- was 3.5 % for GLS and 3.8 % for RLS. The ROC analyses revealed higher AUC values than the three other studies (Table 2).

One study incorporating strain measurements at rest and during dobutamine stress (GE equipment)
In the study of Ng et al. [28] 177 consecutive patients were identified from a database as had been evaluated for stable CAD. Exclusion criteria was LVEF < 40 % or moderate to severe valvular disease. The time lapse between echocardiography and coronary angiography was up to 6 months, and 30 % of the patients had a history

of MI. However, in view of its interesting findings including strain measurements during dobutamine stress echocardiography (DSE) the study was included as a compromise. A derivation study population that comprised 62 patients and a validation study population of 40 patients underwent clinically indicated DSE performed < 8 days before coronary angiography. Patients with AMI < 4 weeks, heart failure, cardiomyopathy or severe valvular heart disease had been excluded. The mean difference for GLS in the derivation group was 2.8 % as opposed to 6.0 % during peak stress with the respective figures in the validation group being 1.5 % and 3.0 %. The diagnostic accuracy as judged from the ROC analysis of GLS at peak stress in the derivation group was excellent with an optimal cutoff at - 20.0 (Table 3), being similar to wall motion score index. No such data was presented from the validation group, and RLS was not measured in this study. In conclusion the introduction of GLS strain measurements during DSE resulted in a far better diagnostic accuracy for CAD than of the resting values, especially in the derivation subgroup.

Summary of results
In these 6 studies 778 patients with suspected CAD were examined with speckle tracking echocardiography and coronary angiography; 397 (51 %) had CAD+ and 381 (49 %) had CAD- judged from the angiographic criteria applied. The majority, of patients included had no evidence of obvious CAD on presentation. The most uniform measurements were GLS at rest. Table 4 shows the combined mean and pooled SD in the CAD+ and CAD- populations respectively as each study included is added. The diagram in Fig. 2 shows the differences in GLS measured at rest in the CAD+ and CAD- patients in the six studies and the combined mean and SD for the six studies together. GLS values from the study of Sarvari et al. [23] have been assessed from the endocardial layer. Summarizing these results by methods previously described, patients with CAD+ (n = 397) had on average GLS −17.2 (±2.6)% as opposed to −19.2 (±2.8)% among those with CAD- (n = 381). The average mean difference in GLS between the two groups was 2.7 (interstudy range 1.7-3.9).

Although 4 studies reported RLS measurements, the heterogeneous methodology applied did not allow any direct inter-study comparison. The individual studies and their respective mean and SD for RLS in the CAD+/CAD-groups are presented in Fig. 3. In two of the studies ROC analysis of GLS at rest was not presented [23, 28].

The area under curve in 4 studies for predicting CAD+ ranged from 0.68 to 0.80. The cut-off level for prediction of CAD+ in the ROC analysis varied between −17.4 % and −19.7 % with a sensitivity from 51 % to 81 %) and specifcity between 58 % and −81 %.

Table 3 GLS measurements at rest and during PDS for identification of significant CAD on CAG

Study	Strain masurements	Derivation group, n = 62		p-value	Validation Group n = 40		p-value
		CAD- n = 14	CAD+ n = 48		CAD- n = 15	CAD+ n = 25	
Ng [28]							
	GLS at rest	−19.1 ± 2.9	−16.3 ± 2.4	0.001	−19.0 ± 2.8	−17.5 ± 2.4	n.s.
	GLS at PDS	−21.7 ± 3.0	−15.7 ± 2.9	<0.001	−20.7 ± 0.8	−17.7 ± 2.7	<0.05
	ROC analysis		Optimal cut-		Sensitivity	Specicity	Accuracy
		AUC	off for GLS		(%)	(%)	(%)
	Peak stress	0.93, p < 0,001	−20 %		84	88	85

mean ± SD

n.s not significant, PDS Peak dobutamine stress, otherwise as in Table 1

Discussion

In this review of a limited number of patients recruited from 6 heterogeneous studies, measurements of GLS and RLS revealed significantly higher values (less negative) among patients with CAD+ than in those with CAD-. However, the overlap in distribution of GLS values between the CAD+ and CAD- groups was considerable both in the individual studies and in our analysis of the combined samples. This implies that it is difficult to correctly identify a patient as CAD+ or CAD- using GLS values at rest alone, and stresses the point that statistical significance does not equal clinical relevance.

It should be noted that our analysis of the combined samples does present some methodological problems. It assumes implicitly that all studies used the same inclusion criteria, and that no selection bias was present in any of the studies. This is a problem with many combined analysis of several studies and also in this case. Furthermore, it disregards various possible measurement biases that may stem from the use of different equipment and measurement methods and/or skills. Also, the assumption of normality in distribution of GLS values for CAD+ and CAD- patients may or may not hold

(without access to raw data, this assumption could not be subjected to statistical tests).

We still argue that even with these challenges present, the analysis still provides useful insight as to the clinical relevance of GLS at rest in this context. This is because the estimated degree of overlap between GLS values of CAD+ and CAD- patients is so significant that the overall picture would most likely remain the same even if several possible biases were adjusted for (note also that the individual studies produce similar degrees of overlap). As for the assumption of normality, the significant degree of overlap does not rely on the distributions being exactly normal, as is evident in Fig. 2. Substantial changes to skewness and/or kurtosis will still produce overlap with the same clinical implications. Hence we argue that the value of GLS at rest to identify CAD+ patients with chest pain from those with CAD- is only moderate.

Interestingly, in one study [28] a subgroup that underwent DSE demonstrated that this overlap was nearly eliminated when GLS was calculated during peak stress. On the other hand, such a difference was not as pronounced in another subgroup that underwent DSE in the same study. In one study [23], using layer specific

Table 4 Table showing the combined mean and pooled SD at rest in the CAD - and CAD + populations respectively as each study included is added

	CAD +						CAD -					
Study	n (% of total weight)	Cumulative n	Mean GLS, %	SD	Combined mean	Pooled SD	n (% of total weight)	Cumulative n	Mean GLS, %	SD	Combined Mean	Pooled SD
Ng	48 (12 %)		−16,3	2,4			14 (4 %)		−19,1	2,9		
Ng	25 (6 %)	73	−17,5	2,4	−16,7	2,5	15 (4 %)	29	−19	2,8	−19,0	2,8
Montgo	56 (14 %)	129	−16,8	3,2	−16,7	2,8	67 (18 %)	96	−19,1	3,4	−19,1	3,2
Smedsr	43 (11 %)	172	−17,7	3	−17,0	2,9	43 (11 %)	139	−19,5	2,6	−19,2	3,1
Shimon	69 (17 %)	241	−17,3	2,4	−17,1	2,8	28 (7 %)	167	−20,8	2,3	−19,5	3,0
B-Sørens	107 (27 %)	348	−17,3	2,5	−17,1	2,7	186 (49 %)	353	−18,9	2,6	−19,2	2,8
Sarvari	49 (12 %)	397	−17,3	2,2	−17,2	2,6	28 (7 %)	381	−19,2	2,2	−19,2	2,8

The study by Ng has two lines because it was divided into one validation and one derivation group

Abbreviations: CAD+ coronary artery disease, CAD- no coronary artery disease, SD standard deviation, GLS slobal longitudinal strain

Cumulative n describes the total number of pateints as each study is added on

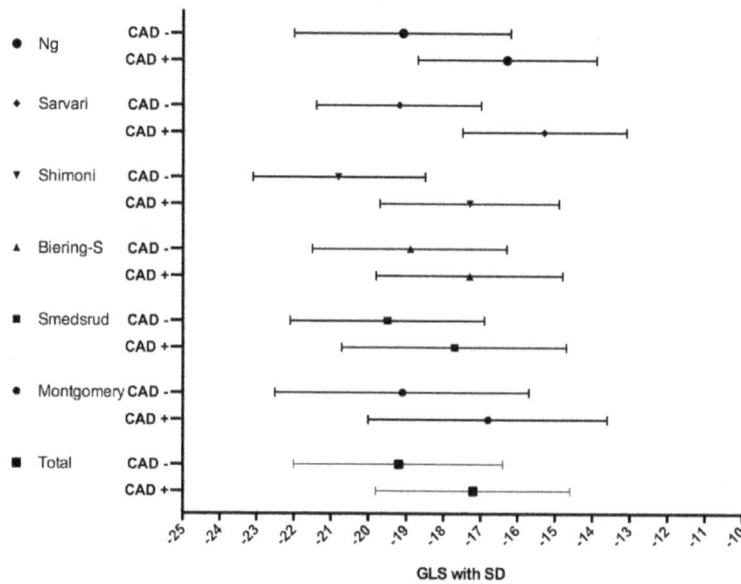

Fig. 2 Six included studies with results of mean GLS with SD in their CAD +/CAD- groups. Abbreviations: CAD+: Coronary artery disease. CAD-: No significant coronary artery disease. GLS: Global longitudinal strain. SD: standard deviation

measurements of both GLS, RLS and circumferential strain at rest, a very high diagnostic accuracy was observed for the endocardial and mid-myocardial layers.

Since CAD is primarily a regional problem and GLS is a global assessment the present findings were perhaps not surprising. The study of Sarvari et al. [23] using layer-specific regional strain and the study of Shimoni et al. [27] using the least negative strain value during systole for the segmental division of three major coronary arteries introduced by Cerquira et al. [29] both showed a

lesser degree of overlap of the strain values in the CAD +/CAD-groups and thereby better potential (Fig. 3). However, in the two other studies that reported RLS, the overlap was significant and did not appear to be better than for GLS.

The different methods used for obtaining regional strain results represent a problem. In 1989 the American Society of Echocardiography recommended a 16-segment model for LV segmentation [31]. In 2002 they introduced a 17-segment model in an attempt to establish segmentation

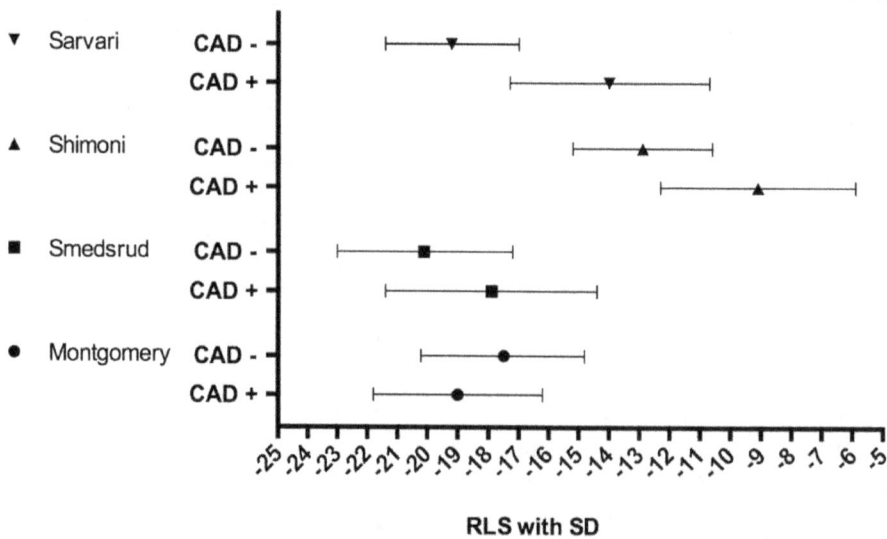

Fig. 3 Four included studies with results of mean RLS with SD in their CAD +/CAD- groups. Abbreviations: CAD+: Coronary artery disease. CAD-: No significant coronary artery disease. RLS: regional longitudinal strain. SD: standard deviation

standards applicable to all types of imaging. The new segment was the apical cap [29]. This model should be used for myocardial perfusion studies and the 16-segment model is appropriate for studies assessing wall-motion abnormalities. The Bulls-Eye used for RLS assessment is derived from the latter for both GE and Toshiba equipment. In the 2002 recommendations individual segments were clustered and combined assigned to specific coronary artery territories, although there is individual variability in the coronary blood supply to myocardial segments. Most studies in this review including RLS have incorporated this model, but two studies used the average of all segments in one territory [23, 25], one used the lowest strain value a single segment [27], one assessed the average values in the LAD segment only [24] and one did not incorporate RLS measurements at all. In the large Danish study [26], in contrast to the others, ischemic segments were not assigned to prespecified vascular territories because they obtained information about how significant stenosis in the three main coronary arteries affected regional LS in each segment.

Until a standard and well established approach is generally adopted, measurements today of RLS is hampered by the use of an arbitrary anatomical model that does not necessarily reflect the individual coronary artery distribution, and the need for proper standardization of how to uniformly obtain RLS data is obvious.

Patients studied were principally without LV dysfunction, overt heart failure, left bundle branch block or heart failure, and only a minority had evidence of previous CAD, most of whom had been revascularized. With that reservation in mind, the results observed are probably representative for most patients presenting with chest pain and without previously known CAD.

It seems to be that the number of patients hospitalized for non-coronary chest pain (NCCP) is increasing [1–3]. This group consists of patients both with and without established CAD. Interestingly, only two of the studies [23, 27] evaluated LS measurements in patients hospitalized for acute chest pain. The 56 CAD- patients in these studies most probably represent NCCP. Dahlslett et al. recently published a study that explored the value of LS measurements at rest and during stress to predict the absence of CAD [22]. Because the study was designed to "rule out" CAD rather than detect it, it was not included in this review. Interestingly they found that strain measurements may be helpful in excluding significant CAD among NCCP patients. Clearly, larger "rule out studies" are needed in order to further evaluate the role of LV strain measurements this increasing group of patients that represent a huge burden to contemporary health care. There are at present no established guidelines for management of such patients, and a simple, fast method to exclude those without CAD beyond the information

obtained from ECG and cardiac markers would be highly welcome. Strain measurements by STE at rest are fast and simple to apply, without any discomfort to the patients. If this method appears to be of value in the classification of patients with unexplained chest pain to CAD+ or CAD- it may obtain acceptance for a more common use in clinical practice.

The results from this review, however, were somewhat disappointing both in the acute and elective evaluation of suspected CAD, confirming that GLS at rest is not sensitive enough to detect regional CAD. The influence of afterload and diastolic function on GLS may have contributed to these findings, but these parameters were not addressed in this review.

The overlap may be overcome by the introduction of layer specific measurements [23].

For patients with stable CAD the addition of STE to simple stress test that is fast and easy to perform may be of value in this context. The improved diagnostic accuracy of an ordinary exercise test added to GLS measurements in the study of Biering-Sørensen et al. [26] is interesting, but requires considerable time and resources. The findings of Ng et al. [28] were somewhat disturbing, with different diagnostic accuracy of DSE with strain in the two subgroups studied. The use of DSE with strain is further hampered by the limited availability of DSE in many smaller hospitals. This procedure requires highly trained staff, good machine capacity and a considerable volume of examinations. Therefore, a proven clinical value of strain measurements at rest would be highly beneficial to many cardiologists in everyday practice. As with exercise testing, adding pretest probability is essential and a model including this and loading conditions along with strain measurements would possibly improve the benefit of STE in clinical practice.

Study limitations
Selection bias is present in studies selected for this review, represented by the different number of patients with obvious CAD on inclusion. Knowledge of previous CAD might influence the measurements because the technique is not fully automated and thereby operator dependent. The presence of established CAD would require previous strain images for comparison, like the assessment of a new ECG requires old ECGs for the evaluation of new changes in patients with established CAD. At the present stage, it seems unrealistic to assume that most patients with CAD have previous strain measurements for comparison. Therefore, we aimed to comprise patients without previously established CAD when admitted with chest pain.

It ought to be emphasized that we only included studies where coronary angiography was performed, hence selection bias is presented and the results cannot be applied to the large group of patients with chest pain and CAD ranging from stable angina to ACS.

In addition, selection bias may be unavoidable when different selection criteria for "good quality images" are being applied. Due to operational bias, better results may be expected in studies with the most experienced and competent echocardiographers. Differences in the time lapse between the two examinations may also have an influence across studies, not only within them.

Most studies had used GE Vingmed equipment. The problem of manufacturer bias is already introduced with the inclusion of the study using Artida Toshiba system, and more will follow. It will present a challenge for the medical community and the various manufacturers to introduce uniform principles for strain measurements in the future. Operator bias in the review cannot be excluded, since no study reported the level of expertise of the actual Using too strict inclusion criteria for studies may have precluded this present review. Therefore, a more extended validation of the strain method may have been missed. Only 15 full articles were assessed after the performing the previously described search and there is always a chance that important studies were left out of although no additional citations could be found from screening the reference lists of these articles and reviews included in the search.

Conclusions

Based upon the findings GLS measurements at rest only have modest diagnostic accuracy in predicting CAD+ among patients presenting with acute or stable chest pain. GLS measurements during peak DSE and showed better accuracy in two separate studies, but these findings have to be verified in larger studies. RLS showed greater potential in detecting CAD, but the heterogeneity for obtaining regional data and different terminology remains a challenge. Clearly, more refined strain measurements at rest are needed to identify patients with vs. without significant coronary heart disease, and the introduction of models including pretest probability and possibly also afterload/diastolic function should be developed.

Abbreviations

ACS: Acute coronary syndrome; AUC: Area under curve; CAD+: Significant coronary artery stenosis; CAD-: No significant coronary artery stenosis; CTA: Coronary computed tomography angiography; DSE: Dobutamine stress echocardiography; GCS: Global circumferential strain; GLS: Global longitudinal strain; LS: Longitudinal strain; LV: Left ventricular; MI: Myocardial infarction; NCCP: Non coronary chest pain; NPV: Negative predictive value; PCI: Percutaneous coronary intervention; PPV: Positive predictive value; ROC: Receiver operating characteristics; SD: Standard deviation; STE: Speckle tracking echocardiography; RLS: Regional longitudinal strain.

Competing interests

The authors have no competing interests.

Authors' contributions

IBN: Design of study, data collection, analysis and interpretation of data, drafting the manuscript, critical revision of the manuscript, final approval of the manuscript submitted. VR: Analysis and interpretation of data, critical revision of the manuscript, final approval of the manuscript submitted. TE: Analysis and interpretation of data, critical revision of the manuscript, final approval of the manuscript submitted. JEO: Design of study, data collection, analysis and interpretation of data, drafting the manuscript, critical revision of the manuscript, final approval of the manuscript submitted.

Acknowledgements

We thank Mariann Mathisen, librerian at Vestfold Hospital Trust, who helped with the literarture search and Hallvard Billehaug Norum for statistical analysis.

Author details

[1]Department of Cardiology, Vestfold Hospital Trust, Pb 2168, 3103 Tønsberg, Norway. [2]University of Oslo, Faculty of Medicine, Pb 1078 Blindern, 0316 Oslo, Norway. [3]Department of Cardiology, Oslo University Hospital, Rikshospitalet, Pb 4950Nydalen, 0424 Oslo, Norway.

References

1. Aune E, Hjelmesaeth J, Fox KA, Endresen K, Otterstad JE. High mortality rate in conservatively managed patients with acute coronary syndrome. Scand Cardiovasc J. 2006;40:137–44.
2. Narallah N, Steiner H, Hasin Y. The challenge of chest pain in the emergency room: now and in the future. Eur Heart J. 2011;32:656.
3. Ruddox V, Mathisen M, Otterstad JE. Prevalence and prognosis of non-specific chest pain among patients hospitalized for suspected acute coronary syndrome—a systematic literature search. BMC Medicine. 2012;10:58.
4. Damman P, van Geloven N, Walentin L, Lagerqvist B, Fox CA, Clayton T, et al. Timing of angiography with a routine invasive strategy and long-term outcomes in non-ST segment evaluation acute coronary syndrome: a collaborative analysis of individual patient data from the FRISC II (Fragmin an Fast Revascularization During Instability in Coronary Artery Disease), ICTUS (Invasive versus conservative Treatment in Unstable Coronary Syndormes), and RITA-3 (Intervention vs Conservative treatment Strategy in Patients With Unstable Angina or Non-ST elevation Myocardial Infarction) Trial. J Am Coll Cardiol Intv. 2012;5:191–9.
5. Montalescot G, Sechtem U, Achenbach S, Andreotti F, Arden C, Budaj A, et al. ESC guidelines on the management of stable coronary artery disease. European Heart Journal. 2013;2013(34):2949–3003.
6. Hamm CW, Bassand JP, Agewall S, Bax J, Boersma E, Bueno H, et al. ESC Guidelines for the management of acute coronary syndromes in patients presenting without persistent ST-segment elevation: The Task Force for the management of acute coronary syndromen (ACS) in patients presenting without persistent ST-segment elevation of the European Society of Cardiology. European Heart Journal. 2011;32:2999–3054.
7. Hare JL, Brown JK, Leano R, Jenkins C, Woodward N, Marwick TH. Use of myocardial deformation imaging to detect preclinical myocardial dysfunction before conventional measures in patients undergoing breast cancer treatment with trastuzumab. Am Heart J. 2009;158:294–301.
8. Sarvari SI, Gjesdal O, Gude E, Arora S, Andreassen AK, Gullestad L, et al. Early postoperative left ventricular function by echocardiographic strain is a predictor of 1-year mortality in heart transplant recipients. J Am Soc Echocardiogr. 2012;25:1007–14.
9. Edvardsen T, Skulstad H, Aakhus S, Urheim S. Regional myocardial systolic function during acute myocardial ischemia assessed by strain Doppler echocardiography. J Am Coll Cardiol. 2001;37:726–30.
10. Sutherland G, De Salvo G, Claus P, D'Hooge J, Bijnens B. Strain and strain rate imaging: a new clinical approach to quantifying regional myocardial function. J Am Soc Echocardiogr. 2004;17:788–802.

11. Gjesdahl O, Helle-Valle T, Hopp E, Lunde K, Vartdal T, Aakhus S, et al. Nonivasive separation of large, medium, and small myocardial infarcts in survivors of reperfused ST-elevation myocardial infarction. Circ Cardiovasc Imaging. 2008;1:189–96.

12. Feigenbaum H, Mastouri R, Sawada S. A practical approach to using strain echocardiography to evaluate the left ventricle. Circ J. 2012;76:1550–5.

13. Grenne B, Eek C, Sjøli B, Skulstad H, Aakhus S, Smiseth OA, et al. Changes of myocardial function in patients with non-ST-elevation acute cornary syndrome awaiting coronary angiography. Am J Cardiol. 2010;105:1212–8.

14. Grenne B, Eek C, Sjøli B, Dahlslett T, Ucto M, Hol PK, et al. Acute coronary occlusion in non-ST-elevation acute coronary syndrome: outcome and early identification by strain echocardiography. Heart. 2010;96:1550–6.

15. Eek C, Grenne B, Brunvand H, Aakhus S, Endresen K, Smiseth OA, et al. Strain echocardiography predicts acute coronary occlusion in patients with non-ST-segment elevation acute coronary syndrome. Eur J Echocardiogr. 2010;11:501–8.

16. Choi J-O, Cho SW, Song YB, Cho SJ, Song BG, Lee SC, et al. Longitudinal 2D strain at rest predicts the presence of left main and three vessel coronary artery disease in patients without regional wall motion abnormality. Eur J Echocardiogr. 2009;10:695–701.

17. Celutkiene J, Zakaralte D, Skorniakov V, Zvironaite V, Grabauskiene V, Burca J, et al. Quantitative approach using multiple single parameters versus visual assessment in dobutamine stress echocardiography. Cardiovasc Ultrasound. 2012;10:31.

18. Stanton T, Leano R, Marwick T. Prediction of all-cause mortality from global longitudinal speckle strain. Circ Cardiovasc Imaging. 2009;2:356–64.

19. Nucifora G, Schuijf JD, Delgado V, Bertini M, Scholte AJ, Ng AC, et al. Incremental value of subclinical left ventricular systolic dysfunction for the identification of patients with obstructive coronary artery disease. Am Heart J. 2010;159:148–57.

20. Hanekom L, Cho G-Y, Leano R, Jeffries L, Marwick T. Comparison of two-dimensional speckle and tissure Doppler strain measurements during dobutamine strain echocardiography: an angiographic correlation. Eur Heart J. 2007;28:1765–72.

21. Anwar AM. Accuarcy of two-dimensional speckle tracking echocardiography for the detection of significant coronary stenosis. J Cardiovasc Ultrasound. 2013;21:177–82.

22. Dahlslett T, Karlsen S, Grenne B, Eek C, Sjøli B, Smiseth OA, et al. Early assessment of strain echocardiography can accurately exclude significant coronary artery stenosis in suspected non-ST-segment elevation acute coronary syndrome. J Am Soc Echocardiogr. 2014;27:512–9.

23. Sarvari S, Haugaa KH, Zahid W, Bendz B, Aakhus S, Aaberge L, et al. Layer-specific quantitatification of myocardial deformation by strain echocardiography nay reveal significant CAD in patients with non-segment elevation acute coronary syndromes. J Am Coll Cardiovasc Imaging. 2011;6:535–44.

24. Montgomery DE, Puthumana JJ, Fox JM, Ogunyakin KO. Global longitudinal strain aids the detection of non-obstructive coronary artery disease in the resting echocardiogram. Eur Heart J – Cardiovasc Imaging. 2012;13:579–87.

25. Smedsrud MK, Sarvari S, Haugaa KH, Gjesdal O, Ørn S, Aaberge L, et al. Duration of myocardial early systolic lengthening predicts the presence of significant coronary artery disease. J Am Coll Cardiol. 2012;60:1086–93.

26. Biering-Sørensen T, Hoffman S, Mogelvang R, Zeeberg Iversen A, Galatius S, Fritz-Hansen T, et al. Myocardial strain analysis by 2-Dimensional speckle tracking echocardiography improves diagnostics of coronary artery stenosis in stable angina pectoris. Circ Cardiovasc Imaging. 2014;7:58–65.

27. Shimoni S, Gendelmann G, Ayzenberg O, Smirin N, Lysyansky P, Edri O, et al. Differential effects of coronary artery stenosis of myocardial function: The value of myocardial strain analysis for the detection of coronary artery disease. J Am Soc Echocardiogr. 2011;24:748–57.

28. Ng AC, Sitges M, Pham PN, Tran da T, Delgado V, Bertini M, et al. Incremental value of 2-dimensional speckle treacking strain imaging to wall motion analysis for detection of coronary artery disease in patients undergoing dobutamine stress echocardiography. Am Heart J. 2009;158:836–44.

29. Cerquieira MD, Weissman NJ, Dilsizian V, Jacobs AK, Kaul S, Laskey WK, et al. Standardized myocardial segmentation and nomenclature for tomographic imaging of the heart: a statement for heartcare professionals from the Cardiac Imaging Committee of the Council on Clinical Cardiology of the American Heart Association. Circulation. 2002;105:539–42.

30. Lang RM, Bierig M, Devereux RB. Recommendations for chamber quantification: a report from the American Society of Echocardiography's guideines and standards committee and the chamber quantification writing group, developed in conjunction with the European association of echocardiography, a branch of the European society of Cardiology. J Am Soc Echocardiography. 2005;18:1440–63.

31. Schiller NB, Shah PM, Crawford M, DeMaria A, Devereux R, Feigenbaum H, et al. Recommendations for quantitation of the left ventricle by two-dimensional echocardiography: American Society of Echocardiography committee on standards, subcommittee on quantitation of two-dimensional echocardiograms. J Am Soc Echocardiogr. 1989;2:358–67.

4

Regression models for analyzing radiological visual grading studies

S. Ehsan Saffari[1,2], Áskell Löve[3,4], Mats Fredrikson[5] and Örjan Smedby[1,6]*

Abstract

Background: For optimizing and evaluating image quality in medical imaging, one can use visual grading experiments, where observers rate some aspect of image quality on an ordinal scale. To analyze the grading data, several regression methods are available, and this study aimed at empirically comparing such techniques, in particular when including random effects in the models, which is appropriate for observers and patients.

Methods: Data were taken from a previous study where 6 observers graded or ranked in 40 patients the image quality of four imaging protocols, differing in radiation dose and image reconstruction method. The models tested included linear regression, the proportional odds model for ordinal logistic regression, the partial proportional odds model, the stereotype logistic regression model and rank-order logistic regression (for ranking data). In the first two models, random effects as well as fixed effects could be included; in the remaining three, only fixed effects.

Results: In general, the goodness of fit (AIC and McFadden's Pseudo R^2) showed small differences between the models with fixed effects only. For the mixed-effects models, higher AIC and lower Pseudo R^2 was obtained, which may be related to the different number of parameters in these models. The estimated potential for dose reduction by new image reconstruction methods varied only slightly between models.

Conclusions: The authors suggest that the most suitable approach may be to use ordinal logistic regression, which can handle ordinal data and random effects appropriately.

Keywords: Image quality, Visual grading, Ordinal data, Regression models, Fixed effects, Random effects

Background

When evaluating medical imaging methods, the most relevant performance measures of a procedure are related to its ability to produce correct answers to a diagnostic problem. This is typically done with concepts such as sensitivity, specificity and receiver operating characteristic (ROC) analysis. When developing a new method, however, it is often necessary to fine-tune numerous parameters that need to be specified in modern imaging equipment in order to obtain as much diagnostic information as possible at the minimum cost in radiation dose (effective dose) to the patient. In this optimization process, a common approach is to perform *visual grading experiments*, where a group of observers (e.g. radiologists) assess the fulfillment of certain well-defined image quality criteria using an ordinal scale [1]. As the data are given on an ordinal scale, the data analysis methods should be chosen accordingly, using techniques that are appropriate for such data. Still, a number of studies have been published where ordinal data from visual grading experiments are analyzed with ANOVA and similar linear models, although these build on assumptions of interval scale data, homoscedasticity and so forth.

In earlier publications, our group has proposed to use ordinal regression models in these situations to compare alternative imaging procedures [2]. Using such models, and an assumption of the relationship between the effective dose to the patient and the image quality, it is also possible to estimate the potential for dose reduction

* Correspondence: orjan.smedby@sth.kth.se
[1]Department of Medical and Health Sciences (IMH), Linköping University, Linköping, Sweden
[6]KTH Royal Institute of Technology, School of Technology and Health, Alfred Nobels allé 10, SE-141 52 Huddinge, Stockholm, Sweden
Full list of author information is available at the end of the article

that may be expected when a new technique is introduced [3]. Based on an experiment where both the imaging technique and the effective dose are varied, the estimated dose reduction is obtained from the ratio between two regression coefficients in the regression equation. Since two of the experimental factors, the patient and the observer, are not interesting *per se*, but can be seen as samples from two underlying populations, it may be appropriate to treat them as random effects, which can also be done with ordinal regression models [4].

In addition to the most common form of ordinal regression, the proportional odds model [5], alternative approaches for analyzing ordinal data with regression models include the partial proportional odds model [6] and the stereotype logistic model [7]. These do not seem to have been applied to visual grading data before. In addition, random effects models have not been systematically compared to models with only fixed effects. Finally, it is not known to what extent the results of ordinal regression models differ from those of the simpler linear models.

Thus, the aim of the present study was to review regression models potentially suitable for analyzing visual grading studies and to empirically compare them on already available data, in particular to study the effect of including random effects in the model.

Material and methods
Data
The data used were taken from a previously published study on image quality and radiation dose in brain Computed Tomography (CT) which evaluated two new reconstruction algorithms, i.e. methods for creating images from the acquired raw data [8]. It has been suggested that new reconstruction algorithms (in particular iterative algorithms) may improve image quality to such an extent that the radiation dose to the patient may be reduced without impairing the image quality, which otherwise occurs when the radiation dose is reduced. Six neuroradiologists evaluated image quality in images acquired from 40 patients, each of whom underwent two consecutive brain CT examinations with two different effective dose levels. Images from all 80 examinations were reconstructed using four different image reconstruction methods: the traditional filtered back projection algorithm using the full dose (CTDI$_{vol}$) of 57 mGy (*fd*), which served as the reference, the same algorithm using a reduced dose of 40 mGy (*rd*), and two different levels of iterative reconstruction algorithms (*id2* and *id4*), also using the reduced dose. In the visual evaluation, each observer individually graded three image quality criteria – gray-white-matter discrimination (GW), basal ganglia delineation (BG) and general image quality (GQ) – using a four-grade ordinal scale ranging from 1 (poor) to 4 (excellent). In addition, each observer

ranked each set of four reconstructions, i.e. sorted the four image stacks in order from 1 (best) to 4 (worst) for each of the image quality criteria.

Thus the grading data comprises 3 image quality scores (*GWscore*, *BGscore* and *GQscore*) and 3 image quality ranks (*GWrank*, *BGrank* and *GQrank*) for each imaging protocol, observer and patient. As there were 6 observers and 40 patients, and we considered 4 imaging protocols (*nd*, *rd*, *id2* and *id4*), the dataset consists of 6 × 40 × 4 = 960 observations. The data were stored in *Stata* format, and *Stata* 13.1 (StataCorp, College Station, TX, USA) was used for all analyses.

The ethical approval of the acquisition of data for the original publication [8] was given by the regional research ethics committee in Lund, Sweden (decision nr. 2010/594, date Nov. 11, 2010). Written informed consent was obtained from each patient before examination, and the study was performed in compliance with the Helsinki Declaration.

Analysis of absolute grading scores
In this section, different regression models will be discussed. In all models, the response variable is *GWscore*, which is treated as an interval scale variable. We assume that the influence of dose is best modeled via the logarithm of the dose rather than the dose itself [2]. Thus, there are five covariates in the regression models: log(*CTDI*), *id2*, *id4*, patient and observer, the two last of which are nominal, whereas *id2* and *id4* are dummy variables indicating whether an iterative reconstruction method was used.

Regression models with fixed effects
We suppose in this section that all covariates are fixed effects in the regression models. We start the analysis with the most fundamental regression model, i.e. the linear regression model, and will then discuss the logistic regression models, which are the main concern of this paper.

Linear model In a linear regression model, it is supposed that the relationship between the dependent variable and the vector of regressors is linear; thus the model takes the following form:

$$GWscore = \beta_0 + \beta_1 \log(CTDI) + \beta_2 \, id2 \qquad (1)$$
$$+ \beta_3 \, id4 + \beta_{4,p} + \beta_{5,o} + \epsilon$$

where β_i's are the regression coefficients, and ϵ is an error term from the population. This was achieved with the following Stata command:

   regress GWscore logCTDI id2 id4 i.patient i.observer

Ordinal logistic regression The ordinal logistic regression model (proportional odds model) is used when the dependent variable is ordinal. The cumulative probability of this regression model can be expressed in this form:

$$P(GWscore \leq i \,|\, \boldsymbol{x}) = \frac{e^{\beta_{0i} - \boldsymbol{\beta}' \boldsymbol{x}}}{1 + e^{\beta_{0i} - \boldsymbol{\beta}' \boldsymbol{x}}} , i = 2, \; 3, \; 4$$

(2)

or

$$logit(P(GWscore \leq i \,|\, \boldsymbol{x})) = \; log \frac{P(GWscore \leq i \,|\, \boldsymbol{x})}{1 - P(GWscore \leq i \,|\, \boldsymbol{x})}$$
$$= \beta_{0i} - \boldsymbol{\beta}' \boldsymbol{x} , i = 2, \; 3, \; 4$$

(3)

where $\boldsymbol{x}$ is the vector of covariates, β_{0i} is a parameter that depends on i, and $\boldsymbol{\beta}'$ (transposed $\boldsymbol{\beta}$) is the coefficient vector which is constant for all i. According to equations (2) and (3), there is only one set of coefficients ($\boldsymbol{\beta}'$) in the ordinal logistic regression model, and due to the same relationship between each pair of outcome groups, the ordinal logistic model will make the parallel regression assumption [7, 9]. Since only the β_{0i} differ across values of $i = 2, 3, 4$, the three regression lines are all parallel. The following *Stata* command was used for this model:

ologit GWscore logCTDI id2 id4 i.patient i.observer

Partial proportional odds model In situations where the parallel regression assumption is violated, the ordinal logistic regression model is no longer an appropriate model. In this case, an alternative may be the partial proportional odds model, in which some of the β coefficients can be the same for all values of i, while others can differ (γ_i). Thus, this model is represented in the following form:

$$P(GWscore > i \,|\, \boldsymbol{x}) = \frac{1}{1 + e^{-\beta_{0i} + \boldsymbol{\beta}' \boldsymbol{x} + \gamma_i' T}} , i = 2, \; 3$$

(4)

or

$$logit \, (P(GWscore > i \,|\, \boldsymbol{x})) = \beta_{0i} - \boldsymbol{\beta}' \boldsymbol{x} - \gamma_i' T , i = 2, \; 3$$

(5)

where $\boldsymbol{x}$ and T are the covariates. This model is more difficult to interpret than the ordinal logistic regression model, since there will be many more parameters to consider and some effects might be statistically insignificant due to the increased number of parameters [6, 10].

We have used the *gologit2* command in *Stata* for this model as follows:

xi : gologit2 GWscore logCTDI id2 id4 i.observer
i.patient, pl(i.patient) difficult

Stereotype logistic model An alternative model is to consider the response variable as categorical, rather than ordinal, i.e., we are unsure of the relevance of the ordering in the response variable in this case. Also, a multinomial logistic regression model may be suggested when the assumptions of the proportional odds model are not satisfied. Thus, the stereotype ordinal regression model can be considered as imposing ordering constraints on a multinomial model, which is a form of ordinal regression model. Unlike ordered logistic models, stereotype logistic models do not impose the proportional-odds assumption [6, 11]. A full multinomial model can be represented by:

$$P(GWscore = s \,|\, \boldsymbol{x}) = \frac{\exp\left(\beta_{0s} - \boldsymbol{\beta}_s' \boldsymbol{x}\right)}{\sum_{t=2}^{4} \exp\left(\beta_{0t} - \boldsymbol{\beta}_t' \boldsymbol{x}\right)},$$

(6)

where $s = 2, \; 4,$ and $\beta_{00} \equiv 0$ and $\beta_0 \equiv 0$. In the multinomial logistic model, the number of parameter vectors to estimate is m-1, where m is the number of levels in the response variable. Based on the restriction on the multinomial model by the stereotype logistic model, the number of parameter vectors is between one and min (m-1, p), where p is the number of covariates [12]. Thus, replacing $\beta_s = \phi_s \; \beta$, the stereotype ordinal regression model can be written as follows:

$$P(GWscore = s \,|\, \boldsymbol{x}) = \frac{\exp\left(\beta_{0s} - \phi_s \boldsymbol{\beta}' \boldsymbol{x}\right)}{\sum_{t=2}^{4} \exp\left(\beta_{0t} - \phi_t \boldsymbol{\beta}' \boldsymbol{x}\right)},$$

(7)

where $\beta_{00} = \phi_0 \equiv 0$. This was achieved with the following *Stata* command:

slogit GWscore logCTDI id2 id4 i.patient i.observer

Regression models with random effects
In this section, it is supposed that three covariates including log(*CTDI*), id2 and id4 are considered as fixed effects and two covariates including *patient* and *observer* are specified as crossed random effects. The basic concept of a random effects model is that the variation across entities is assumed to be random and uncorrelated with the covariates, unlike the fixed effects model. The mixed linear model as well as the mixed-effects ordered logistic regression model will be discussed to

analyze the data when there are both fixed and random effects in the model.

Mixed linear model The simplest model to analyze a data set with both fixed effects and random effects is a mixed linear model, which can be written in the following form:

$$GWscore = \boldsymbol{\beta}'\boldsymbol{x} + \boldsymbol{b}'\boldsymbol{z} + \epsilon, \tag{8}$$

where $\boldsymbol{x}$ is the model matrix for *id2*, *id4* and *nd* as fixed effects, $\boldsymbol{z}$ is the model matrix for *patient* and *observer* as random effects, $\boldsymbol{\beta}$ is the vector of fixed-effects coefficients, $\boldsymbol{b}$ is the vector of random-effects coefficients, and ⊠ is an error term [13]. We have used the *mixed* command in *Stata* for a mixed linear model including crossed random effects as follows:

> *mixed GWscore id2 id4 logCTDI || _all*
> *: R.observer|| _all : R.patient*

Mixed-effects ordered logistic regression A model that can handle random effects where the response variable is ordinal is the mixed-effects ordered logistic regression [14]. In contrast to the ordinal logistic model, the model with random effects has the form:

$$P(GWscore_{ij} \leq t \,|\, \boldsymbol{x}_{ij}, \boldsymbol{z}_{ij}) = \frac{\exp(\alpha_t - \boldsymbol{\beta}'\boldsymbol{x}_{ij} - \boldsymbol{u}_i'\boldsymbol{z}_{ij})}{1 + \exp(\alpha_t - \boldsymbol{\beta}'\boldsymbol{x}_{ij} - \boldsymbol{u}_i'\boldsymbol{z}_{ij})} \,, \; t = 2, 3, \tag{9}$$

or

$$logit \, P(GWscore_{ij} \leq t \,|\, \boldsymbol{x}_{ij}, \boldsymbol{z}_{ij}) = \alpha_t - \boldsymbol{\beta}'\boldsymbol{x}_{ij} - \boldsymbol{u}_i'\boldsymbol{z}_{ij}, \tag{10}$$

where $\boldsymbol{z}_{ij}$ refers to a vector of covariates for the random effects (*patient* and *observer*) and $\boldsymbol{u}_i$ is the vector of random-effects coefficients [14]. In *Stata*, the *meologit* command can be used for the ordinal logistic regression model with crossed random effects as follows:

> *meologit GWscore logCTDI id2 id4 || _all*
> *: R.observer|| _all : R.patient*

Goodness of fit The metrics used to compare the methods were the pseudo R^2 and Akaike's information criterion (AIC). The *Pseudo R^2*, also called McFadden's R^2, [15], defined by

$$R_{McF}^2 = 1 - \frac{\log \hat{L}(M_{Full})}{\log \hat{L}(M_{intercept})} \tag{11}$$

is one of several approximations of the R^2 for linear regression. None of these are interpreted as the R^2 for linear regression, and they all give different result [16]. An advantage of the McFadden R^2, in addition to its simple definition, is that it can be used for all models estimated by maximum likelihood. Since all models used in this study are based on maximum likelihood, the McFadden R^2 is calculated in the same way for all models, and they can therefore be compared with respect to R^2. The model with the largest R^2 is the one that best fits the data.

However, for comparing models differing in the number of parameters, AIC [17] is more suitable:

$$AIC = \frac{-2 \log \hat{L}(M_k) + 2p}{N} \tag{12}$$

The most common alternative to AIC is the Bayesian information criterion (BIC). However, BIC takes the number of parameters (the degrees of freedom) into account in a way that makes it less appropriate than AIC for selecting between models with different number of parameters. The model with the smallest AIC value is considered to be the best [17].

Estimation of potential for dose reduction To estimate the dose reduction (in percent) that might come about by the application of *id2* and *id4*, we have used the technique proposed in our earlier publication [3], which relates the effect of replacing the reconstruction method to that of changing the effective dose. This involves forming the ratio between two regression coefficients and computing the confidence limits of the final expression using the delta method [18]. The required *Stata* commands to be applied after fitting the regression model are as follows:

> *nlcom $\left(dosereduction\_id2 : \; 1 - exp \left(- \left(\_b[id2] / \_b[logCTDI] \right) \right) \right)$*

> *nlcom $\left(dosereduction\_id4 : \; 1 - exp \left(- \left(\_b[id4] / \_b[logCTDI] \right) \right) \right)$*

Analysis of ranking data

Rank-order data differ in certain respects from grading data where each case is graded on the same absolute scale. One way of understanding ranking is to regard it as a sequence of choices. Then, there is gradually less freedom in the choice of grades, since the earlier choices constrain the available ranks for subsequent cases to those not used previously. This motivates the introduction of dedicated regression techniques for situations with rank-order data.

All regression models discussed in the previous section (including the linear model, ordinal logistic regression, partial proportional odds model, stereotype logistic model, mixed linear model and mixed-effects ordered logistic regression) can be applied to the data in which the response variable is *GWrank*. Besides these regression models, the rank-ordered logistic regression model can be an appropriate model since there is some extra information about the ranking of outcomes.

We define the response of respondent i by the vector $y_i = (y_{i1}, ..., y_{iJ})'$, where y_{ij} denotes the rank that individual i gives to item j. Let $GWrank_{ij} = 1$ represent the event that respondent i most prefers alternative j. This leads to the following expression for the probability that item j is most preferred by individual i:

$$P(GWrank_{ij} = 1 \mid x_{ij}) = \frac{\exp\left(x_i' \beta_j\right)}{\sum_{t=1}^{J} \exp\left(x_i' \beta_t\right)} \qquad (13)$$

where $\beta = \{\beta_1, ..., \beta_J\}$ and β_J is considered as zero for identification [19]. We have used the *rologit* command in *Stata*, which is specifically designed for ranking data, as follows:

rologit GWrank logCTDI id2 id4 , group(groupid)

where *groupid* is an identifier variable that links the alternatives. Since the default for the *rologit* command is that higher values represent more attractive alternatives, we have recoded the *GWrank* variable to have a higher value indicating better quality. In this case, the *Stata* output is the same as when the *reverse* option in *rologit* is used, which specifies that in the preference order, a higher number means a less attractive alternative in the original data [10].

Results
Absolute scores
The results of the different regression models for *GWscore*, *BGscore* and *GQscore* are presented in Tables 1, 2 and 3, respectively. The intercepts are excluded from the reported results in these tables due to different parameterization of the regression models. The analyses have been made using fixed effects models as well as fixed and random effects models, as explained in the previous section. All regression coefficients are statistically significant at the 0.01 level, except when contrasting categories 1 & 2 with category 3 (highest image quality) in the second panel with the partial proportional odds model for *id2* with *GWscore* (Table 1), and for both *id2* and *id4* with *BGscore* and *GQscore* (Tables 2 and 3). The confidence intervals of the coefficients are reported in parentheses in Tables 1, 2 and 3.

In the linear model (*regress*), the regression equation of *GWscore* can be obtained using the coefficients reported in Table 1. The relationship between the covariates and the response variable is assumed to be linear, and an increase in the independent variables – i.e. increasing the effective dose as well as replacing the standard reconstruction with *id2* or *id4* – results in an increase in the *GWscore*, since the signs of all regression coefficients are positive.

In the ordinal logistic model (*ologit*), a log(*CTDI*) coefficient of 8.825 implies that a doubling of the *CTDI* for

Table 1 Estimated parameters, goodness-of-fit statistics and estimated dose reduction for GWscore

Model	Coefficient						Goodness-of-fit		Dose reduction	
	logCTDI		id2		id4		AIC	Pseudo R²	id2	id4
	Est.	P-value	Est.	P-value	Est.	P-value				
regress[a]	1.459	<0.001	0.158	<0.001	0.208	<0.001	-	0.4160	10.29 %	13.31 %
	(1.244, 1.674)		(0.082, 0.234)		(0.132, 0.284)				(6.14 %, 14.43 %)	(9.37 %, 17.24 %)
ologit[a]	8.825	<0.001	0.966	<0.001	1.271	<0.001	1124.35	0.4172	10.37 %	13.41 %
	(7.354, 10.295)		(0.512, 1.419)		(0.812, 1.730)				(6.35 %, 14.39 %)	(9.60 %, 17.23 %)
gologit2[a] =2	9.487	<0.001	1.262	<0.001	1.465	<0.001	1184.56	0.4342	12.45 %	14.31 %
	(7.213, 11.761)		(0.682, 1.842)		(0.873, 2.058)				(7.44 %, 17.46 %)	(9.25 %, 19.37 %)
gologit2[a] =3	8.165	<0.001	0.521	0.172	0.985	0.008			6.18 %	11.37 %
	(6.143, 10.189)		(−.227, 1.269)		(0.260, 1.711)				(−1.62 %, 13.98 %)	(4.87 %, 17.86 %)
slogit[a]	17.447	<0.001	1.887	<0.001	2.433	<0.001	1123.27	0.4201	10.25 %	13.05 %
	(14.460, 20.435)		(1.028, 2.746)		(1.555, 3.310)				(6.35 %, 14.15 %)	(9.23 %, 16.80 %)
mixed[b]	1.459	<0.001	0.158	<0.001	0.208	<0.001	1225.30	0.2748	10.29 %	13.31 %
	(1.244, 1.673)		(0.082, 0.234)		(0.132, 0.284)				(6.14 %, 14.43 %)	(9.38 %, 17.24 %)
meologit[b]	8.433	<0.001	0.922	<0.001	1.213	<0.001	1215.96	0.2751	10.36 %	13.4 %
	(6.685, 10.180)		(0.452, 1.392)		(0.735, 1.692)				(6.21 %, 14.51 %)	(9.49 %, 17.32 %)

95 % confidence limits of each estimate given in parentheses
[a]regression model with fixed effects only
[b]regression model with fixed and random effects

Table 2 Estimated parameters, goodness-of-fit statistics and estimated dose reduction for BGscore

Model	Coefficient						Goodness-of-fit		Dose reduction	
	logCTDI		id2		id4		AIC	Pseudo R²	id2	id4
	Est.	P-value	Est.	P-value	Est.	P-value				
regress[a]	1.329	<0.001	0.129	0.001	0.183	<0.001	-	0.3645	9.26 %	12.88 %
	(1.113, 1.546)		(0.052, 0.206)		(0.107, 0.260)				(4.58 %, 13.94 %)	(8.50 %, 17.26 %)
ologit[a]	8.249	<0.001	0.760	0.001	1.071	<0.001	1135.11	0.3705	8.80 %	12.17 %
	(6.766, 9.732)		(0.321, 1.200)		(0.623, 1.520)				(4.44 %, 13.17 %)	(8.00 %, 16.35 %)
gologit2[a]	7.804	<0.001	0.883	0.001	1.431	<0.001	1190.70	0.3915	10.69 %	16.76 %
=2	(5.807, 9.801)		(0.368, 1.398)		(0.877, 1.986)				(5.18 %, 16.21 %)	(10.97 %, 22.55 %)
gologit2[a]	7.842	<0.001	0.505	0.261	0.408	0.369			6.24 %	5.07 %
=3	(5.577, 10.107)		(−.376, 1.387)		(−.481, 1.298)				(−3.27 %, 15.76 %)	(−4.86 %, 15.00 %)
slogit[a]	15.378	<0.001	1.337	0.001	2.036	<0.001	1124.99	0.3791	8.33 %	12.40 %
	(12.340, 18.42)		(0.577, 2.098)		(1.246, 2.826)				(4.17 %, 12.48 %)	(8.30 %, 16.50 %)
mixed[b]	1.329	<0.001	0.129	0.001	0.183	<0.001	1224.58	0.2207	9.26 %	12.88 %
	(1.114,1.545)		(0.053, 0.206)		(0.107, 0.260)				(4.59 %, 13.93 %)	(8.51 %, 17.26 %)
meologit[b]	7.806	<0.001	0.736	<0.001	1.031	<0.001	1216.93	0.2230	9.00 %	12.38 %
	(6.733, 8.879)		(0.327, 1.146)		(.618, 1.445)				(4.52 %, 13.48 %)	(8.09 %, 16.67 %)

95 % confidence limits of each estimate given in parentheses
[a]regression model with fixed effects only
[b]regression model with fixed and random effects

one of the image stacks in the comparison would lead to a huge increase by a factor of $2^{8.825} = 453.513$ in the odds for a higher score for that stack. The coefficient regression for *id*2 and *id*4 are 0.966 and 1.271, respectively, and they can be interpreted to the odds being multiplied by $e^{0.966} = 2.627$ and $e^{1.271} = 3.564$, respectively, when the

corresponding iterative reconstruction method is used instead of the standard method.

For the partial proportional logistic model (*gologit2*), the first panel contrasts *GWscore* = 1 with categories 2 and 3, whereas the second panel contrasts with category 4. Hence, positive coefficients indicate

Table 3 Estimated parameters, goodness-of-fit statistics and estimated dose reduction for GQscore

Model	Coefficient						Goodness-of-fit		Dose Reduction	
	logCTDI		id2		id4		AIC	Pseudo R²	id2	id4
	Est.	P-value	Est.	P-value	Est.	P-value				
regress[a]	1.424	<0.001	0.158	<0.001	0.175	<0.001	-	0.3560	10.53 %	11.57 %
	(1.217, 1.630)		(0.085, 0.232)		(0.102, 0.248)				(6.46 %, 14.59 %)	(7.58 %, 15.56 %)
ologit[a]	9.626	<0.001	1.011	<0.001	1.133	<0.001	1060.25	0.3573	9.97 %	11.10 %
	(8.020, 11.232)		(0.547, 1.476)		(0.665, 1.600)				(6.13 %, 13.17 %)	(7.32 %, 14.88 %)
gologit2[a]	8.627	<0.001	1.092	<0.001	1.484	<0.001	1113.99	0.3816	11.89 %	15.80 %
=2	(6.519, 10.735)		(0.558, 1.625)		(0.924, 2.044)				(6.74 %, 17.03 %)	(10.48 %, 21.12 %)
gologit2[a] =3	9.652	<0.001	0.964	0.073	0.387	0.507			9.50 %	3.93 %
	(6.915, 12.388)		(−0.091, 2.019)		(−0.756, 1.529)				(1.29 %, 17.72 %)	(−6.76 %, 14.61 %)
slogit[a]	18.523	<0.001	1.867	<0.001	2.148	<0.001	1061.13	0.3594	9.59 %	10.95 %
	(15.277,21.769)		(0.997, 2.738)		(1.275, 3.022)				(5.80 %, 13.38 %)	(7.23 %, 14.67 %)
mixed[b]	1.424	<0.001	0.158	<0.001	0.175	<0.001	1119.97	0.1857	10.53 %	11.57 %
	(1.218, 1.630)		(0.085, 0.231)		(0.102, 0.248)				(6.47 %, 14.59 %)	(7.58 %, 15.55 %)
meologit[b]	9.179	<0.001	0.967	<0.001	1.085	<0.001	1123.66	0.1853	10.00 %	11.15 %
	(7.031, 11.328)		(0.468, 1.467)		(0.578, 1.592)				(6.03 %, 13.98 %)	(7.25 %, 15.05 %)

95 % confidence limits of each estimate given in parentheses
[a]regression model with fixed effects only
[b]regression model with fixed and random effects

that higher values on the independent variable make it more likely that the respondent will be in a higher category of *GWscore* than the current one.

Since the stereotype model (*slogit*) is a type of an ordinal logistic regression model, the interpretation of its coefficients is similar to the ordinal logistic model. For the *id*2 and *id*4 variables, the odds of the highest image quality versus lowest image quality increased by a factor of $e^{1.887} = 6.6$ and $e^{2.433} = 11.4$, respectively, holding all other variables constant. As discussed in the previous section, there is another parameter in the stereotype model and that is ϕ_s. Since the response variable has only three categories in this case, it is supposed that $\phi_0 \equiv 0$, $\phi_2 \equiv 1$, and the estimate of ϕ_1 is equal to 0.431. Since we have $\phi_0 < \phi_1 < \phi_2$, we conclude that the stereotype logistic model confirms that the subjective assessment of the dependent variable is indeed ordered, and the groups (*GWscore* categories) are distinguishable.

For the mixed linear model (*mixed*), the regression coefficients are similar to the linear regression model with fixed effects (*regress*) and the only difference is that the *patient* and *observer* variables have been considered as random effects in the mixed linear model.

Also the regression coefficients of the mixed-effects ordered logistic regression (*meologit*) are very close to the ordinal logistic regression model (*ologit*). The estimates of the variance of the random intercept at the *observer* and *patient* level are 0.689 and 4.478, respectively.

The goodness-of-fit statistics (*AIC* and *Pseudo* R^2) of all regression models are also given in Tables 1, 2 and 3. In Tables 1 and 2 the *slogit* model, and in Table 3 the *ologit* model, present the smallest *AIC* among all fixed effects models, although the differences are small. The *gologit2* model represents the largest *Pseudo* R^2 among all fixed effects models in Tables 1, 2 and 3.

The estimated potential for reduction of the *CTDI* settings (dose reduction) for *GQscore*, *BGscore* and *GQscore* are reported in Tables 1, 2 and 3, respectively. The confidence limits of the dose reductions, calculated using the delta method, are also presented. The proposed percentage of dose reduction for *id*2 (around 10 %, with confidence intervals around (6 %, 14 %), for *GWscore*) is very similar for all regression models in Table 1, except for the partial proportional odds model. This is also true for the estimated percentages of dose reduction for *id*4 (around 13 %, with a confidence interval around 9 %, 17 %). The results thus indicate smaller dose reductions for *id*2 than for *id*4, although the confidence intervals overlap to a large extent.

To compare the effect of *id*2 with *id*4 on the response variable, we restricted the analysis to observations using *id*2 or *id*4 and considered only one covariate (*id*2) in the regression models. The estimates thus obtained and their confidence intervals are reported in Table 4 for

Table 4 Parameter estimation of id2 versus id4

Model	GWscore		GQscore		BGscore	
	Est.	P-value	Est.	P-value	Est.	P-value
regress[a]	−0.050	0.199	−0.017	0.641	−0.054	0.141
	(−0.126, 0.026)		(−0.087, 0.054)		(−0.126, 0.018)	
ologit[a]	−0.322	0.164	−0.13	0.603	−0.374	0.127
	(−0.775, 0.131)		(−0.621, 0.361)		(−0.854, 0.107)	
gologit2[a] =2	−0.215	0.488	−0.393	0.185	−0.596	0.046
	(−0.823, 0.392)		(−0.975, 0.189)		(−1.182, −0.010)	
gologit2[a] =3	−0.472	0.182	0.629	0.228	0.104	0.82
	(−1.166, 0.221)		(−0.394, 1.653)		(−0.788, 0.996)	
slogit[a]	−0.592	0.194	−0.408	0.281	−0.743	0.052
	(−1.485, 0.301)		(−1.150, 0.334)		(−1.491, 0.005)	
mixed[b]	−0.050	0.176	−0.017	0.640	−0.054	0.14
	(−0.122, .022)		(−0.087, 0.053)		(−0.126, 0.018)	
meologit[b]	−0.3217	0.164	−0.126	0.598	−0.336	0.152
	(−0.775, 0.131)		(−0.597, 0.344)		(−0.794, 0.123)	

95 % confidence limits given in parentheses
[a]regression model with fixed effects only
[b]regression model with fixed and random effects

GWscore, *BGscore* and *GQscore*. It was found that the coefficients are all statistically insignificant at the 0.01 level.

Ranking data

The rank-ordered logistic regression model was applied with *GWrank*, which represents the ranked order between the four imaging protocols, as the response variable. The regression coefficients, goodness-of-fit statistics and the estimates of dose reduction for linear models (fixed effects and mixed effects), ordinal logistic regression models (fixed effects and mixed effects) as well as the rank-ordered logistic model are reported in Table 5. All regression coefficients are statistically significant at the 0.01 level. The rank-ordered logistic model, which is designed specifically for analyzing rank-order data, presents the best performance among all models in terms of the goodness-of-fit measures (*AIC* and *Pseudo* R^2). Unlike the results of *GWscore*, the estimated dose reduction figures for *id*2 (around 18 %) were greater than for *id*4 (around 15 %) while working with *GWrank*. The corresponding finding was also made for *BGrank* and *GQrank*. (Tables 6 and 7) In all cases, though, there was considerable overlap of the confidence intervals.

Discussion

In the present study, we did not find any dramatic differences in the results between the tested regression models. Overall, the goodness-of-fit statistics in Tables 1,

Table 5 Estimated parameters, Goodness-of-fit statistics and dose reduction of GWrank

Model	Coefficient						Goodness-of-fit		Dose Reduction	
	logCTDI		id2		id4		AIC	Pseudo R^2	id2	id4
	Est.	P-value	Est.	P-value	Est.	P-value				
regress[a]	4.482	<0.001	0.850	<0.001	0.696	<0.001	-	0.0959	17.27 %	14.38 %
	(3.981, 4.983)		(0.673, 1.027)		(0.518, 0.873)				(14.44 %, 20.11 %)	(11.44 %, 17.32 %)
ologit[a]	9.247	<0.001	1.780	<0.001	1.531	<0.001	2462.68	0.1138	17.51 %	15.26 %
	(8.126, 10.368)		(1.428, 2.132)		(1.168, 1.894)				(14.99 %, 20.02 %)	(12.51 %, 18.01 %)
rologit[a]	5.537	<0.001	1.232	<0.001	0.932	<0.001	1303.66	0.1493	19.95 %	15.49 %
	(4.734, 6.340)		(0.969, 1.495)		(0.666, 1.197)				(17.06 %, 22.84 %)	(12.24 %, 18.74 %)
mixed[b]	4.482	<0.001	0.850	<0.001	0.696	<0.001	2670.66	0.0000	17.27 %	14.38 %
	(3.995, 4.970)		(0.677, 1.023)		(0.523, 0.869)				(14.51 %, 20.04 %)	(11.51 %, 17.24 %)
meologit[b]	9.267	<0.001	1.751	<0.001	1.549	<0.001	2452.89	0.0320	17.22 %	15.40 %
	(8.991, 9.543)		(1.416, 2.086)		(1.214, 1.885)				(14.36 %, 20.07 %)	(12.43 %, 18.36 %)

95 % confidence limits of each estimate given in parentheses
[a]regression model with fixed effects only
[b]regression model with fixed and random effects

2 and 3 were similar in magnitude for all the tested models, with the exception of the *Pseudo R^2* values for the mixed effects models (*mixed* and *meologit*), which were considerably lower than for the models with fixed effects only. This is most likely due to the different numbers of parameters in the models. However, also with *AIC*, which is supposed to compensate for differences in the number of fitted parameters, slightly worse fit was found for the models including random effects.

The original study using the same data [8] applied a linear mixed model, corresponding to the analysis here described by the command *mixed*. The findings were basically the same in the new analysis, with significant differences between the normal dose reconstructions and all other schemes, as well as significant effects of the iterative algorithms applied to reduced-dose data, for all

the tested image quality criteria. In this study, we also added the estimation of potential dose reductions, which is important for clinical application of the results.

As for the regression coefficients, their values from the linear models should not be directly compared with those from the logistic models, due to entirely different principles for parametrization. It may be noted, though, that the addition of random effects in the linear models (*mixed* vs. *regress*) had no effect on the coefficient estimates and hardly any on the confidence limits. Among the logistic models, the most striking finding was the fact that with *gologit2*, different estimates were obtained when contrasting the two best categories than when contrasting the two worst categories (second vs. first *gologit2* panel in Tables 1, 2 and 3). This suggests that the proportional odds assumption may not have been

Table 6 Estimated parameters, Goodness-of-fit statistics and dose reduction of BGrank

Model	Coefficient						Goodness-of-fit		Dose Reduction	
	logCTDI		id2		id4		AIC	Pseudo R^2	id2	id4
	Est.	P-value	Est.	P-value	Est.	P-value				
regress[a]	−4.812	<0.001	−0.863	<0.001	−0.683	<0.001	-	0.1141	16.41 %	13.24 %
	(−5.299, −4.324)		(−1.035, −0.690)		(−0.856, −0.511)				(13.82 %, 19.00 %)	(10.53 %, 15.95 %)
ologit[a]	−9.793	<0.001	−1.734	<0.001	−1.424	<0.001	2420.57	0.1297	16.23 %	13.53 %
	(−10.916, −8.671)		(−2.081, −1.387)		(−1.780, −1.067)				(13.80 %, 18.65 %)	(10.86 %, 16.20 %)
rologit[a]	−5.344	<0.001	−0.881	<0.001	−0.836	<0.001	1308.64	0.1461	15.20 %	14.48 %
	(−6.116, −4.571)		(−1.117. −0.645)		(−1.081, −0.592)				(12.01 %, 18.40 %)	(11.10 %, 17.87 %)
mixed[b]	−4.812	<0.001	−0.862	<0.001	−0.683	<0.001	2617. 17	0.000	16.41 %	13.24 %
	(−5.286, −4.337)		(−1.030, −0.694)		(−0.851, −0.515)				(13.88 %, 18.94 %)	(10.60 %, 15.88 %)
meologit[b]	−10.460	<0.001	−1.861	<0.001	−1.545	<0.001	2355.74	0.0086	16.30 %	13.73 %
	(−10.633, −10.288)		(−2.144, −1.579)		(−1.846, −1.245)				(14.01 %, 18.59 %)	(11.24 %, 16.23 %)

95 % confidence limits of each estimate given in parentheses
[a]regression model with fixed effects only
[b]regression model with fixed and random effects

Table 7 Estimated parameters, Goodness-of-fit statistics and dose reduction of GQrank

Model	Coefficient						Goodness-of-fit		Dose Reduction	
	logCTDI		id2		id4		AIC	Pseudo R^2	id2	id4
	Est.	P-value	Est.	P-value	Est.	P-value				
regress[a]	−4.671	<0.001	−0.817	<0.001	−0.463	<0.001	-	0.1134	16.04 %	9.43 %
	(−5.158, −4.183)		(−.989, −.644)		(−0.635, −0.290)				(13.36 %, 18.73 %)	(6.44 %, 12.42 %)
ologit[a]	−9.433	<0.001	−1.691	<0.001	−1.033	<0.001	2427.97	0.1269	16.41 %	10.37 %
	(−10.550, −8.317)		(−2.039, −1.343)		(−1.395, −0.672)				(13.93 %, 18.88 %)	(7.39 %, 13.36 %)
rologit[a]	−4.766	<0.001	−0.709	<0.001	−0.576	<0.001	1337.79	0.1270	13.81 %	11.38 %
	(−5.516, −4.015)		(−0.940, −0.477)		(−0.823, −0.328)				(10.23 %, 17.40 %)	(7.35 %, 15.41 %)
mixed[b]	−4.671	<0.001	−0.8167	<0.001	−0.4625	<0.001	2619.45	0.0000	16.04 %	9.43 %
	(−5.145, −4.196)		(−0.985, −0.648)		(−0.631, −0.294)				(13.42 %, 18.66 %)	(6.51 %, 12.34 %)
meologit[b]	−9.380	<0.001	−1.680	<0.001	−1.027	<0.001	2367.96	0.0105	16.40 %	13.37 %
	(−9.506, −9.255)		(−1.956, −1.405)		(−1.331, −0.723)				(13.91 %, 18.89 %)	(7.45 %, 13.29 %)

95 % confidence limits of each estimate given in parentheses
[a]regression model with fixed effects only
[b]regression model with fixed and random effects

appropriate for these data. To test this, the commonly recommended procedure is to apply Brant's test [20]. Unfortunately, the *Stata* implementation of Brant's test (which only works with *ologit*) does not allow nominal or random effects, so we were not able to carry out a formal test of this assumption. Also, when comparing the logistic models *ologit* and *meologit*, the addition of random effects had only a minute effect on the estimates. It should be kept in mind that when there are two crossed random effects in the model (in this case *patient* and *observer*), the integration method used by *Stata* is Laplacian integration, in which the parameter estimates are biased. In the variance components, the bias of the estimates tends to be more prominent than in the estimates of the fixed effects due to the Laplacian approximation [14].

For all the tested models (except *gologit2* at the highest level), the regression coefficients had larger values for *id4* than for *id2*, which was expected from previous knowledge about the algorithms, with *id4* differing more from the standard algorithm than *id2*. The confidence intervals, though, overlapped to a large extent. The difference between *id4* and *id2* was also not significant when tested formally (Table 4).

More interesting from an application point of view are probably the estimates of potential dose reductions. Here all the regression models that summarize the different image quality levels gave similar results for the three image quality scores, with somewhat larger estimates for *id4* than for *id2*, as expected, but widely overlapping confidence intervals. For *gologit2*, contrasting the highest quality levels gave smaller estimates than contrasting the lowest levels for both *id4* and *id2*. A possible interpretation is that it will be more difficult to maintain the probability of producing images of excellent

quality by applying the new reconstruction algorithms while reducing the radiation dose than to maintain the probability of producing images of clinically acceptable quality. Thus, the somewhat different results for the two levels seem, to some extent, to answer different research questions. The fact that, in general, non-significant results were obtained when contrasting the highest quality levels may be related both to the weaker effect at this level and to a loss of power when more parameters are estimated from the same data.

When analyzing the rank-order data (Tables 5–7), the regression model specifically designed for this type of data, *rologit*, yielded much better fit (lower *AIC* and higher *Pseudo R^2*). A surprising finding was that with the ranking data, larger effects, and thus larger dose reduction estimates, were found for *id2* than for *id4*. The difference was even greater with *rologit*. However, again the two confidence intervals overlap.

Broadly speaking, the results of our comparison did not give any clear-cut empirical evidence for selecting the most appropriate regression model for analyzing visual grading data in medical imaging, except for choosing *rologit* when analyzing rank data. Thus, the selection of model must be based on other considerations.

The use of linear models for analyzing ordinal scale data is generally discouraged in statistical textbooks. Also, on theoretical grounds, it is commonly recommended to handle variables such as *patient* and *observer* in our study as random effects, since they both represent samples from larger populations. This would speak in favor of the *meologit* approach when analyzing absolute scores. The greatest problem of this model appears to be the proportional odds assumption (parallel regression assumption), which may well have been violated by our data. Using instead *gologit2* might resolve this problem, but at the expense of more complex results that are less straightforward to interpret. Still, there are situations where the relevant research questions may motivate this more complex model. It is more difficult to weigh the importance of handling violations of the proportional odds assumption (*gologit2*) against correctly controlling random effects (*meologit*). Also for *slogit*, the results are more complex and possibly difficult for an applied researcher to interpret. The main finding from *slogit* in our study was the confirmation of the ordinal structure that had been defined beforehand.

Conclusions

In conclusion, a number of logistic regression methods are available for handling ordinal data from visual grading experiments in medical imaging. Our study did not provide any empirical support for selecting a different regression model than the one we would recommend on theoretical grounds, i.e. the ordinal logistic regression model with mixed effects, which is appropriate for handling random effects when the response variable is ordinal. For rank-order data, the rank-ordered logistic regression model appears to be most appropriate, since this model can handle the rank-order data correctly and because of its better performance in terms of the goodness-of-fit among the tested regression models.

Abbreviations
AIC: Akaike information criterion; ANOVA: Analysis of variance; BG: Basal ganglia delineation; CT: Computed tomography; CTDI$_{vol}$: Volume computed tomography dose index; fd: Full dose; gologit2: Generalized ordered logit/ partial proportional odds; GQ: General image quality; GW: Gray-white-matter discrimination; id2: Iterative reconstruction with noise reduction level 2; id4: Iterative reconstruction with noise reduction level 4; meologit: Mixed-effects ordered logistic regression; ologit: Ordinal logistic regression; rd: Reduced dose; ROC: Receiver operating characteristic; rologit: Rank-ordered logistic regression; slogit: Stereotype logistic regression.

Competing interests
The authors declare that they have no competing interests.

Authors' contributions
AL designed and carried out the visual grading experiments. ÖS designed the current study and proposed the statistical methodology. SES performed the statistical analysis under the supervision of MF. SES prepared the first draft of the manuscript, and all authors took part in its final formulation

Acknowledgements
No specific funding was received for this study.

Author details
^{1}Department of Medical and Health Sciences (IMH), Linköping University, Linköping, Sweden. ^{2}Sabzevar University of Medical Sciences, Sabzevar, Iran. ^{3}Department of Diagnostic Radiology, Lund University, Clinical Sciences, Lund, Sweden. ^{4}Department of Radiology, Landspitali University Hospital, Reykjavik and Faculty of Medicine, University of Iceland, Reykjavik, Iceland. ^{5}Department of Clinical and Experimental Medicine, Linköping University, Linköping, Sweden. ^{6}KTH Royal Institute of Technology, School of Technology and Health, Alfred Nobels allé 10, SE-141 52 Huddinge, Stockholm, Sweden.

References
1. Månsson LG. Methods for the evaluation of image quality: a review. Radiat Prot Dosim. 2000;90:89–99.
2. Smedby Ö, Fredrikson M. Visual grading regression: analysing data from visual grading experiments with regression models. Br J Radiol. 2010;83:767–75. doi:10.1259/bjr/35254923.
3. Smedby Ö, Fredrikson M, De Geer J, Borgen L, Sandborg M. Quantifying the potential for dose reduction with visual grading regression. Br J Radiol. 2013;86:20110784. doi:10.1259/bjr/31197714.
4. Smedby Ö, Fredrikson M, De Geer J, Sandborg M. Visual grading regression with random effects. Proc SPIE. 2012;8318:831805. doi:10.1117/12.913650.
5. McCullagh P. Regression models for ordinal data. J R Stat Soc B. 1980;42:109–42.
6. Williams R. Generalized ordered logit/ partial proportional odds models for ordinal dependent variables. Stata J. 2006;6(1):58–82.
7. Anderson JA. Regression and ordered categorical variables. J R Stat Soc Ser B. 1984;46:1–40.
8. Löve Á, Siemund R, Höglund P, Van Westen D, Stenberg L, Petersen C, et al. Hybrid iterative reconstruction algorithm in brain CT: a radiation dose reduction and image quality assessment study. Acta Radiol. 2014;55(2):208–17. doi:10.1177/0284185113494980.
9. Agresti A. Analysis of ordinal categorical data. 2nd ed. Hoboken, NJ: Wiley; 2010. p. 9–24.
10. Long JS, Freese J. Regression models for categorical dependent variables using stata. 2nd ed. College Station, TX, USA: Stata Press; 2003.
11. Lunt M. Stereotype ordinal regression. Stata Tech Bull. 2001;61:12–8.
12. Ahn J, Mukherjee B, Banerjee M, Cooney KA. Bayesian inference for the stereotype regression model: application to a case–control study of prostate cancer. Stat Med. 2009;28:3139–57. doi:10.1002/sim.3693.
13. Laird NM, Ware JH. Random-effects models for longitudinal data. Biometrics. 1982;38:963–74.
14. Rabe-Hesketh S, Skrondal A. Multilevel and longitudinal modeling using stata. 3rd ed. College Station, TX, USA: Stata Press; 2012. p. 575–90.
15. McFadden D. Conditional logit analysis of qualitative choice behavior. In: Zarembka P, editor. Frontiers in econometrics. New York: Academic; 1974. p. 105–42.
16. Hardin J, Hilbe J. Generalized linear models and extensions. College Station, TX, USA: Stata Press; 2001.
17. Akaike H. A new look at the statistical model identification. Autom Contr IEEE Trans. 1974;19(6):716–23. doi:10.1109/tac.1974.1100705.
18. Oehlert GW. A note on the delta method. Am Stat. 1992;46:27–9.
19. Hair JF, Black JWC, Babin BJ, Anderson RE. Multivariate data analysis. 7th ed. Upper Saddle River, NJ: Pearson; 2010.
20. Brant R. Assessing proportionality in the proportional odds model for ordinal logistic regression. Biometrics. 1990;46:1171–8.

5

A computer aided measurement method for unstable pelvic fractures based on standardized radiographs

Jing-xin Zhao[1,2†], Zhe Zhao[2,3†], Li-cheng Zhang[2], Xiu-yun Su[2,4], Hai-long Du[2], Li-ning Zhang[2], Li-hai Zhang[2*] and Pei-fu Tang[2*]

Abstract

Background: To set up a method for measuring radiographic displacement of unstable pelvic ring fractures based on standardized X-ray images and then test its reliability and validity using a software-based measurement technique.

Methods: Twenty-five patients that were diagnosed as AO/OTA type B or C pelvic fractures with unilateral pelvis fractured and dislocated were eligible for inclusion by a review of medical records in our clinical centre. Based on the input pelvic preoperative CT data, the standardized X-ray images, including inlet, outlet, and anterior-posterior (AP) radiographs, were simulated using Armira software (Visage Imaging GmbH, Berlin, Germany). After representative anatomic landmarks were marked on the standardized X-ray images, the 2-dimensional (2D) coordinates of these points could be revealed in Digimizer software (Model: Mitutoyo Corp., Tokyo, Japan). Subsequently, we developed a formula that indicated the translational and rotational displacement patterns of the injured hemipelvis. Five separate observers calculated the displacement outcomes using the established formula and determined the rotational patterns using a 3D-CT model based on their overall impression. We performed 3D reconstruction of all the fractured pelvises using Mimics (Materialise, Haasrode, Belgium) and determined the translational and rotational displacement using 3-matic suite. The interobserver reliability of the new method was assessed by comparing the continuous measure and categorical outcomes using intraclass correlation coefficient (ICC) and kappa statistic, respectively.

Result: The interobserver reliability of the new method for translational and rotational measurement was high, with both ICCs above 0.9. Rotational outcome assessed by the new method was the same as that concluded by 3-matic software. The agreement for rotational outcome among orthopaedic surgeons based on overall impression was poor (kappa statistic, 0.250 to 0.426). Compared with the 3D reconstruction outcome, the interobserver reliability of the formula method for translational and rotational measures was perfect with both ICCs more than 0.9.

Conclusions: The new method for measuring displacement using a formula was reliable, and could minimise the measurement errors and maximise the precision of pelvic fracture description. Furthermore, this study was useful for standardising the operative plan and establishing a theoretical basis for robot-assisted pelvic fracture surgery based on 2-D radiographs.

Keywords: Unstable pelvic fractures, Radiographic assessment, Software-based measurement, Reliability study

* Correspondence: zhanglihai301@gmail.com; pftang301@163.com
†Equal contributors
2Department of Orthopedics, Chinese PLA General Hospital, No.28 Fuxing Road, Beijing, Haidian District 100853, People's Republic of China
Full list of author information is available at the end of the article

Background

The most severe injury observed in an orthopaedic trauma centre are disruptions of the pelvic ring, especially unstable pelvic ring fractures, which are characterized as a posterior pelvic ring fracture with the partial or total displacement of unilateral or bilateral pelvis. In cases of increased displacement and the incidence of complications from fractured pelvis, it is much more difficult to manage these types of complicated fractures. Traditionally, the fracture displacement is assessed using radiological tools, including roentgenography and CT scans. As radiographic assessment remains the standard for preoperative assessment, the first step of management is rapid and precise measurement and the determination of the displacement of the injured pelvis. For a long time, CT based measurements method of pelvic displacements was considered as the "gold standard" [1, 2]. However, regarding the higher cost and patients' radiation exposure of CT scan, the imaging examinations based on the radiographs were still the most available and convenient tools in most clinical settings.

A review of the literature revealed that displacement assessments of the pelvis relied on three-direction roentgenography, including inlet, outlet and anterior-posterior (AP) plain radiographs [3–9]. As with other outcome measurement tools, reliability and validity of radiographic measurement methods are of utmost importance if there is an intention or attempt to use them to conduct pre- or post-operative assessment and to correlate them with an operation's outcome. However, the reliability and validity of current measurement techniques are not strong [8, 10], because of patient factors (the presence of overlapping osseous structures, bowel gas and intestinal contrast materials) and technical factors (unstandardized technique, deficiency of validation) [2].

Nystrom et al. used the Sawbones model to simulate unstable pelvic ring fracture patterns and reconstructed the 3-dimensional (3D) model based on CT scan data [11]. After measuring the pelvic displacement using 3 previous established methods, they found that the measurement of vertical translation and sacroiliac (SI) joint separation as described by Henderson et al. was reliable [3], and the measurement of SI joint displacement as described by Matta et al. was difficult to make and unreliable [7]. Previous measurement techniques mainly focused on translational displacement of the pelvis, whereas unstable pelvic ring fractures often lead to translational or rotational displacement of the pelvis in different planes in 3D space. Solely measuring translational displacement without considering rotational displacements not only increased the measurement error but also neglected important anatomic information, which underlied the following treatment plan.

We simulated standardized X-ray images using Armira software and hypothesized that some formulas can be developed to precisely measure and indicate the translational and rotational displacements of the injured hemipelvis in each plane based on the 2D coordinate information of those representative anatomic landmarks. Ideally, this study could be used to standardize the operative plan and establish a theoretical basis for robot-assisted surgery based on 2D radiographs.

Methods

Design and setting

The study was a medical imaging investigation approved by the Ethics Committee of Chinese PLA General Hospital. Due to its retrospective nature and the anonymous patient data, a waiver of patients' informed consent was granted. Data were obtained on patients with pelvic fractures who were admitted to the Department of Orthopaedics and Trauma at the Chinese PLA General Hospital between March 2012 and March 2013.

A review of plain radiographs revealed that 25 patients with unilateral pelvis injury and dislocation had minimal or no displacement of the contralateral segment. We collected the CT Digital-Imaging-and-Communications-in-Medicine (DICOM) data. All CT scans were performed with a Somatom sensation open CT System (Siemens AG, Erlangen, Germany) with slice thicknesses of 1.5 mm.

Pelvis specific coordination system

To better illustrate the rotational and translational displacement types, the pelvis specific coordination system was set up, in which the definition of all rotation types and the X/Y/Z coordinate system were defined (Fig. 1). In this system, the X/Z and X/Y planes represented the standard inlet and outlet radiographs of pelvis, respectively.

To present the relationship of the anatomic points between the intact and the injured hemipelvis, the standard radiographs have to be established at first. In this study, we imported the CT-DICOM data into Armira software (Visage Imaging GmbH, Berlin, Germany) to simulate the standard inlet, outlet, and AP radiographs of pelvises, which was defined as the standardized X-ray group.

Representative anatomic landmarks

Several representative anatomic landmarks were selected using Digimizer 4.1.1.0 software (Model: Mitutoyo Corp., Tokyo, Japan) to measure and indicate the displacement type in inlet, outlet and AP images. In AP radiographs anterior superior iliac spine (ASIS) and ischial tubercle were marked to determine the rotation direction around the X-axis in the sagittal plane (Fig. 2). In inlet radiographs, the anterior SI joint (iliac side), ASIS and centre of sacral endplate were selected to determine the X-axis

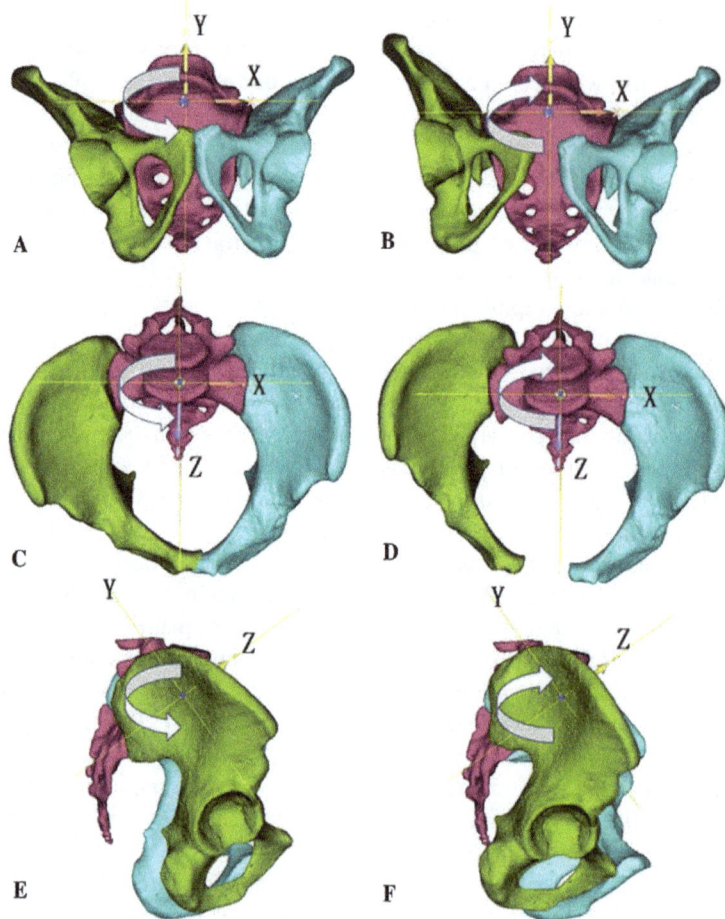

Fig. 1 The rotational direction of the right hemipelvis is indicated by the curved arrow symbol in each pelvis, and the coordinate systems are denoted by the capital letters of X, Y and Z. **a** and **b** represent the varus and valgus of hemipelvis around the Z-axis in the outlet plane, respectively. **c** and **d** represent the internal and external rotation of the hemipelvis around the Y-axis in the inlet plane, respectively. **e** and **f** represent the flexion and extension of the hemipelvis around the X-axis in the sagittal plane, respectively

transverse and the Z axis AP displacement (Fig. 3). In outlet radiographs, the superior point of iliac wing was used to determine the vertical displacement, and ASIS and ischial tubercle were used to calculate the varus or valgus of the hemipelvis (Fig. 4).

Standardization of the evaluation process

As the diameter of the intact femoral head in each case was different from the others, it was necessary to measure it using 3-matic (Materialise) in order to establish the relationship between pixel and actual distance, which could be used as the reference to set the size of the corresponding femoral head in each standardized radiograph. One independent investigator imported the CT scan data into Mimics 16 software (Materialise, Haasrode, Belgium) to create the 3D models of the fractured pelvises and measure the diameter of each femoral head, independently.

The formulas for the translational and rotational displacement

The 2D coordinates of the previous mentioned anatomic landmarks in all three standard radiographs were acquired using Digimizer software and recorded in a Microsoft Excel file (Table 1). The following formulas were used as Excel commands and input into corresponding blanks, which could indicate the direction of displacement and calculate the actual parameters (Table 2). The translational displacement parameters of fractured hemipelvis were as follows.

Y-axis vertical displacement in outlet radiographs: $|Y'_C-Y_S|-|Y_C-Y_S|$.

Z-axis AP displacement in inlet radiographs: $|Y'_H-Y_S|-|Y_H-Y_S|$.

X-axis transverse displacement in inlet radiographs: $|X'_H-X_S|-|X_H-X_S|$.

The established inequalities to indicate the direction of rotation were based on the relative spatial positions

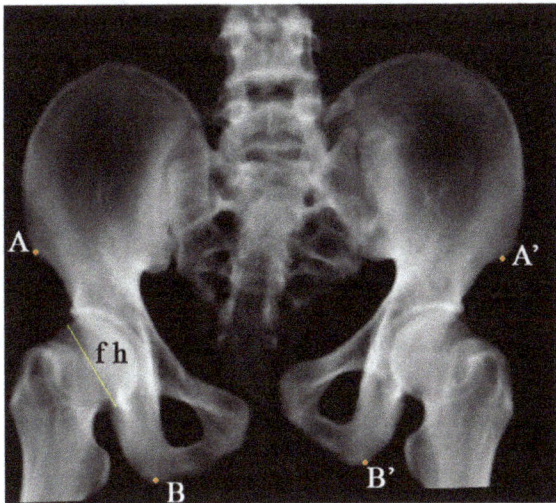

Fig. 2 Anatomic landmarks in AP view: ASIS (A and A'), ischial tuberosity (B and B'). The right femoral head diameter is indicated by and was measured using line "fh"

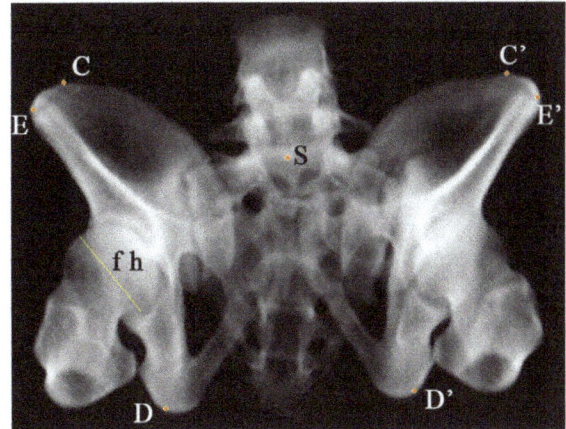

Fig. 4 Anatomic landmarks in outlet view: ASIS (G and G'), anterior SI joint (iliac side) (H and H'), center of sacral endplate (S). The right femoral head diameter is indicated by and was measured using line "fh"

between bilateral corresponding anatomic landmarks in 3D space during the movement of hemipelvis in a special direction (Table 2).

In the AP view, the vertical distance between ASIS and the ischial tubercle in the injured side smaller than that of the intact side could indicate extension of the injured hemipelvis in the sagittal plane, and vice versa. The difference between the vertical distances between ASIS and ischial tubercle in the injured side and that in the intact side could be used as an indicator of the sagittal rotational displacement of the injured hemipelvis (Fig. 2).

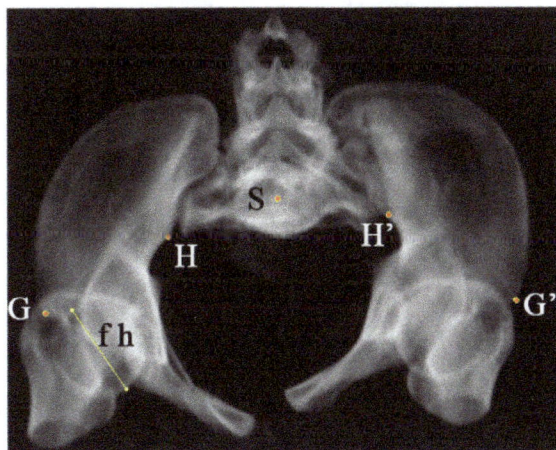

Fig. 3 Anatomic landmarks in inlet view: ASIS (E and E'), superior point of iliac wing (C and C'), ischial tuberosity (D and D') and centre of sacral endplate (S). The right femoral head diameter is indicated by and was measured using line "fh"

In the inlet view or the X/Z plane, the transverse distance between ASIS and the anterior SI joint (iliac side) in the injured side, smaller than that of the intact side, indicated internal rotation of the injured hemipelvis, and vice versa. The difference between the transverse distance between ASIS and the anterior SI joint (iliac side) in the injured side and that in the intact side could be used as an indicator of the rotational displacement of the injured hemipelvis in the inlet plane (Fig. 3).

In the outlet view or the X/Y plane, the transverse distance between ASIS and the ischial tubercle in the injured side smaller than that of the intact side indicated valgus of the injured hemipelvis, and vice versa. The difference between the transverse distance between ASIS and the ischial tubercle in the injured side and that in the intact side could be used as an indicator of the degree of varus and valgus of the injured hemipelvis in the outlet plane (Fig. 4).

Table 1 The representative anatomic landmarks used to measure the displacement of the hemipelvis in each projection

Radiographs	Anatomic landmarks	Intact side	Injured side
AP view	ASIS	X_A,Y_A	X'_A,Y'_A
	ischial tuberosity	X_B,Y_B	X'_B,Y'_B
Outlet view	superior point of iliac wing	X_C,Y_C	X'_C,Y'_C
	ischial tuberosity	X_D,Y_D	X'_D,Y'_D
	ASIS	X_E,Y_E	X'_E,Y'_E
	center of sacral endplate	X_S,Y_S	
Inlet view	ASIS	X_G,Y_G	X'_G,Y'_G
	anterior SI joint (iliac side)	X_H,Y_H	X'_H,Y'_H
	center of sacral endplate	X_S,Y_S	

AP anterior-posterior; ASIS anterior superior iliac spine

Table 2 Formulas to determine the displacement type

Type	Plane	Formulas and parameters	Direction	Related axes
Translational	Outlet	$|Y'_C-Y_S|-|Y_C-Y_S| > 0$	Cephlad	Y
		$|Y'_C-Y_S|-|Y_C-Y_S| < 0$	Caudad	Y
	Inlet	$|Y'_H-Y_S|-|Y_H-Y_S| > 0$	Anterior	Z
		$|Y'_H-Y_S|-|Y_H-Y_S| < 0$	Posterior	Z
		$|X'_H-X_S|-|X_H-X_S| > 0$	Lateral	X
		$|X'_H-X_S|-|X_H-X_S| < 0$	Medial	X
Rotational	Sagittal	$|Y_A-Y_B|-|Y'_A-Y'_B| < -2$	Flexion	X
		$-2 \leq |Y_A-Y_B|-|Y'_A-Y'_B| \leq 2$	Neutral	X
		$|Y_A-Y_B|-|Y'_A-Y'_B| > 2$	Extension	X
	Inlet	$|X_G-X_H|-|X'_G-X'_H| < -2$	External rotation	Y
		$-2 \leq |X_G-X_H|-|X'_G-X'_H| \leq 2$	Neutral	Y
		$|X_G-X_H|-|X'_G-X'_H| > 2$	Internal rotation	Y
	Outlet	$|X_E-X_D|-|X'_E-X'_D| < -2$	Valgus	Z
		$-2 \leq |X_E-X_D|-|X'_E-X'_D| \leq 2$	Neutral	Z
		$|X_E-X_D|-|X'_E-X'_D| > 2$	Varus	Z

Reliability study

Five separate observers, including 2 full-time orthopaedic trauma surgeons (LHZ and XYS) and 3 orthopaedic trauma fellows (ZZ, LCZ and HLD), were recruited to perform this study.

Before actual measurements were performed, premeasurement assessment of the rotational direction in each plane using the 3D CT data was based on overall impression. Observers were asked to look through the AP views of all 3D CT reconstruction models of the pelvic fracture in a random order and an independent manner. It was stressed that this was their impression of the rotation direction, not based on actual measurement. They were asked not to change their answer after the measurements had been taken. After at least 3 days, the previously mentioned anatomic landmarks in all the standardized X-ray images in a random order were marked and determined the translational and rotational displacement using the established formulas by the same 5 doctors in an independent manner.

To compare the outcomes based on the standardized X-ray images, all 3D models of the fractured pelvises were reconstructed using Mimics software and the inlet, outlet, and AP views were simulated using 3-Matic software by one doctor (LNZ). The measurement outcomes were considered as the standard to test the standardized X-ray groups' outcomes.

One orthopaedic surgeon (JXZ) simulated the inlet, outlet, and AP view and completed the calculation, independently. The methods of calculating the translational

and rotational displacement in the outlet plane and the translational displacement in the inlet plane were the same as that used in the radiographic measurement (Figs. 5 and 6). In the inlet plane, posterior superior iliac spine was introduced and marked with the ASIS to indicate the internal or external rotational displacement in the same calculation method. (Figs. 5) In the sagittal plane, the flexion and extension around the X-axis were indicated by the relationship between bilateral lines extending from the respective iliac superior point and ischial tubercle (Fig. 7). The 2D indicator of the sagittal rotational displacement was also calculated in the AP view (Fig. 8).

Statistical analysis

Agreement between observers for categorical and continuous outcomes was calculated using kappa statistic [12] and intraclass correlation coefficient (ICC) by Minitab 16 (Minitab Inc., State College, PA, USA) and SPSS 20 software (SPSS Inc., Chicago, IL, USA), respectively. According to Shrout et al. [13], the two-way random model of ICC was selected to assess the interobserver reliability. In both instances, the strength of agreement was determined based on a standardized Landis-Koch scale (0, poor; 0 to 0.2, slight; 0.21 to 0.40, fair; 0.41 to 0.60, moderate; 0.61 to 0.80, substantial; 0.81 to 1.0, almost perfect) [14].

Results

The 25 patients included in this study were of a mean age of 37.4 years at the time of injury, with 17 men and 8 women. The case series included AO/OTA type C

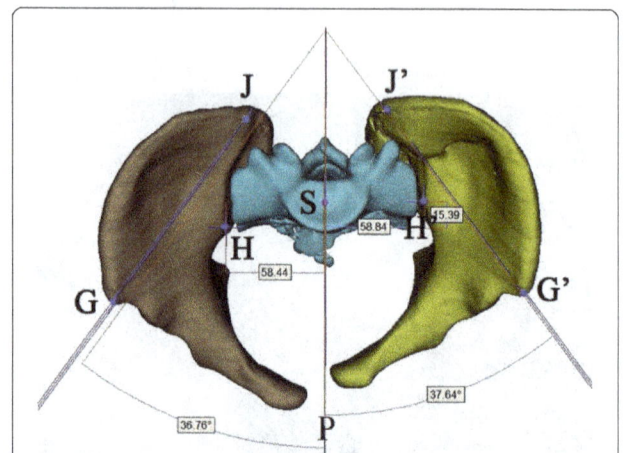

Fig. 5 Anatomic landmarks in inlet view of 3D reconstruction model: anterior superior iliac spine (ASIS, G and G') posterior superior iliac spine (PSIS, J and J') anterior SI joint (iliac side) (H and H') and centre of sacral endplate (S). The transverse and AP displacements and the degrees of internal and external rotation were measured using 3-matic measurement tool. The capital P represents the sagittal plane

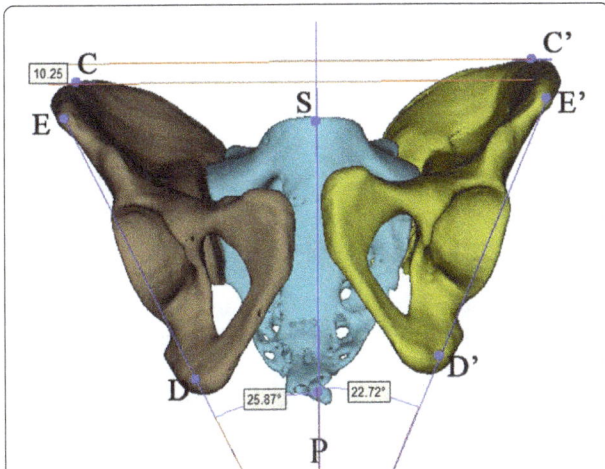

Fig. 6 Anatomic landmarks in outlet view of 3D reconstruction model: ASIS (E and E'), centre of sacral endplate (S), ischial tuberosity (D and D'), and the software measurement method of vertical translational displacement and the degree of varus and valgus. The capital P represents the sagittal plane

(vertical shear) and type B (AP or lateral compression) with unilateral pelvis injured and dislocated.

The evaluation of the translational measurement outcome of the standardized X-rays showed an overall very good agreement between observers with an ICC of 0.9 and 95 % confidential interval greater than 0.75, as seen in Table 3. Table 4 showed that the agreement of rotational measurement outcomes of the standardized X-rays with an ICC of 0.9 (almost perfect). The interobserver reliability of the reader's impression of the rotational results based on the 3D-CT model was fair overall with a kappa statistic between 0.265 and 0.426 (Table 5), among which the agreement of full-time orthopaedic trauma surgeons was higher than that of orthopaedic trauma fellows, with average kappa statistics of 0.428 and 0.162, respectively (not shown in table).

As the Majeed scale defines 0–2 mm displacement as the anatomic reduction of a fractured hemipelvis [15], we defined the absolute value of rotational parameter between 0 and 2 calculated in 3D model by 3-matic as neutral position. Based on this precondition, the assessment of the rotational parameters between the impression outcome of the 3D model and the displacement measurement calculated by 3-matic showed that the interobserver reliability was in a wide range between 0.634 and 0.169 (Table 6). It can be seen that the agreement of full-time orthopaedic trauma surgeons (number 1–3) was higher than that of orthopaedic trauma fellows (number 4, 5) (Table 6).

As the rotational direction assessed in the standardized X-rays was the same as that of 3D reconstruction group, the interobserver agreement between both groups was evaluated using rotational displacement parameters calculated by formula. Table 7 and 8 showed the interobserver agreement of rotational and translational displacement

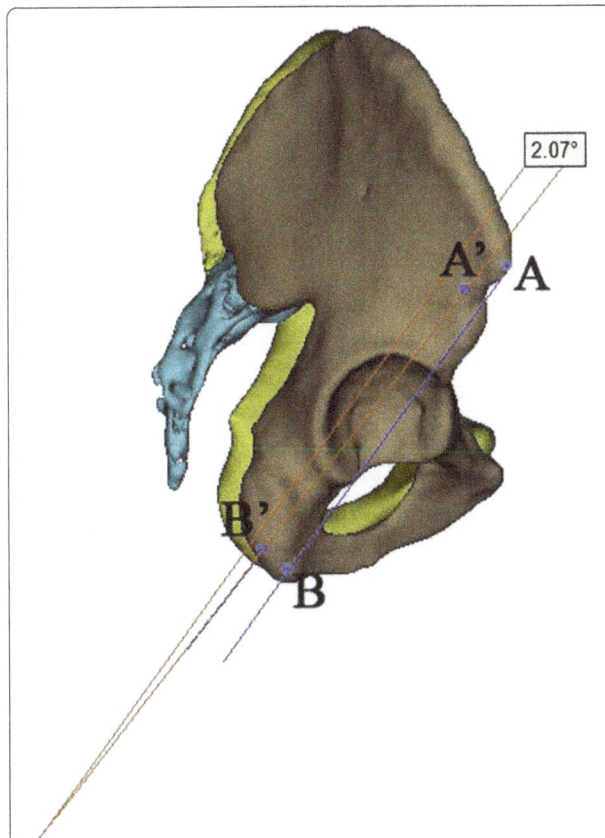

Fig. 7 Anatomic landmarks in lateral view of 3D reconstruction model: ASIS (A and A'), ischial tuberosity (B and B'), and the measurement method of the degree of flexion or extension rotation using software tool

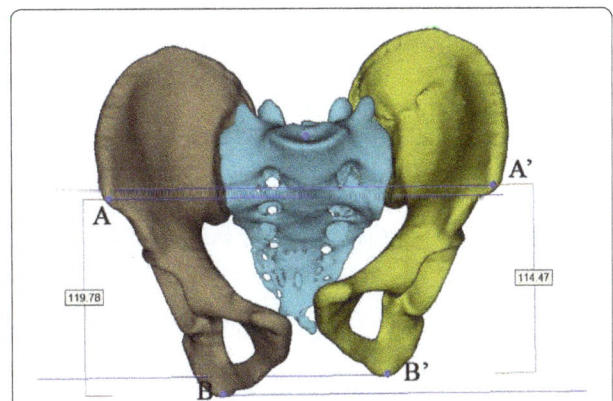

Fig. 8 Anatomic landmarks in AP view of 3D reconstruction model: ASIS (A and A'), ischial tuberosity (B and B'), and the measurement results of parameters of flexion and extension rotation using 3-matic software

Table 3 ICC for translational displacement in the standardized X-ray

Displacement	ICC Coefficient	95 % CI
Vertical	0.920	0.856–0.963
AP	0.934	0.878–0.974
Transverse	0.945	0.893–0.972

AP anterior-posterior; ICC intraclass correlation coefficient

parameters with both the ICCs being higher than 0.9 (almost perfect).

Discussion

Currently, radiographic assessment remains the standard for preoperative assessment and the most frequently used outcome measure during studies of the pelvis. As with other outcome measurement tools, reproducibility, reliability and validity of radiographic measurement techniques are of utmost importance if there is an intention to use these to assess outcome. However, many authors argue that the current measurement methods for fractured pelvises lack standardization, well-accepted reliability, and validity [8, 10].

A literature review by Mataliotakis et al. on the radiographic measurement of pelvic fractures showed various measurement systems introduced by different authors [16]. Radiological evaluation on vertical pelvic displacement was mainly dependent on AP view of the pelvis [3, 7–9]. Matta et al. and Dickson et al. measured the vertical displacement as the difference in the height of the femoral heads in AP view [4, 7]. Henderson et al. and Griffin et al. also used the AP view to measure the perpendicular difference between the most superior points of the bilateral iliac wings as the vertical displacement [3, 17]. Sagi et al. modified the method of Matta and Tornetta and used the superior edge of the femoral head in the outlet radiograph to determine the vertical displacement of the displaced hemipelvis [18]. Lefaivre et al. used the top of the iliac crests in the outlet film to determine the vertical displacement of the displaced hemipelvis relative to its counterpart [8].

Almost all methods for the vertical displacement measurement used by authors were dependent on the pelvic AP X-ray. Actually, both the AP and the outlet

Table 4 ICC for rotational displacement in different planes in the standardized X-ray

Displacement	ICC Coefficient	95 % CI
Sagittal	0.947	0.872–0.997
Inlet	0.925	0.887–0.976
Outlet	0.903	0.861–0.957

ICC intraclass correlation coefficient

Table 5 Agreement for rotational displacement based on the first impression of the AP view of 3D CT images

Displacement	Kappa	P value
Sagittal	0.250	<0.001
Inlet	0.426	<0.001
Outlet	0.265	<0.001

radiographs could be used to measure the vertical displacement of the pelvis. The main difference is that which reference system is selected beforehand. With regard to the movements in 3D space, the best method to depict and determine it is to establish a Cartesian coordinate system which includes three mutually orthogonal axes, such as the X, Y and Z axes. If the vertical displacement of the pelvis is measured on the AP radiograph, it means that the vertical axis is considered as an axis of the rotational or translational movements, and another two axes have to be determined using the transverse and the body's anterior-posterior axes. However, the types of open and close book of the pelvic injuries are the most frequently mentioned type of pelvic injuries which compose almost all the Young-Burgess lateral compression type of pelvic injuries. The open and close book of the pelvic injuries are mainly determined and better demonstrated on the inlet radiographs, which could be considered as the external or internal rotation of the displaced hemipelvis around the axis across the centre of the sacrum and perpendicular to the inlet plane. Based on this precondition, another two axes could be established perpendicular to this axis at the

Table 6 Agreement for rotational displacement between the first impression of the 3D CT images and the measurements of the 3D reconstruction models

Doctor	Displacement plane	Kappa	P value
1	Sagittal	0.269	0.030
	Inlet	0.202	0.088
	Outlet	0.307	0.022
2	Sagittal	0.384	<0.001
	Inlet	0.540	<0.001
	Outlet	0.340	0.008
3	Sagittal	0.211	0.069
	Inlet	0.169	0.125
	Outlet	0.196	0.104
4	Sagittal	0.634	<0.001
	Inlet	0.493	<0.001
	Outlet	0.438	0.001
5	Sagittal	0.451	<0.001
	Inlet	0.549	<0.001
	Outlet	0.454	<0.001

Table 7 Agreement for rotational displacement between the standardized X-ray and 3D reconstruction

Doctor	Displacement plane	ICC	95 % CI
1	Sagittal	0.929	0.877–0.964
	Inlet	0.913	0.891–0.995
	Outlet	0.947	0.896–0.981
2	Sagittal	0.911	0.843–0.945
	Inlet	0.903	0.865–0.957
	Outlet	0.939	0.867–0.978
3	Sagittal	0.977	0.941–0.997
	Inlet	0.935	0.899–0.971
	Outlet	0.933	0.871–0.973
4	Sagittal	0.929	0.874–0.969
	Inlet	0.957	0.902–0.995
	Outlet	0.907	0.885–0.959
5	Sagittal	0.918	0.871–0.961
	Inlet	0.971	0.931–0.996
	Outlet	0.951	0.895–0.979

ICC intraclass correlation coefficient

same time, which are the body's transverse axis and the axis perpendicular to the outlet plane.

Another reason why the physiologic coordination is not chosen is that the oblique degrees of the pelvis are inconsistent among people and vary with a range between 40° and 60° [19], but the pelvis specific coordination could be considered as a relative objective reference system to depict and measure the movement type of the pelvis itself.

Table 8 ICC for translational displacement between the standardized X-ray and 3D reconstruction

Doctor	Displacement direction	ICC Coefficient	95 % CI
1	Vertical	0.994	0.984–0.998
	AP	0.943	0.898–0.974
	Transverse	0.977	0.967–0.998
2	Vertical	0.987	0.958–0.994
	AP	0.957	0.935–0.984
	Transverse	0.961	0.931–0.985
3	Vertical	0.953	0.936–0.989
	AP	0.945	0.907–0.977
	Transverse	0.911	0.887–0.953
4	Vertical	0.932	0.897–0.976
	AP	0.935	0.895–0.965
	Transverse	0.959	0.941–0.989
5	Vertical	0.928	0.887–0.978
	AP	0.974	0.947–0.996
	Transverse	0.985	0.975–0.992

AP anterior-posterior; ICC intraclass correlation coefficient

Thus, although almost all methods for the vertical displacement measurement used by authors were dependent on the pelvic AP X-ray, the measurement results based on the AP view might not correspond to the true one. Boontanapibul et al. compared hemipelvic vertical displacement measurements results based on the pelvic outlet and AP radiographs, and concluded that pelvic outlet radiograph could provide efficient measurements of hemipelvic vertical displacement, but the measurements results based on the AP radiographs were inconsistent [20].

In addition, as severe complications and multiple injuries are common in high-energy pelvic fractures, compared to the hip joint, which is easy to implicate and fracture, the iliac crest seems to be a more consistent anatomic landmark to use as the reference to measure the displacement. Consequently, it is more reliable and precise to reflect the vertical displacement of hemipelvis by measuring the positions of bilateral iliac crests' superior points in outlet view rather than measuring the hip joints' positions in the AP view.

For the measurement of AP displacement of pelvis, Henderson et al. used both ischial spine positions in the inlet view as the bony landmark [3]. Sagi et al. also used the inlet radiograph for the AP displacement [18]. Lindahl et al. used pelvic CT scans' axial sections for the measurement of the AP displacement, even though no details of measurement methods were available [21].

Regarding the rotational displacement, current inconsistent evaluation methods mainly focused on the rotation in the unilateral plane. Lefaivre et al. evaluated the rotational displacement of the hemipelvis in the horizontal plane by measuring the pubic symphysis diastasis in AP X-rays. Dickson et al. measured the difference between the width of bilateral ischiums as the reference reflecting the rotational direction of hemipelvis, and measured the angle between the midline and the quadrilateral plate of the injured side in the CT scan axial section to represent the rotational angle of the hemipelvis [4]. Sagi et al. measured the perpendicular distances between the acetabulum and sacrum in inlet and outlet views, separately, and evaluated the asymmetry of the pelvis in inlet and outlet views by calculating the ratio between the bilateral distances in the respective plane, which was also named as the inlet/outlet ratio method [18]. Keshishyan et al. evaluated the pelvic asymmetry by calculating the ratio between the distances of the inferior aspect of the sacroiliac joint to the inferior aspect of the contralateral teardrop on both sides of the pelvis. As the pelvis represents a three-dimensional structure, any rotational measurements applied should be as representative as possible to its three dimensions. Although the present different methods for rotation displacement were complicated, there has not been a well-accepted validated method thus far. Nystrom et al. developed a rotational assessment method based on the computer-reconstructed radiographs [1]. However, in their study, the pelvic rotational displacements were only measured around two axes perpendicular to the inlet and sagittal planes, respectively.

Lefaivre et al. analyzed almost all the radiographic measurement methods for the rotational displacement of the pelvic fracture and concluded three most reliable methods [22], including the Sagi, the Keshishyan or Smith and the Lefaivre methods [8, 18, 23, 24]. Hereafter, they performed a comparative study to test the interobserver reliability of three commonly used radiographic measurement methods [10]. The cross measurement technique of Keshishyan showed that overall there is very good agreement between observers, with an ICC coefficient above 0.9 [24]. The inlet and outlet ratio method of Sagi showed less interobserver reliability with a coefficient between 0.5 and 0.8 [18]. The absolute displacement methods described by Lefaivre et al. showed the poorest interobserver agreement [8]. The authors analyzed and noted that the more reference lines or marks and the more steps used, the poorer the agreement would be concluded and the greater the error would be magnified.

The aim of this study was to set up a measurement system, which could allow observers to complete the measurement of displacement in a more convenient manner within as few steps as possible. Ideally, it could minimize the disagreement and errors brought by multiple steps and precisely indicate the rotational direction in different planes, which could be used as the basis for preoperative assessment and treatment plan.

As unstable pelvic fractures are classified as a pelvis with the complete disruption of the posterior osseous ligamentous structure, the posterior pelvic ring was the keystone for preoperative assessment and treatment plans. Thus, the measurement technique of the pelvic translational displacement should focus on the area around the SI joint or posterior pelvic ring. Furthermore, we studied the relationship between the positions of bilateral corresponding anatomic landmarks in 3D coordinate systems and the motion of the hemipelvis in different directions, set up a series of formulas to indicate the rotational displacement around three mutually perpendicular axes, and calculated the associated displacement parameters. Regarding the three-dimensional structure of pelvis, to minimize the measurement error, we selected three landmarks with different 3D coordinates dispersed far away from each other, such as ASIS, the iliac aspect of the SI joint, and ischial tubercle. By comparing with the coordinates of the corresponding anatomic landmarks in bilateral hemipelvis, we concluded a series of formulas that could indicate the rotational direction of the injured hemipelvis, based on the variation of the difference between the distance between

landmarks of the injured side in one plane and the distance between the same corresponding landmarks of the intact side in the same plane, following the rotation of injured hemipelvis in the same specified plane. For example, if the injured hemipelvis flexed in the sagittal plane, the distance between the ASIS and ischial tubercle would be reduced compared with the distance between corresponding points on the opposite side, and vice versa. The same situation happened in other types of motions in the corresponding plane.

After the previous step where the formula is established, we also need the ratio between the actual distance and the measurement on the X-ray images, by acquiring and setting each femoral head diameter through measuring its 3D model using 3-matic software, and the relationship between the measurement on the X-ray images and the distance between pixels on the 2D coordination system. In the end, the process of all relevant cumbersome calculations could be simplified by the acquisition of special anatomic landmarks' 2D coordinates in the corresponding planes and carried out in a few mouse clicks. Ideally, this method could reflect the actual spatial rotational displacements of injured hemipelvis more precisely, and direct the manual reduction manipulations in the clinical practices. However, as was the case in most previous measurement methods, the premise of the current measurement system is that the injured hemipelvis was relatively intact. The proposed measurement method could be used by all the researchers, medical students, radiologists and orthopedic surgeons who are familiar with the pelvic anatomic morphology and landmarks and the injury mechanisms, including AO/OTA and Young-Burgess classifications, and displacements characteristics of the unstable pelvic fractures.

Viegas et al. demonstrated that the three-dimensional CT scan reconstruction technique could provide the bone measurement a volumetric accuracy of 94 % and a linear accuracy of 97 % [25]. Nystrom et al. also tested and verified the validity of CT based measurements of fracture displacement [11]. Thus, the measurement on the 3D CT model was regarded as the standard to test the measurements on the standardized X-ray images. According to the results, interobserver reliability of either translational or rotational measurement was high as both ICCs were higher than 0.9, which means the agreement was nearly perfect and would allow subsequent authors to repeat it.

Conclusion

The new method for measuring translational and rotational displacement based on the established formula is reliable and can minimize the errors in pelvic fracture measurements. Furthermore, this study was possible for the standardization of the preoperative plan and used as the theoretical basis for initiating a process of robot-assisted pelvic fracture surgery based on two-dimensional radiographs.

Abbreviations
AP: Anterior-posterior; 2D: 2-dimensional; 3D: 3-dimensional; ICC: Intraclass correlation coefficient; SI: Sacroiliac; DICOM: Digital-imaging-and-communications-in-medicine; ASIS: Anterior superior iliac spine.

Competing interests
The authors declare that they have no competing interests.

Authors' contributions
Five authors, including 2 full-time orthopaedic trauma surgeons (LHZ and XYS) and 3 orthopaedic trauma fellows (ZZ, LNZ and HLD) carried out the reliability study. ZZ drafted the manuscript. JXZ and LCZ revised the manuscript. LHZ and PFT conceived of the study, and participated in its design and coordination. Statistical analysis was done by JXZ. All authors read and approved the final manuscript.

Acknowledgements
The authors acknowledge the support from the radiography department of Chinese PLA General Hospital. This research received no specific grant from any funding agency in the public, commercial, or not-for-profit sectors.

Author details
[1]Department of Orthopedics, Chinese PLA 82nd Hospital, No.100 East Jiankang Road, Qinghe District, Huai'an, Jiangsu Province 223001, People's Republic of China. [2]Department of Orthopedics, Chinese PLA General Hospital, No.28 Fuxing Road, Beijing, Haidian District 100853, People's Republic of China. [3]Department of Orthopedics, Beijing Tsinghua Chang Gung Hospital, No.1 Block Tiantongyuan North, Beijing 102218, People's Republic of China. [4]Department of Orthopedics, Affiliated Hospital of the Academy of Military Medical Sciences, No.8 Dongdajie Road, Beijing 100071, People's Republic of China.

References
1. Nystrom LM, McKinley TO, Marsh JL. Radiographic Measurement of Rotational Deformity in Pelvic Fractures: A Novel Method With Validity and Reliability Testing. J Orthop Trauma. 2015;29(8):365–9. doi:10.1097/BOT.0000000000000306.
2. Boulay C, Tardieu C, Benaim C, Hecquet J, Marty C, Prat-Pradal D, et al. Three-dimensional study of pelvic asymmetry on anatomical specimens and its clinical perspectives. J Anat. 2006;208(1):21–33. doi:10.1111/j.1469-7580.2006.00513.x.
3. Henderson RC. The long-term results of nonoperatively treated major pelvic disruptions. J Orthop Trauma. 1989;3(1):41–7.
4. Dickson KF, Matta JM. Skeletal deformity after anterior external fixation of the pelvis. J Orthop Trauma. 2009;23(5):327–32. doi:10.1097/BOT.0b013e3181a23f5b.
5. Dujardin FH, Hossenbaccus M, Duparc F, Biga N, Thomine JM. Long-term functional prognosis of posterior injuries in high-energy pelvic disruption. J Orthop Trauma. 1998;12(3):145–50. discussion 50–1.
6. Lefaivre KA, Starr AJ, Reinert CM. Reduction of displaced pelvic ring disruptions using a pelvic reduction frame. J Orthop Trauma. 2009;23(4):299–308. doi:10.1097/BOT.0b013e3181a1407d.
7. Matta JM, Tornetta 3rd P. Internal fixation of unstable pelvic ring injuries. Clin Orthop Relat Res. 1996;329:129–40.
8. Lefaivre KA, Starr AJ, Barker BP, Overturf S, Reinert CM. Early experience with reduction of displaced disruption of the pelvic ring using a pelvic reduction frame. J Bone Joint Surg (Br). 2009;91(9):1201–7. doi:10.1302/0301-620x.91b9.22093.
9. Lindahl J, Hirvensalo E, Bostman O, Santavirta S. Failure of reduction with an external fixator in the management of injuries of the pelvic ring. Long-term evaluation of 110 patients. J Bone Joint Surg (Br). 1999;81(6):955–62.
10. Lefaivre KA, Blachut PA, Starr AJ, Slobogean GP, O'Brien PJ. Radiographic displacement in pelvic ring disruption: reliability of 3 previously described measurement techniques. J Orthop Trauma. 2014;28(3):160–6. doi:10.1097/BOT.0b013e31829efcc5.
11. Nystrom LM, McKinley TO, Marsh JL. Accuracy in radiographic assessment of pelvic ring fracture deformity: analysis of current methods. J Orthop Trauma. 2013;27(12):708–15. doi:10.1097/BOT.0b013e318298e6cf.
12. Cohen J. A Coefficient of Agreement for Nominal Scales. Educ Psychol Meas. 1960;20(1):37–46. doi:10.1177/001316446002000104.
13. Shrout PE, Fleiss JL. Intraclass correlations: uses in assessing rater reliability. Psychol Bull. 1979;86(2):420–8.
14. Borrelli Jr J, Peelle M, McFarland E, Evanoff B, Ricci WM. Computer-reconstructed radiographs are as good as plain radiographs for assessment of acetabular fractures. Am J Orthop (Belle Mead NJ). 2008;37(9):455–9. discussion 60.
15. Majeed SA. External fixation of the injured pelvis. The functional outcome. J Bone Joint Surg (Br). 1990;72(4):612–4.
16. Mataliotakis GI, Giannoudis PV. Radiological measurements for postoperative evaluation of quality of reduction of unstable pelvic ring fractures: Advantages and limitations. Injury. 2011;42(12):1395–401. doi:10.1016/j.injury.2011.10.012.
17. Griffin DR, Starr AJ, Reinert CM, Jones AL, Whitlock S. Vertically unstable pelvic fractures fixed with percutaneous iliosacral screws: does posterior injury pattern predict fixation failure? J Orthop Trauma. 2006;20(1):S30–6. discussion S6.
18. Sagi HC, Militano U, Caron T, Lindvall E. A comprehensive analysis with minimum 1-year follow-up of vertically unstable transforaminal sacral fractures treated with triangular osteosynthesis. J Orthop Trauma. 2009;23(5):313–9. doi:10.1097/BOT.0b013e3181a32b91. discussion 9–21.
19. Ricci WM, Mamczak C, Tynan M, Streubel P, Gardner M. Pelvic inlet and outlet radiographs redefined. J Bone Joint Surg Am. 2010;92(10):1947–53. doi:10.2106/jbjs.i.01580.
20. Boontanapibul K, Harnroongroj T, Sudjai N, Harnroongroj T. Vertical pelvic ring displacement in pelvic ring injury: Measurements in pelvic outlet radiograph and in cadavers. Indian J Orthop. 2015;49(4):425–8. doi:10.4103/0019-5413.159634.
21. Lindahl J, Hirvensalo E. Outcome of operatively treated type-C injuries of the pelvic ring. Acta Orthop. 2005;76(5):667–78. doi:10.1080/17453670510041754.
22. Lefaivre KA, Slobogean G, Starr AJ, Guy P, O'Brien PJ, Macadam SA. Methodology and interpretation of radiographic outcomes in surgically treated pelvic fractures: a systematic review. J Orthop Trauma. 2012;26(8):474–81. doi:10.1097/BOT.0b013e3182323aa2.
23. Smith W, Shurnas P, Morgan S, Agudelo J, Luszko G, Knox EC, et al. Clinical outcomes of unstable pelvic fractures in skeletally immature patients. J Bone Joint Surg Am. 2005;87(11):2423–31. doi:10.2106/JBJS.C.01244v.
24. Keshishyan RA, Rozinov VM, Malakhov OA, Kuznetsov LE, Strunin EG, Chogovadze GA, et al. Pelvic polyfractures in children. Radiographic diagnosis and treatment. Clin Orthop Relat Res. 1995;320:28–33.
25. Viegas SF, Hillman GR, Elder K, Stoner D, Patterson RM. Measurement of carpal bone geometry by computer analysis of three-dimensional CT images. J Hand Surg [Am]. 1993;18(2):341–9. doi:10.1016/0363-5023(93)90372-A.

6

How to measure renal artery stenosis - a retrospective comparison of morphological measurement approaches in relation to hemodynamic significance

Malin Andersson[1,2†], Karl Jägervall[1,2†], Per Eriksson[3], Anders Persson[1,2], Göran Granerus[4], Chunliang Wang[1,2,5] and Örjan Smedby[1,2,5*]

Abstract

Background: Although it is well known that renal artery stenosis may cause renovascular hypertension, it is unclear how the degree of stenosis should best be measured in morphological images. The aim of this study was to determine which morphological measures from Computed Tomography Angiography (CTA) and Magnetic Resonance Angiography (MRA) are best in predicting whether a renal artery stenosis is hemodynamically significant or not.

Methods: Forty-seven patients with hypertension and a clinical suspicion of renovascular hypertension were examined with CTA, MRA, captopril-enhanced renography (CER) and captopril test (Ctest). CTA and MRA images of the renal arteries were analyzed by two readers using interactive vessel segmentation software. The measures included minimum diameter, minimum area, diameter reduction and area reduction. In addition, two radiologists visually judged the diameter reduction without automated segmentation. The results were then compared using limits of agreement and intra-class correlation, and correlated with the results from CER combined with Ctest (which were used as standard of reference) using receiver operating characteristics (ROC) analysis.

Results: A total of 68 kidneys had all three investigations (CTA, MRA and CER + Ctest), where 11 kidneys (16.2 %) got a positive result on the CER + Ctest. The greatest area under ROC curve (AUROC) was found for the area reduction on MRA, with a value of 0.91 (95 % confidence interval 0.82–0.99), excluding accessory renal arteries. As comparison, the AUROC for the radiologists' visual assessments on CTA and MRA were 0.90 (0.82–0.98) and 0.91 (0.83–0.99) respectively. None of the differences were statistically significant.

Conclusions: No significant differences were found between the morphological measures in their ability to predict hemodynamically significant stenosis, but a tendency of MRA having higher AUROC than CTA. There was no significant difference between measurements made by the radiologists and measurements made with fuzzy connectedness segmentation. Further studies are required to definitely identify the optimal measurement approach.

Keywords: Renal artery stenosis, Computed tomography angiography, Magnetic resonance angiography, Renography, Fuzzy connectedness segmentation, Vessel diameter, Cross-sectional area

* Correspondence: orjan.smedby@sth.kth.se
†Equal contributors
[1]Center for Medical Image Science and Visualization (CMIV), Linköping University, Linköping, Sweden
[2]Department of Radiology and Department of Medical and Health Sciences, Linköping University, Linköping, Sweden
Full list of author information is available at the end of the article

Background

Renal artery stenosis (RAS), most commonly due to atherosclerosis, is an important cause of hypertension and accounts for 1–5 % of all hypertension cases in the general population, but when at-risk patients are identified through clinical selection criteria, the estimated prevalence of renovascular-induced hypertension increases to 20–40 % [1]. Currently, there is much debate over how to best treat these patients and the value of percutaneous transluminal renal angioplasty (PTRA) in renal artery stenosis is not completely known [2, 3]. The recently published CORAL study even found that renal artery stenting does not significantly improve clinical outcome [4]. It is therefore important to have reliable diagnostic methods in order to identify patients that could benefit from treatment.

The most commonly available methods to diagnose RAS are computed tomography angiography (CTA), magnetic resonance angiography (MRA), captopril-enhanced renography (CER), captopril test (Ctest), ultrasonography and invasive intra-arterial renal angiography (IARA) [1]. IARA has long been considered the gold standard for diagnosing RAS [5], but it is not an ideal method. It relies strictly on lumen morphology and thus gives only indirect information about the hemodynamic consequences of the stenosis [6]. Besides, the invasive nature also means a risk of severe complications [7–10]. It can sometimes be combined with measurement of the pressure drop through the stenosis, which may indicate more reliably hemodynamically significant RAS [11], although the presence of a catheter in the artery might disturb the measurements [12]. Rapid progress in spatial resolution and image quality has allowed MRA and CTA to replace the invasive examinations as the standard diagnostic methods [1, 13]. Although a major prospective study, conducted between 1998 and 2001 and published in 2004 (the RADISH-trial), concluded that neither CTA nor MRA are reproducible or sensitive enough to replace IARA as the diagnostic gold standard [14], randomized trials comparing CTA and MRA to IARA have shown a sensitivity of 94–95 % and a specificity of 92–93 % for CTA [15, 16], and a sensitivity of 90–100 % and a specificity of 94–98 % for MRA [15, 17].

Renography is a method for functional evaluation of the kidney. The use of angiotensin converting enzyme (ACE) inhibitors, such as captopril, in conjunction with radionuclide renography has been shown to enhance sensitivity and specificity for detecting renovascular hypertension [18, 19]. CER has been reported to have a sensitivity of 87–95 % and specificity of 93–100 % when the reference is whether there is a reduction in blood pressure following intervention [20, 21]. That makes CER a valuable method for detecting hemodynamically significant stenoses. However, in cases with potential bilateral stenosis, as well as in severe renal failure, its value is doubtful [19]. In cases of intermediate test results on CER, the captopril test (Ctest), which includes analysis of the plasma concentration of renin before and after ingestion of captopril, has been applied to strengthen the diagnosis [6].

The advances of computer post-processing techniques enable researchers to obtain detailed quantitative information about different morphological measures of the vessels, such as minimum diameter, diameter reduction, minimum area and area reduction, from CTA and MRA. A diameter reduction of >50 % has been considered hemodynamically significant by many authors [13, 22, 23], whereas others have advocated higher threshold values [24], but this is not necessarily equivalent to a decrease in function of one or both kidneys [6]. There is therefore a need to investigate how to measure RAS on MRA and CTA to find the best predictive measure of the hemodynamic significance of the stenosis. Although Schoenberg et al. have shown that measurements of the area of the stenosis on MRA might be a better predictor of hemodynamically significant stenosis than the diameter [23], there is not much information about how different morphological measures correlate with renal functional tests. Thus, the aim of our study was to compare different morphological measurements describing renal artery stenoses in CTA and MRA images with respect to their ability to predict a hemodynamically significant stenosis as defined by captopril-enhanced renography.

Methods

Patients

For this study, the patient material from an earlier study [6] was used. The ethical approval of the acquisition of data for the original publication was given by the regional research ethics committee in Linköping, Sweden (decision nr. 03–412 and M90-05, dated Nov. 4, 2003 and Aug. 10, 2005). Written informed consent was obtained from each patient before examination, and the study was performed in compliance with the Helsinki Declaration. Forty-seven patients of both genders, 18–80 years old, with a screening serum creatinine of 150–300 μmol/L, hypertension and clinical suspicion of renovascular hypertension were consecutively recruited for the study and examined with MRA, CTA, CER and Ctest. Inclusion and exclusion criteria as well as demographic characteristics are described in [6].

Morphological investigations

The imaging technique for the CTA and MRA examinations has been published previously [6]. The acquisition protocol for CTA specified a voxel size of $0.75 \times 0.5 \times 0.5$ mm^3, and that for MRA a voxel size of $2.0 \times 0.7 \times 0.7$ mm^3. However, in eight of the patients, CTA data with a higher slice thickness of up to

3 mm had to be used, due to incomplete archiving. In one case, CTA data were missing.

Evaluation of CTA and MRA data was made with OsiriX (v.3.6.1 32-bits) [25] and the semi-automated CTA plug-in (CMIV CTA tools) [26] (Fig. 1a and b). The plug-in uses a competing fuzzy-connectedness tree algorithm to segment vessels and extract vessel centerlines [27]. The studied arteries were visualized using curved plane reformatting and the measurements were performed with in a cross-section view of the vessel. The vessel cross-sections were automatically segmented using a thresholding-based level-set method [28]. Some parameters that had to be set in the algorithm were selected after testing and visually assessing the results of alternative settings. The curvature scale was set to 10 to eliminate the effects of noise and keep the vessel contour smooth. A lower threshold (LT) value had to be defined for both MRA and CTA, and for CTA, an upper threshold (UT) was also needed, since calcified plaques have an attenuation exceeding that of contrast-mixed blood.

The LT was set using a grey-scale value in between the value contrast agent and background. The value of contrast agent was determined by measuring the maximum values of ROIs in aorta. The final value is calculated as the mean values from three cross-sections of the aorta (the cross-section of the abdominal aorta giving the greatest mean value and the corresponding slices 10 mm proximal and 10 mm distal to the maximum value). A background grey-scale value was determined by measuring the mean value of ROIs in non-contrast-filled areas. In CTA, four regions of interests (ROIs) were placed in the psoas muscles, and in MRA, three ROIs were placed in the vertebral bodies. For both modalities, the LT was then calculated for each patient with the formula $LT = (aorta + 2*background)/3$, which visually was the most reliable in a pilot-group of seven patients. The UT for CTA was calculated as the mean value of the maximum value of the cross-section slices of the abdominal aorta and the corresponding maximum values 10 mm proximal and 10 mm distal to the maximum value.

The CMIV CTA tools of the OsiriX software was in most cases able to automatically define the centerline of the vessel. When not possible, or when the automatically created centerline was obviously false, the centerlines had to be drawn manually.

Two segments in each renal artery were measured. The first segment was limited by the aorta and the most proximal bifurcation, while the second segment was defined as the largest branch from the first bifurcation to the second bifurcation. In each segment, the minimum diameter (MinD), the minimum area (MinA), the maximum diameter (MaxD) and the maximum area (MaxA) were measured and the relative diameter reduction (Dred) was calculated as

$$Dred = (1 - MinD/MaxD) \times 100\%$$

and the relative area reduction (Ared) was calculated as

$$Ared = (1 - MinA/MaxA) \times 100\%$$

To make sure that the MaxD and the MaxA were not affected by the bifurcation geometry, rules were set prohibiting the readers from measuring the MaxD and MaxA (i) less than 10 mm from the aorta and (ii) less than 5 mm proximal or distal to a bifurcation. When the rules made it impossible to measure the maximum values (e.g. in cases with very short distances between the branches) they were visually obtained.

The measurements of the renal arteries were made by two medical students, each blinded for the other's result and for the results of the other modalities. The morphological measures were calculated as the mean value of the two reader's observations, except for the analysis of the inter-observer agreement. In those cases where only one reader considered a segment measurable, that reader's measurements were used.

Since two segments were measured in each artery, and each kidney might have more than one artery, several measurements were obtained from each kidney. However, for correlation with the CER + Ctest, only one segment had to be chosen. Three different measurement approaches were used to summarize the results from the two segments of each artery to only one result for the whole kidney (i) the most pronounced stenosis (defined as the segment with the largest Dred) in the first segment, or first segments if the patient had accessory renal arteries (referred to as First), (ii) the most pronounced stenosis in any segment on one side (Tightest), and (iii) the most pronounced stenosis in the main artery (the artery with the largest maximum diameter) (Main).

Visual assessment was performed by two radiologists with at least 20 years of clinical experience [6]. The degree of stenosis was defined for both CTA and MRA on a six-grade scale: normal, diameter reduction >10 % but ≤ 30 %, diameter reduction >30 % but ≤ 50 %, diameter reduction >50 % but ≤ 70 %, diameter reduction >70 %, and occlusion. Those results were obtained from the previous study [6].

Functional investigations

The result from the CER + Ctest was considered to be the reference for defining hemodynamically significant stenoses. A 2-day protocol with a baseline renogram Day 1 and a captopril-stimulated renogram Day 2 was followed [6]. The interpretation of the CER was based on the criteria in [19]. Six patients got an intermediate test result on the CER. In those cases, adding the result of a Ctest made the final interpretation [6]. Two of the 6

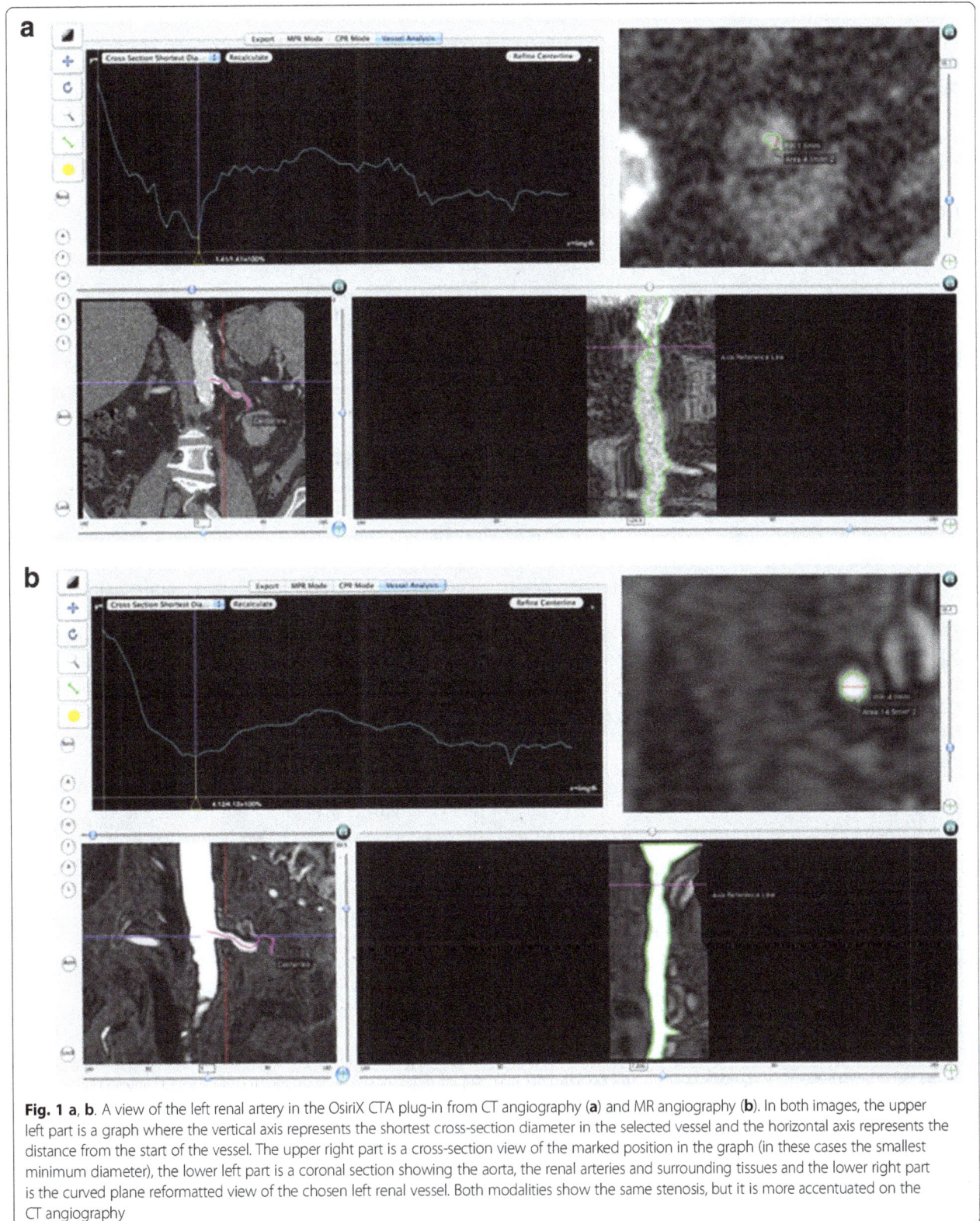

Fig. 1 a, **b**. A view of the left renal artery in the OsiriX CTA plug-in from CT angiography (**a**) and MR angiography (**b**). In both images, the upper left part is a graph where the vertical axis represents the shortest cross-section diameter in the selected vessel and the horizontal axis represents the distance from the start of the vessel. The upper right part is a cross-section view of the marked position in the graph (in these cases the smallest minimum diameter), the lower left part is a coronal section showing the aorta, the renal arteries and surrounding tissues and the lower right part is the curved plane reformatted view of the chosen left renal vessel. Both modalities show the same stenosis, but it is more accentuated on the CT angiography

intermediate results were judged positive after the Ctest, and 4 were considered negative.

Statistics

For descriptive purposes, the mean and standard deviation (SD) were used. The inter-observer agreement refers to the difference between the two readers' results for the same morphological measurement. It was calculated from all vessels judged measurable by both readers. The inter-method agreement refers to the difference between the mean value of the two readers' CTA measurements and the mean value of the two readers' MRA measurements. It was calculated at kidney level using the three different measurement approaches described above. The inter-observer and inter-method agreement was described as the 95 % limits of agreements (the mean value of the difference ± 2 SD [29]. In addition, the intraclass correlation (ICC) was computed, treating both cases (kidneys or vessels) and observers as random effects [30]. All these calculations were made with SPSS 19.0.0 (SPSS Inc., Chicago, IL, USA).

To evaluate the morphological methods' ability to predict hemodynamically significant stenosis as defined by the CER + Ctest, receiver operating characteristic curves (ROC curves) were created for each measurement, as well as for the radiologists' measurement from the previous study, using the statistical software JMP 9.0 (SAS Inc., Cary, NC, USA). The areas under the ROC curves (AUROCs) of the different measurements in relation to the CER + Ctest were compared using Stata 10.1 (StataCorp, College Station, TX, USA).

Results

In the 47 patients, where 16 patients had more than one artery per kidney, 104 first segments and 99 second segments of the arteries were considered measurable (by at least one observer) for CTA, and for MRA, 92 first segments and 68 second segments were considered measureable. For CTA, 92 % of the measurable first segments ($n = 96$), and 73 % of the second segments ($n = 72$) were considered measurable by both readers, and for MRA, 90 % of the measureable first segments ($n = 83$) and 67 % of the second segments ($n = 46$) were considered measurable by both readers. The mean values and the standard deviations of the measured segments at artery level are given in Table 1. In general, both the absolute measures (MinD an MinA) and the relative measures (Dred and Ared) gave roughly similar values regardless of whether they were computed from CTA or MRA images.

Our material consisted of 47 patients, hence 94 kidneys. Only patients who had all three investigations (MRA, CTA and CER + Ctest) were included. Eleven kidneys got a positive result on the CER + Ctest, and the kidneys contralateral to the positive results were excluded since

the method is unable to give useful information in such cases. Four kidneys were excluded because their vessels were non-measurable on either CTA or MRA. One of the kidneys that were non-measureable on MRA had a positive result on the CER + Ctest and the contralateral kidney was thereby excluded. Thus, the analyses were made on 68 kidneys, where 11 kidneys (16.2 %) had a positive result on the CER + Ctest and 57 kidneys (83.8 %) had a negative result. The mean values and standard deviations of the vascular morphology measures for the 68 kidneys using the three different measurement approaches are found in Table 1. Again, no obvious difference was found between CTA and MRA. The smallest MinD and MinA and largest Dred and Ared were found for both CTA and MRA in the Tightest approach, while the largest MinD and MinA and smallest Dred and Ared were found with the First approach.

Inter-observer agreement

The inter-observer differences in the measurements from CTA and MRA are shown in Table 2. There was excellent agreement for all measurements in the first segment (ICC values between 0.91 and 0.98), while the agreement was lower for the second segment (ICC values between 0.48 and 0.87). For each measurement, the agreement was significantly higher for the first segment than for the second segment. On CTA and on the first segment in MRA there seems to be no systematic under- or overestimation by any reader, but on the MRA of the second segment, the negative mean differences between reader 1 and reader 2 imply that reader 2 measured more severe stenoses than reader 1. Figure 2 shows Bland-Altman plots illustrating the difference in agreement between the two segments, here shown for MRA Ared.

Inter-method agreement

The inter-method analysis was made using the 68 vessels that were compared with the CER + Ctest. The result of the statistical analysis of the agreement between CTA and MRA is shown in Table 3. Although all measurements have an excellent agreement, there is generally a higher agreement for the measurements of the area than for the measurements of the diameter, with the highest ICC being found for MinA of First. For all measurement approaches, Dred, which is the traditionally most used measure, has the lowest agreement. When comparing the three measurement approaches, the agreement is generally highest for First and lowest for Tightest.

Comparison of morphological and functional investigations

There was a tendency of MRA having higher predictive ability (AUROC) than CTA (Table 4); however, there were

Table 1 Descriptive statistics of stenosis measurements (Mean ± SD). Most prominent stenosis defined in three different ways: most pronounced stenosis in proximal vessel segment (*First*), segment with most pronounced stenosis (*Tightest*) and most pronounced stenosis in main renal artery (*Main*)

Modality	Measure	All arteries		Most prominent stenosis for each kidney		
		Segment 1	Segment 2	First	Tightest	Main
CTA	MinD (mm)	2.65 ± 1.46	2.82 ± 1.01	2.93 ± 1.55	2.68 ± 1.44	2.79 ± 1.35
	MinA (mm^2)	10.56 ± 8.41	9.49 ± 6.08	12.61 ± 9.05	10.86 ± 7.84	11.24 ± 7.55
	Dred (%)	46.7 ± 25.5	24.7 ± 14.7	44.8 ± 26.2	48.4 ± 24.9	46.3 ± 23.2
	Ared (%)	58.4 ± 25.5	36.3 ± 17.6	55.5 ± 26.0	59.3 ± 24.0	57.7 ± 22.9
	n	96	72	68	68	68
MRA	MinD (mm)	2.88 ± 1.76	2.78 ± 1.37	3.06 ± 1.74	2.62 ± 1.64	2.64 ± 1.62
	MinA (mm^2)	11.63 ± 9.49	9.66 ± 7.01	12.90 ± 9.61	10.54 ± 8.53	10.58 ± 8.49
	Dred (%)	45.4 ± 30.8	33.1 ± 25.5	43.6 ± 29.3	50.2 ± 28.2	49.2 ± 27.6
	Ared (%)	55.8 ± 29.4	44.1 ± 25.9	53.3 ± 28.1	60.0 ± 26.0	59.3 ± 25.5
	n	83	46	68	68	68

no significant differences between them. The highest AUROC of all measurements made with the computer-assisted vessel analysis tool was found for *Ared* on *Main* in MRA (0.91) and the highest value for CTA was found for the *Dred* on *Main* (0.88). The lowest AUROC was found for *MinA* and *Ared* on CTA in *Tightest* (0.81), while the lowest AUROC for MRA was *Dred* in *First* (0.84). For the radiologists' visual assessment on a six-grade ordinal scale, the AUROC were 0.90 for CTA and 0.91 for MRA. The absolute measures had highest AUROC in *First* while the relative measures had the highest AUROC in *Main*. *Ared* had higher AUROC than *Dred* for MRA, but lower on the CTA. There were no significant differences between any of the AUROC values.

Discussion

A central finding in this study is the excellent ICC values for the inter-method agreement and for the inter-observer agreement of the first segments, which indicate good reproducibility for measuring RAS with the computer-assisted vessel analysis tool. The high reproducibility is probably due to the low influence of individual arbitrariness because of the highly automated work-flow. The formula for the threshold values, the well-defined measuring rules, the automatically generated vessel centerlines and the use of the graph in the CMIV CTA plug-in all make it easy to extract the minimum and maximum values.

As the differences in AUROC were not significant, it cannot be concluded whether measurements from the software tool or visual assessments by radiologists are the best predictors of a hemodynamically significant stenosis. In spite of a tendency for AUROC in general being higher for the visually assessed measurements than for the computer-assisted vessel analysis tool, there were no, or only slight, differences when the best measures with the software on MRA and CTA were used in comparison with

Table 2 The inter-observer agreement of morphological measures described as the mean difference Reader 1 – Reader 2 and the 95 % limits of agreement (mean –2SD; mean + 2SD), as well as the intraclass correlation and its 95 % confidence limits, n = 68

Measure	Segment 1		Segment 2	
	Mean difference (95 % limits of agreement)	Intraclass correlation (95 % confidence limits)	Mean difference (95 % limits of agreement)	Intraclass correlation (95 % confidence limits)
CTA MinD (mm)	−0.11(−1.09; 0.86)	0.97 (0.95–0.98)	−0.11(1.57; 1.35)	0.86 (0.78–0.92)
CTA MinA (mm^2)	0.08(−5.68; 5.83)	0.97 (0.95–0.98)	−0.48(−9.27; 8.31)	0.87 (0.80–0.92)
CTA Dred (%)	2.46(−22.08; 26.99)	0.94 (0.91–0.96)	2.40(−31.10; 35.90)	0.57 (0.32–0.73)
CTA Ared (%)	−2.03(−33.01; 28.94)	0.91 (0.86–0.94)	−1.91(−41.02; 37.19)	0.64 (0.42–0.78)
MRA MinD (mm)	−0.07(−1.16; 1.03)	0.97 (0.96–0.98)	0.15(−2.32; 2.63)	0.70 (0.47–0.84)
MRA MinA (mm^2)	−0.23(−8.25; 7.79)	0.95 (0.93–0.97)	0.40(−10.52; 11.32)	0.76 (0.57–0.87)
MRA Dred (%)	0.97(−17.65; 19.59)	0.98 (0.96–0.98)	−6.90(−64.87; 51.07)	0.48 (0.08–0.71)
MRA Ared (%)	−0.58(−16.81; 15.64)	0.98 (0.97–0.99)	−8.35(−64.59; 47.90)	0.54 (0.19–0.74)

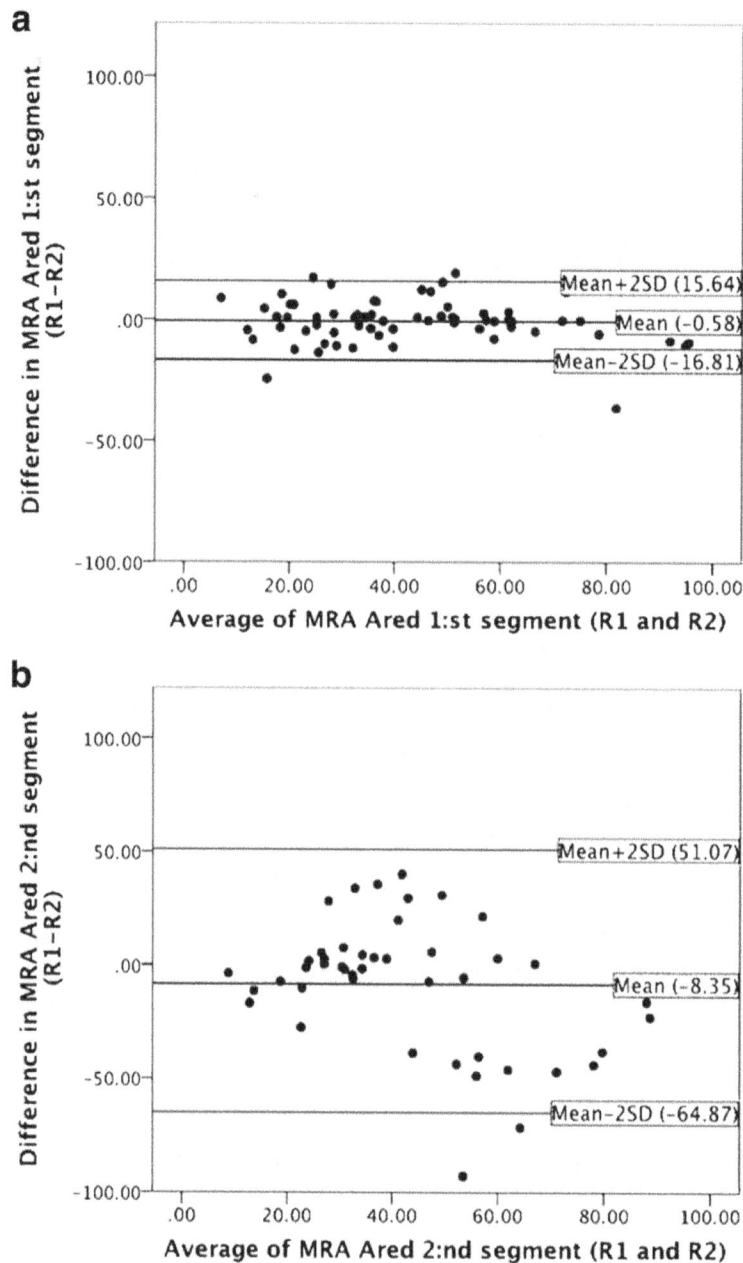

a

b

Fig. 2 a, b. Bland-Altman plots showing the agreement between the two readers (R1 and R2) for *Ared* in MR angiography for the first (**a**) and second (**b**) segment. The agreement is highest for the first segment as it has the narrowest limits of agreement

the visually assessed measurements (0.91 vs. 0.91 for MRA and 0.88 vs. 0.90 for CTA). It is, however, interesting to notice that users without extensive training (medical students) using the computer-assisted vessel analysis tool were able to attain AUROC values very close to those of the visual assessments of experienced radiologists. Since the influence of individual arbitrariness is minimized when measuring renal arteries with the standardized algorithm in a much automated process, the level of education

may be a minor problem for obtaining adequate results. Also, with an excellent inter-observer agreement for the first segments and an excellent inter-method agreement, the reproducibility for the method appears satisfactory. The good reproducibility and AUROCs fairly similar to the radiologists' measurements suggest that computer-assisted vessel segmentation is a promising method for analyzing RAS, even though definite conclusions about the clinical utility cannot be drawn.

Table 3 The inter-method agreement of morphological measures described as the mean difference of Reader 1 – Reader 2 and the 95 % limits of agreement (mean −2SD; mean + 2SD), as well as the intraclass correlation and its 95 % confidence limits. $n = 68$

Measure	Mean difference (95 % limits of agreement)	Intraclass correlation (95 % confidence limits)
MinD first	−0.14(−2.30; 2.03)	0.88 (0.80–0.93)
MinA first	−0.29(−9.85; 9.27)	0.93 (0.89–0.96)
Dred first	1.25(−40.31; 42.81)	0.84 (0.74.0.90)
Ared first	2.12(−29.95; 34.20)	0.90 (0.84–0.94)
MinD tightest	0.06(−2.30; 2.43)	0.83 (0.73–0.90)
MinA tightest	0.32(−10.46; 11.09)	0.88 (0.81–0.93)
Dred tightest	−1.83(−44.20; 40.53)	0.81 (0.70–0.88)
Ared tightest	−0.63(−33.58; 32.32)	0.88 (0.80–0.93)
MinD main	0.15(−2.04; 2.34)	0.84 (0.75–0.90)
MinA main	0.66(−9.55; 10.87)	0.89 (0.82–0.93)
Dred main	−2.93(−42.29; 36.42)	0.83 (0.72–0.89)
Ared main	−1.60(−32.80; 29.60)	0.89 (0.81–0.93)

As mentioned earlier, the inter-observer agreement was excellent for the first segments, but it was considerably lower for the second segments. The inter-method agreement was also lower for the second segment as the highest ICC-value was found in *First*, which is the only measurement approach that excludes the second segments. One reason might be that the second segment was defined as the largest branch from the first bifurcation to the second bifurcation, and in some cases it was not obvious which branch was the largest. This might lead to the two readers measuring different segments, which could lead to a lower agreement. One might speculate that if the second segments were excluded, the measurements would be more accurate and therefore have a higher correlation with the functional

Table 4 Relationship between the morphologic measures and the CER + Ctest expressed as the area under the ROC curve (95 % confidence interval), $n = 68$

Measure	First	Tightest	Main
CTA MinD	0.86 (0.77–0.95)	0.83 (0.71–0.94)	0.86 (0.76–0.96)
CTA MinA	0.86 (0.77–0.95)	0.81 (0.70–0.93)	0.84 (0.74–0-95)
CTA Dred	0.85 (0.76–0.95)	0.84 (0.73–0.95)	0.88 (0.78–0.98)
CTA Ared	0.83 (0.71–0.95)	0.81 (0.67–0.95)	0.83 (0.70–0.97)
MRA MinD	0.90 (0.81–0.99)	0.87 (0.77–0.98)	0.88 (0.78–0.99)
MRA MinA	0.90 (0.80–0.99)	0.87 (0.76–0.98)	0.88 (0.77–0.99)
MRA Dred	0.84 (0.70–0.99)	0.88 (0.78–0.98)	0.89 (0.80–0.99)
MRA Ared	0.86 (0.73–0.99)	0.89 (0.81–0.99)	0.91 (0.82–0.99)

evaluation. However, the highest AUROC was found in *Main*, which includes the second segment. This suggests that despite being more difficult to measure, the most relevant measurements are those that include the second segment (*Main* and *Tightest* rather than *First*).

Since there were no significant differences between any of the morphological measures in their ability to predict a hemodynamically significant stenosis, no definite conclusions can be drawn. However, a tendency of MRA having higher AUROC than CTA was found, but further studies are required to verify this finding. One explanation might have been that one method systematically measured more distinct stenoses than the other; for instance, gadolinium-enhanced MRA is considered to overestimate the degree of RAS [23]. However, since Table 4 shows that there are no systematic differences between CTA and MRA, this does not seem as a likely explanation of our findings. Our impression is that CTA yielded the best spatial resolution but had inferior image-to-noise characteristics, which may be related to X-ray attenuation in surrounding abdominal organs. This might be a possible explanation for tendency to lower AUROC for CTA than for MRA. The lack of significant differences between the morphological measures might indicate that there are no major differences between them, but the fact that we found that *Ared* has the highest AUROC for MRA is in line with the previous result from Schoenberg et al. who have suggested that the cut-off value for a hemodynamically significant renal artery stenosis can be better defined on MRA by measuring the area of the stenosis instead of the diameter [23]. In the coronaries, Zhang et al. found area reduction to be superior to diameter reduction in predicting numerically computed fractional flow reserve [31]. For CTA, on the other hand, the area seems to have a lower concordance with CER + Ctest than the diameter. There is not much information available on the reliability of the different measures on CTA, and, for both modalities, due to the lack of significant results, no definite conclusions can be drawn.

The purpose of applying three different measurement approaches was to investigate whether it is of any importance which segments are included in the measurements. Of the three approaches, the maximum AUROC for both CTA and MRA was found for *Main*, and the minimum AUROC was found for *Tightest*. *Tightest* and *Main* are fairly similar with the only difference being that *Tightest*, in cases of more than 1 artery per kidney, also takes the smaller arteries in account. This result might indicate that stenoses in the main arteries are more crucial than stenoses in smaller arteries, or in other words, a stenosis in a small accessory artery may not affect whole kidney function enough to be detected by CER + Ctest. Another possible explanation is that the larger main arteries are easier to measure as their larger size lead to more accurate measurements.

A common reference when calculating *Dred* and *Ared* seems to be the North American Symptomatic Carotid Endarterectomy Trial (NASCET) criteria [32], which uses a normal vessel segment distal to the stenosis instead of the widest part of the segment, thereby excluding a possible post-stenotic dilatation. Although initially developed for the carotid arteries, it has also been used for measuring the renal arteries [33]. A difficulty with that approach might be that a post-stenotic dilatation extends all the way to the next bifurcation. Another used reference is the diameter and area of the main renal artery immediately proximal to the first bifurcation [34]. In this study, the maximum diameter and the maximum area of the segment were used as reference when calculating the relative reductions (*Dred* and *Ared*), in order to get a more standardized and thus more reproducible process. A limitation of our method is that the *MaxD* and *MaxA* might be measured in a post-stenotic dilation, which might lead to an overestimation of the degree of the stenosis. On the other hand, the presence of post-stenotic dilatations speaks in favor of hemodynamically significant stenoses, and if they were considered when calculating *Dred* and *Ared,* the correlations with CER + Ctest might be better. Another limitation is the fact that we measured stenosis using diameters and cross-sectional areas only, thus ignoring the length of the stenosis, which might also influence arterial blood flow.

When measuring vessels in a 3D dataset, the voxels should be as small as possible and preferably close to isotropic, i.e. have the same size in all three dimensions. With the scanners we had available, this was not feasible, and the MRA voxels ($2.0 \times 0.7 \times 0.7$ mm^3) were larger than the CTA voxels ($0.75 \times 0.5 \times 0.5$ mm^3). The comparatively thicker slices for MRA may have influenced the results for MRA, in particular for *Dred*, which depends heavily on a single diameter measurement. The poorer inter-observer agreement in segment 2 as compared to segment 1 (Table 2) may also be related to the limited spatial resolution.

The ideal method for determining the hemodynamical significance of the stenosis in a clinical context would be to evaluate the outcome of interventions such as PTRA, complemented with information about loss of renal parenchyma. However, the effect of the intervention is confounded by concurrent medical therapy, patient-related preferences and costs [6]. We therefore considered it impractical to use the therapeutic outcome as the reference method. IARA combined with measuring the pressure drop over the stenosis would have been an interesting reference method since it has been shown to correlate with the release of renin behind the stenosed kidney, thus a good indicator of whether the stenosis contributes to

hypertension or not [11]. However, it has the obvious drawback of being an invasive method and it is shown to be associated with a risk of severe complications, including cholesterol embolization, pseudoaneurysm, hematoma [7, 9], arteriovenous fistula and contrast-induced acute renal failure [8, 10]. The presence of a catheter in the artery might also alter the arterial fluid mechanisms, and thereby disturb the measurements; however, using a smaller pressure-sensing guidewire than the conventional catheter might reduce the disturbances [12]. The risks of IARA with measurement of the pressure gradient made it ethically unacceptable to perform an invasive catheterization in those patients where the non-invasive diagnostic methods did not indicate a stenosis, and it was therefore not included in the study protocol. For the same ethical reasons, invasive measurement of renin concentrations in the renal veins [35] was also excluded. Duplex ultrasonography would be another potential reference method. It has the advantage of providing both morphologic and functional assessment of the renal arteries, and it is a fast and inexpensive method, but it is very dependent on the skill of the observer. There are also difficulties in obtaining reproducible results from different sites [18, 19]. Ultrasound was therefore not considered an optimal reference method for the study.

CER + Ctest was chosen because it is a well-known method widely accepted for determining the hemodynamic significance of the stenosis [36]. It has been reported to have good sensitivity (87–95 %) and specificity (93–100 %) for detecting RAS when the reference is whether there is a reduction in blood pressure following intervention [20, 21], suggesting that CER + Ctest is a good predictor of the hemodynamic aspect of the stenosis. Its non-invasive nature also makes it a less harmful procedure compared to IARA. As the aim of the study was to investigate how different morphological measures of a stenosis correlate with the hemodynamic significance, we considered CER + Ctest to be the most suitable reference method. However, the question might be raised whether CER + Ctest is the optimum reference method in this study as the material included patients with moderately reduced renal function (serum creatinine of 150–300 µmol/L), where CER is less sensitive [37]. The sensitivity for detecting RAS with CER in patients with slightly to moderately reduced renal function has been reported between 75 and 87 % [38]. Pedersen [36] draws the conclusion that ACE inhibitor renography seems able to diagnose RAS in patients with reduced renal function as long as the renal function is not severely impaired. Therefore, CER + Ctest was still considered the most suitable reference method for our material despite the moderately reduced renal function of the included patients.

The lack of significance of the results in our study could be explained by the small number of cases, especially the few positive cases (11 kidneys) on CER + Ctest.

Such a small number of positives may give random variations a big impact and therefore results in wide confidence intervals. Because no outlier analysis was made, a few extreme measurements might have severe impacts on the results.

Conclusion

No significant differences were found between different morphological diameter and area measures in their ability to predict hemodynamically significant RAS. However, there is a non-significant tendency of MRA being a better predictor than CTA with the area reduction in the main artery as the best measurement. Automated measurements with the interactive vessel segmentation software showed very good reproducibility and only slightly lower validity than the visually assessed measurements in predicting the outcome of CER + Ctest, suggesting that this segmentation tool might be useful in the diagnosis of RAS. Nevertheless, the diagnostic value of morphological measures of renal artery stenosis is still incompletely known, and further studies using larger materials and scanners permitting higher spatial resolution are needed.

Competing interests
The authors declare that they have no competing interests.

Authors' contributions
PE recruited all patients. ÖS was responsible for MRA examinations and performed visual evaluation of MRA images. AP was responsible for CTA examinations and performed visual evaluation of CTA images. GG was responsible for and evaluated CER + Ctest. CLW wrote the software used for segmentation and measurements. MA and KJ performed the measurements using this software and performed statistical calculations. The manuscript was drafted by MA and KJ, who contributed equally to this project, and all authors read and approved the final manuscript. The main responsibility for the entire process lies with ÖS.

Acknowledgements
The study was supported by the Research Council of South-Eastern Sweden (FORSS) and the Swedish Research Council (VR).

Author details
[1]Center for Medical Image Science and Visualization (CMIV), Linköping University, Linköping, Sweden. [2]Department of Radiology and Department of Medical and Health Sciences, Linköping University, Linköping, Sweden. [3]Department of Nephrology and Department of Medical and Health Sciences, Linköping University, Linköping, Sweden. [4]Department of Clinical Physiology and Department of Medical and Health Sciences, Linköping University, Linköping, Sweden. [5]School of Technology and Health (STH), KTH Royal Institute of Technology, Stockholm, Sweden.

References

1. Chrysochou C, Kalra PA. Epidemiology and natural history of atherosclerotic renovascular disease. Prog Cardiovasc Dis. 2009;52:184–95. doi:10.1016/j.pcad.2009.09.001.

2. Wheatley K, Ives N, Gray R, Kalra PA, Moss JG, Baigent C, et al. Revascularization versus medical therapy for renal-artery stenosis. N Engl J Med. 2009;361:1953–62. doi:10.1056/NEJMoa0905368.

3. Bergqvist D, Björck M, Lundgren F, Troeng T. Invasive treatment for renovascular disease. A twenty year experience from a population based registry. J Cardiovasc Surg (Torino). 2008;49:559–63.

4. Cooper CJ, Murphy TP, Cutlip DE, Jamerson K, Henrich W, Reid DM, et al. Stenting and medical therapy for atherosclerotic renal-artery stenosis. N Engl J Med. 2014;370:13–22. doi:10.1056/NEJMoa1310753.

5. Bosmans JL, De Broe ME. Renovascular hypertension: diagnostic and therapeutic challenges. JBR-BTR. 2004;87:32–5.

6. Eriksson P, Mohammed AA, De Geer J, Kihlberg J, Persson A, Granerus G, et al. Non-invasive investigations of potential renal artery stenosis in renal insufficiency. Nephrol Dial Transplant. 2010;25:3607–14. doi:10.1093/ndt/gfq259.

7. Eklöf H, Ahlström H, Boström A, Bergqvist D, Andrén B, Karacagil S, et al. Renal artery stenosis evaluated with 3D-Gd-magnetic resonance angiography using transstenotic pressure gradient as the standard of reference. A multireader study. Acta Radiol. 2005;46:802–9.

8. Parfrey PS, Griffiths SM, Barrett BJ, Paul MD, Genge M, Withers J, et al. Contrast material-induced renal failure in patients with diabetes mellitus, renal insufficiency, or both. A prospective controlled study. N Engl J Med. 1989;320:143–9. doi:10.1056/NEJM198901193200303.

9. Reiss MD, Bookstein JJ, Bleifer KH. Radiologic aspects of renovascular hypertension. 4. Arteriographic complications. JAMA. 1972;221:375–8.

10. Rihal CS, Textor SC, Grill DE, Berger PB, Ting HH, Best PJ, et al. Incidence and prognostic importance of acute renal failure after percutaneous coronary intervention. Circulation. 2002;105:2259–64.

11. De Bruyne B, Manoharan G, Pijls NH, Verhamme K, Madaric J, Bartunek J, et al. Assessment of renal artery stenosis severity by pressure gradient measurements. J Am Coll Cardiol. 2006;48:1851–5. doi:10.1016/j.jacc.2006.05.074.

12. Colyer Jr WR, Cooper CJ, Burket MW, Thomas WJ. Utility of a 0.014" pressure-sensing guidewire to assess renal artery translesional systolic pressure gradients. Catheter Cardiovasc Interv. 2003;59:372–7. doi:10.1002/ccd.10508.

13. Glockner JF, Vrtiska TJ. Renal MR and CT angiography: current concepts. Abdom Imaging. 2007;32:407–20. doi:10.1007/s00261-006-9066-3.

14. Vasbinder GB, Nelemans PJ, Kessels AG, Kroon AA, Maki JH, Leiner T, et al. Accuracy of computed tomographic angiography and magnetic resonance angiography for diagnosing renal artery stenosis. Ann Intern Med. 2004;141:674–82.

15. Rountas C, Vlychou M, Vassiou K, Liakopoulos V, Kapsalaki E, Koukoulis G, et al. Imaging modalities for renal artery stenosis in suspected renovascular hypertension: prospective intraindividual comparison of color Doppler US, CT angiography, GD-enhanced MR angiography, and digital substraction angiography. Ren Fail. 2007;29:295–302. 0.1080/08860220601166305.

16. Galanski M, Prokop M, Chavan A, Schaefer C, Jandeleit K, Olbricht C. Leistungsfähigkeit der CT-Angiographie beim Nachweis von Nierenarterienstenosen [Accuracy of CT angiography in the diagnosis of renal artery stenosis]. Röfo. 1994;161:519–25. doi:10.1055/s-2008-1032579.

17. Thornton MJ, Thornton F, O'Callaghan J, Varghese JC, O'Brien E, Walshe J, et al. Evaluation of dynamic gadolinium-enhanced breath-hold MR angiography in the diagnosis of renal artery stenosis. AJR Am J Roentgenol. 1999;173:1279–83.

18. Rankin SC, Saunders AJ, Cook GJ, Scoble JE. Renovascular disease. Clin Radiol. 2000;55:1–12. doi:10.1053/crad.1999.0338.

19. Taylor A, Nally J, Aurell M, Blaufox D, Dondi M, Dubovsky E, et al. Consensus report on ACE inhibitor renography for detecting renovascular hypertension. Radionuclides in Nephrourology Group. Consensus Group on ACEI Renography. J Nucl Med. 1996;37:1876–82.

20. Dondi M, Fanti S, De Fabritiis A, Zuccala A, Gaggi R, Mirelli M, et al. Prognostic value of captopril renal scintigraphy in renovascular hypertension. J Nucl Med. 1992;33:2040–4.

21. Mittal BR, Kumar P, Arora P, Kher V, Singhal MK, Maini A, et al. Role of captopril renography in the diagnosis of renovascular hypertension. Am J Kidney Dis. 1996;28:209–13.

22. Salehi N, Firouzi A, Gholoobi A, Shakerian F, Sanati HR, Ahmadabadi MN, et al. Relationship between distribution of coronary artery lesions and renal artery stenosis in patients undergoing simultaneous coronary and renal angiography. Clin Med Insights Cardiol. 2011;5:35–40. doi:10.4137/CMC.S6819.

23. Schoenberg SO, Rieger J, Weber CH, Michaely HJ, Waggershauser T, Ittrich C, et al. High-spatial-resolution MR angiography of renal arteries with

integrated parallel acquisitions: comparison with digital subtraction angiography and US. Radiology. 2005;235:687–98.

24. Textor SC, Novick AC, Tarazi RC, Klimas V, Vidt DG, Pohl M. Critical perfusion pressure for renal function in patients with bilateral atherosclerotic renal vascular disease. Ann Intern Med. 1985;102:308–14. doi:10.7326/0003-4819-102-3-308.

25. Rosset A, Spadola L, Ratib O. OsiriX: an open-source software for navigating in multidimensional DICOM images. J Digit Imaging. 2004;17:205–16.

26. Wang C, Frimmel H, Persson A, Smedby Ö. An interactive software module for visualizing coronary arteries in CT angiography. Int J Comput Assist Radiol Surg. 2008;3:11–8.

27. Wang C, Smedby Ö. Coronary artery segmentation and skeletonization based on competing fuzzy connectedness tree. Med Image Comput Comput Assist Interv. 2007;10:311–8. doi:10.1007/978-3-540-75757-3_38.

28. Ibáñez L, Schroeder W, Ng L. Segmentation. In: ITK software guide. 2nd ed., updated for ITK v2.4. Clifton Park: Insight Software Consortium; 2005. p. 503–604.

29. Bland JM, Altman DG. Statistical methods for assessing agreement between two methods of clinical measurement. Lancet. 1986;327:307–10.

30. Shrout PE, Fleiss JL. Intraclass correlations: Uses in assessing rater reliability. Psychol Bull. 1979;86:420–8. doi:10.1037/0033-2909.86.2.420.

31. Zhang JM, Luo T, Huo Y, Wan M, Chua T, Tan RS, et al. Area stenosis associated with non-invasive fractional flow reserve obtained from coronary CT images. Conf Proc IEEE Eng Med Biol Soc. 2013;2013:3865–8. doi:10.1109/EMBC.2013.6610388.

32. North American Symptomatic Carotid Endarterectomy Trial Collaborators. Beneficial effect of carotid endarterectomy in symptomatic patients with high-grade carotid stenosis. N Engl J Med. 1991;325:445–53.

33. Schoenberg SO, Bock M, Kallinowski F, Just A. Correlation of hemodynamic impact and morphologic degree of renal artery stenosis in a canine model. J Am Soc Nephrol. 2000;11:2190–8.

34. Talenfeld AD, Schwope RB, Alper HJ, Cohen El, Lookstein RA. MDCT angiography of the renal arteries in patients with atherosclerotic renal artery stenosis: implications for renal artery stenting with distal protection. AJR Am J Roentgenol. 2007;188:1652–8. doi:10.2214/AJR.06.1255.

35. Bourgoignie J, Kurz S, Catanzaro FJ, Serirat P, Perry Jr HM. Renal venous renin in hypertension. Am J Med. 1970;48:332–42.

36. Pedersen EB. New tools in diagnosing renal artery stenosis. Kidney Int. 2000;57:2657–77.

37. Soulez G, Oliva VL, Turpin S, Lambert R, Nicolet V, Therasse E. Imaging of renovascular hypertension: respective values of renal scintigraphy, renal Doppler US, and MR angiography. Radiographics. 2000;20:1355–68.

38. McLean AG, Hilson AJ, Scoble JE, Maher ER, Thakrar DS, Moorhead JF, et al. Screening for renovascular disease with captopril-enhanced renography. Nephrol Dial Transplant. 1992;7:211–5.

7

Coronary artery size and origin imaging in children: a comparative study of MRI and trans-thoracic echocardiography

Tarique Hussain[1,2,3*], Sujeev Mathur[2], Sarah A. Peel[1,2], Israel Valverde[1,2], Karolina Bilska[2], Markus Henningsson[1], Rene M. Botnar[1], John Simpson[1,2] and Gerald F. Greil[1,2,3]

Abstract

Background: The purpose of this study was to see how coronary magnetic resonance angiography (CMRA) compared to echocardiography for the detection of coronary artery origins and to compare CMRA measurements for coronary dimensions in children with published echocardiographic reference values.

Methods: Enrolled patients underwent dual cardiac phase CMRA and echocardiography under the same anesthetic. Echocardiographic measurements of the right coronary artery (RCA), left anterior descending (LAD) and left main (LM) were made. CMRA dimensions were assessed manually at the same points as the echocardiographic measurements. The number of proximal LAD branches imaged was also recorded in order to give an estimate of distal coronary tree visualization.

Results: Fifty patients (24 boys, mean age 4.0 years (range 18 days to 18 years)) underwent dual-phase CMRA. Coronary origins were identified in 47/50 cases for CMRA (remaining 3 were infants aged 3, 9 and 11 months). In comparison, origins were identified in 41/50 cases for echo (remaining were all older children).
CMRA performed better than echocardiography in terms of distal visualization of the coronary tree (median 1 LAD branch vs. median 0; $p = 0.001$).
Bland-Altman plots show poor agreement between echocardiography and CMRA for coronary measurements. CMRA measurements did vary according to cardiac phase (systolic mean 1.90, s.d. 0.05 mm vs. diastolic mean 1.84, s.d. 0.05 mm; $p = 0.002$).

Conclusions: Dual-phase CMRA has an excellent (94 %) success rate for the detection of coronary origins in children. Newborn infants remain challenging and echocardiography remains the accepted imaging modality for this age group. Echocardiographic reference ranges are not applicable to CMRA measurements as agreement was poor between modalities. Future coronary reference values, using any imaging modality, should quote the phase in which it was measured.

Keywords: Child, Infant, Newborn, Adolescent, Magnetic resonance imaging, Echocardiography, Coronary vessels

* Correspondence: tarique@doctors.org.uk
[1]Division of Imaging Sciences, King's College London, NIHR Biomedical
Research Centre at Guy's & St Thomas' NHS Foundation Trust, London, UK
[2]Department of Paediatric Cardiology, Evelina London Children's Hospital,
Guy's & St Thomas' NHS Foundation Trust, Westminster Bridge Road, London,
UK
Full list of author information is available at the end of the article

Background

In infants, it is appreciated that currently, echocardiography is the first line imaging method for delineation of the origin and course of the proximal portion of the coronary arteries [1]. However, echocardiographic imaging becomes progressively more difficult in children and adolescents due to patient size and poor transthoracic ultrasound windows.

Normal values exist for coronary dimensions using echocardiography, [2, 3] but no such references exist for coronary magnetic resonance angiography (CMRA). The difficulty exists in producing normal MRI data is that young children and infants would require sedation or general anesthesia. This information, however, may be gained by cross-referencing MRI and echo data, so that MR dimensions can be validated systematically against echo-derived dimensions. This will be important for clinical settings, such as Kawasaki disease (or coronary allograft vasculopathy), where MRI is used for longitudinal follow up of coronary arteries.

In the setting of aneurysmal coronary segments and larger coronary arteries (>3 mm in adults), it has already been shown that CMRA is very accurate [4]. The purpose here is to be able to develop a reference for coronary dimensions in children to identify whether the segment in question is indeed dilated. This is particularly important for longitudinal follow-up and when echocardiographic windows are poor.

Methods

Institutional Review Board approval was obtained for this study (St. Thomas' research ethics committee reference 07/Q0704/3). The inclusion criterion in this prospective study was any patient undergoing a clinical cardiovascular MRI with 3d-whole heart acquisition under general anesthesia at our institution. Written, informed consent was obtained in each case from the patient (if older than 16 years) or from the legal guardian (if patient was younger). Enrolled patients underwent dual phase whole-heart 3D balanced steady state free precession (b-SSFP) imaging and echocardiography under general anesthesia [5].

MRI

Cardiac MRI was performed using a 1.5 Tesla Achieva clinical MR scanner (Philips Healthcare, Best, NL). The 3d whole heart approach, described by Beerbaum et al. [6] was implemented with noticeable changes. It has been recently demonstrated that dual-phase imaging (end-systole and mid-diastole) can improve coronary imaging by providing the ability to retrospectively select the optimum phase to be used for analysis [7]. Hence this approach was used for this study.

As with standard 3D SSFP sequences, the dual-phase sequence is respiratory-gated and ECG-triggered with a fat saturation pre-pulse to null fat signal and a T_2 pre-pulse to improve the myocardium to blood pool contrast [8]. Imaging was acquired in a sagittal orientation (repetition time (TR) /echo time (TE) = 3.4/1.7 ms, flip angle 90°, 60–120 slices, isotropic resolution of 1–1.5 mm^3, reconstructed resolution 0.5–0.75 mm^3, acquisition window of 40–75 ms). For children 15 kg or less, a two-element coil was used (Flex M or Flex S). For children over 15 kg, a five-element cardiac coil was used. Parallel imaging with a SENSitivity Encoding (SENSE) acceleration factor of 2 in the antero-posterior direction was also used [9]. Trigger delays were set for end-systole and mid-diastole. The cardiac rest periods were assessed with a high temporal resolution, balanced steady-state free precession (SSFP), four-chamber cine (TR = 2.8–3.6 ms, TE = 1.4–1.8 ms, no. of lines acquired per heart beat = 3 to 20, flip angle 60°, 6-mm-thick sections, 240–300 mm field of view, 60–80 phases). These parameters were adjusted accordingly to maintain temporal resolution with minimal interpolation. The dual-phase sequence employs navigators for each cardiac phase with a respiratory gating window of 3 mm. Data is only accepted if both navigators, in any given cardiac cycle, fall within this gating window.

In addition, it has been shown that an automated programme is capable of more accurate definitions of cardiac rest periods than visual inspection [10]. It was therefore hoped that clearer definitions for cardiac rest-periods would produce a similar effect. The mid-diastolic period was taken from cessation of movement of RCA (i.e., pause in visible filling of RV) to the beginning of atrial systole. This stringent definition covers both RCA and LAD diastolic rest periods [11]. The end-systolic period was taken from cessation of movement of the RCA (corresponding to lowest RV volume) to just before the beginning of opening of the tricuspid valve. The acquisition window was set according to the shortest rest period. Coronary dimensions were assessed manually at the same points as the echocardiographic measurements. The number of proximal LAD branches imaged was also recorded in order to give an estimate of distal coronary tree visualization.

Coronary origins were classified as abnormal if both echo & MRI observers agreed, without doubt, that they were abnormal. In the case where modalities disagreed, reference was made either to earlier diagnostic catheterization or to previous surgical notes.

Echocardiography

Comprehensive echocardiographic studies were performed using the Philips IE33 ultrasound system (Philips Inc., Andover, MA, USA). 2-Dimensional echocardiography was performed using age appropriate probes (S5-1, S8-3, S12-4). The highest frequency probe yielding adequate depth penetration was employed. The Washington protocol for coronary dimensions was followed [3]. This protocol was chosen in preference as the measurement process is clearly defined. Images of the proximal coronary arteries (right coronary artery (RCA), left mainstem (LM) and left anterior descending (LAD)) were recorded as digital cines using short axis (in preference but alternatively, modified superiorly-tilted long-axis view for LAD was used). Operator assessment of coronary origins was recorded and stored cines were used to assess coronary dimensions.

Measurements of the RCA, LAD and LM were made from inner edge to inner edge, excluding points of branching [12]. LM was measured at its mid-point and the LAD/ RCA was measured 0.2 to 0.5 mm from its origin [3]. Measurements and imaging were performed by three experienced operators (SM, JS and KB, all with >5 years experience in coronary echocardiography in congenital heart disease).

Current echocardiographic data does not specify the point of the cardiac cycle (systole or diastole) over which measurements should be taken [3]. In addition, practically, it is often difficult to get images in both phases. Therefore, only one measurement was taken for each coronary measurement but it was also recorded as to which phase the measurement was taken, in order to compare it fairly to MRI. The number of proximal LAD branches imaged was also recorded in order to give an estimate of distal coronary tree visualization.

Statistical methods

First, bland-Altman plots were used to assess agreement between MRI and echocardiography for coronary dimensions. Using information gleaned from this analysis, regression analyses were planned in order to describe the relationship between MRI and echocardiographic measurements.

Distal coronary visualization, assessed by number of LAD branches visualized, was compared between modalities using Wilcoxon Signed Ranks test.

A repeated measures analysis of variance models for coronary dimensions was constructed in order to assess if the coronary distensibility in children results in different dimensions according to cardiac phase. A repeated measures model was used in order to account for within-subject and between-subject variability arising from testing multiple segments over two phases in each patient. Assumptions of sphericity were formally tested, and accepted, using Mauchly's test. The Bonferroni correction is used to correct for multiple comparisons.

Statistical analyses were performed on SPSS (version 19) 2010. Variables are described using mean ± standard deviation (s.d.).

Results

Subjects

Fifty children participated in this study prospectively with a mean age of 4 ± 4.4 years (range 18 days to 18 years). This included 24 boys (mean age 4.5 ± 4.6 years) and 26 girls (mean age 3.6 ± 4.3 years; no significant age difference according to sex, $p = 0.46$ by independent samples t-test). Mean weight was 15.5 ± 11.6 kg (range 3.7 to 52 kg) and mean height was 94 ± 29 cm. 48 children underwent imaging for follow-up of congenital heart disease, 1 child for cardiomyopathy and 1 for resolved Kawasaki disease.

Reference values

Bland-Altman plots (Figs. 1, 2 and 3) show a systematic bias between echocardiographic and MRI measurements for all coronary measurements (i.e., as the coronary

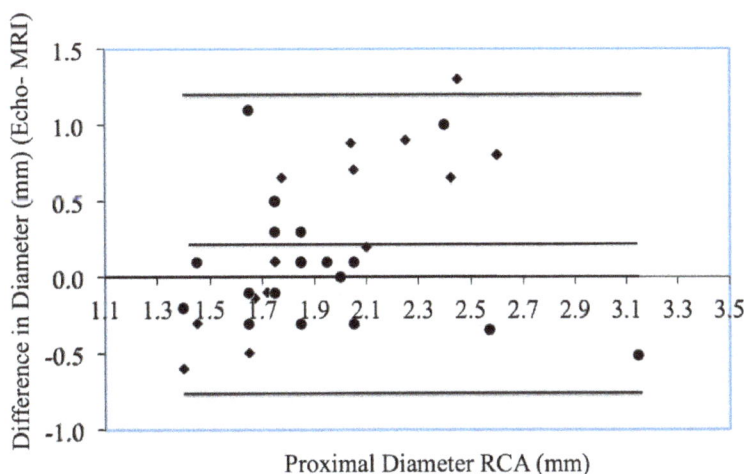

Fig. 1 Bland Altman Mean vs. Difference plots for Echo and MRI RCA measurements. ● Diastolic measurements. ◆ Systolic measurements

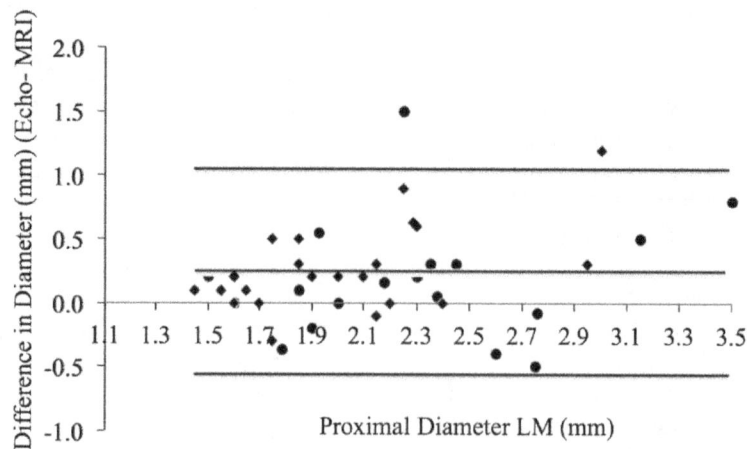

Fig. 2 Bland Altman Mean vs. Difference plots for Echo and MRI LM measurements. ● Diastolic measurements. ♦ Systolic measurements

artery gets larger, the greater the discrepancy between echocardiography and MRI).

However, this may be more usefully summarized by ignoring the segment imaged, removing outliers and pooling data. If this is done we get a simple message: there is indeed a systematic bias for CMRA dimensions between 1 and 2.5 mm. This is demonstrated on the Bland-Altman plot (Fig. 4). More importantly, the accuracy between echo and MRI measurements is not clinically acceptable. The scatter clearly shows that, at dimensions between 1.3 to 2.5 mm, the spread of agreement is more than 0.5 mm at all points. Hence no further analysis was made to describe the correlation (i.e., regression analysis was not felt appropriate due to poor agreement).

CMRA evaluation

Operator certainty regarding the origin of the three main coronary arteries (RCA, LAD and left circumflex (LCx)) was achieved in 47 out of 50 cases for MRI. The three uncertain cases were infant below a year of age (3, 9 and 11 months) and with heart rates >100 bpm. In comparison, certainty was achieved in 41 out of 50 cases for echo. The nine uncertain cases were older patients (mean 4.8 years, range 9 months to 18 years). In two cases, MRI detected abnormalities in coronary origin classified as normal with certainty on echocardiography. These two cases had confirmed abnormalities on surgery. Both were slightly older children (13 months and 8 years age respectively). The 13-month-old child had an anomalous origin of the left circumflex origin from the right coronary artery. The 8-year old child had ventriculo-arterial discordance and had a single coronary artery from left-hand sinus two (Fig. 6).

In total, there were 6 abnormal coronary origins. 5 out of 6 were identified by MRI and the remaining one was classified as unsure. 4 out of 6 were correctly identified on echocardiogram with the remaining two, incorrectly classified as normal as described above. (Sample images: Figs. 5, 6 and 7).

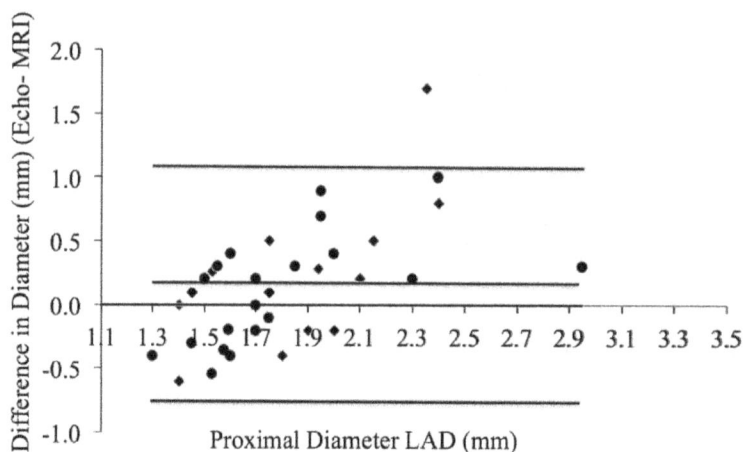

Fig. 3 Bland Altman Mean vs. Difference plots for Echo and MRI LAD measurements. ● Diastolic measurements. ♦ Systolic measurements

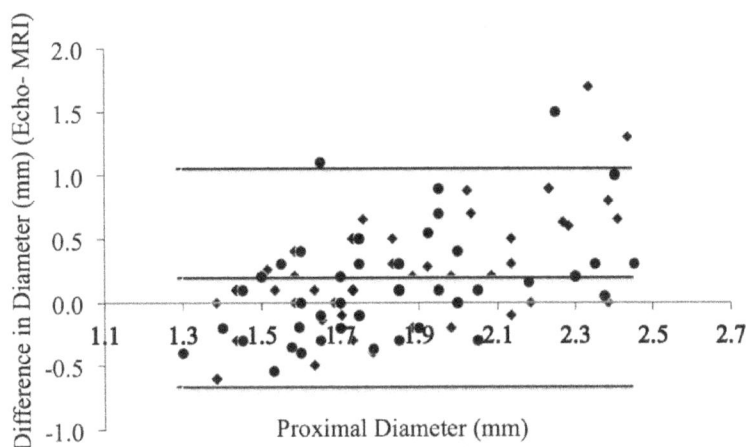

Fig. 4 Bland Altman Mean vs. Difference plots for all Echo and MRI measurements with outliers excluded. ● Diastolic measurements. ◆ Systolic measurements

Overall, CMRA performed better than echocardiography in terms of distal visualization of the coronary tree, as defined by number of proximal LAD branches imaged ($p = 0.001$ by Wilcoxon Signed Ranks test). The median number of LAD branches on MRI was 1 (interquartile range 0 to 2) and on echo was 0 (interquartile range 0 to 1).

CMRA measurements did vary according to cardiac phase. The repeated measures model demonstrates that the systolic coronary dimension (estimated marginal mean 1.90 ± 0.05 mm) is greater than the diastolic measurement (estimated marginal mean 1.84 ± 0.05 mm ($p = 0.002$).

Discussion

This study has important implications for the follow-up of Kawasaki disease in particular. MRI is particularly useful for follow-up of Kawasaki Disease and Coronary Allograft Vasculopathy as anatomic evaluation can be combined with functional evaluation with pharmacological stress testing. Intra- and inter-observer error in coronary measurements for both echocardiography and CMRA have been previously separately investigated and shown to be low for both modalities [3, 7]. However, this

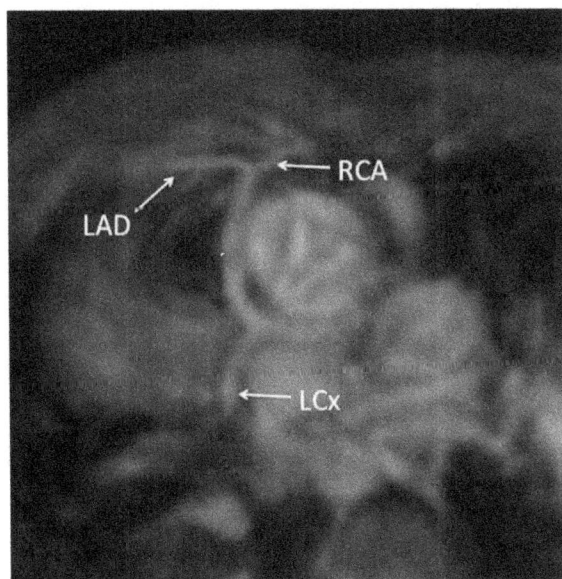

Fig. 5 3-year old girl with Dextrocardia and Tricuspid Atresia. Single Coronary artery imaged with MRA in systole. Echocardiographic data corresponded with MRA findings

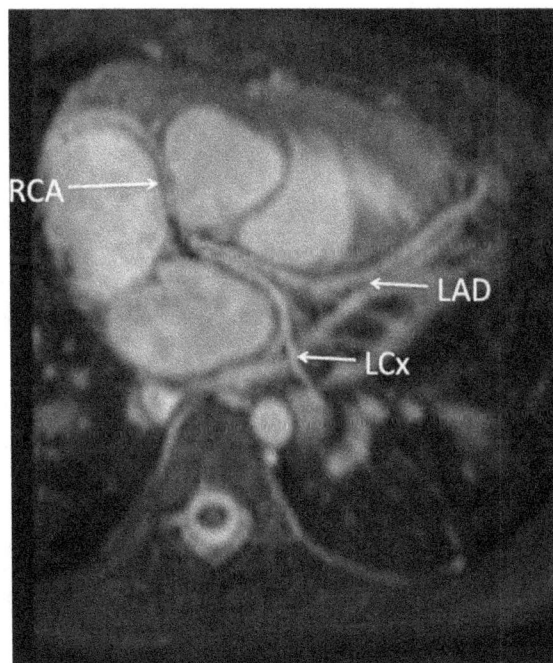

Fig. 6 8-year old boy with ventriculo-arterial discordance showing single coronary artery. Echocardiography was not able to demonstrate this

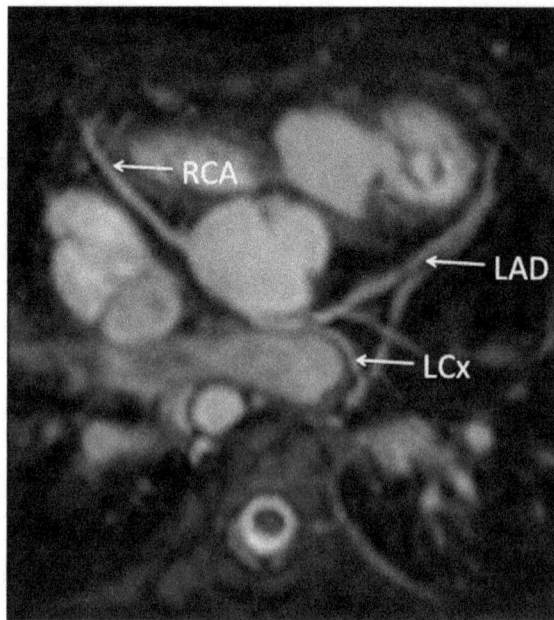

Fig. 7 7-year old girl with repaired pulmonary atresia and ventricular septal defect. RCA arises from posterior non-coronary cusp. Findings were confirmed by echocardiography

study shows poor agreement between techniques. This may be in part, due to the current difficulty achieving sub-millimeter acquired resolution for coronary MRA in small children. The study resolution of 1–1.5 mm^3 acquired (0.5–0.75 mm^3 reconstructed) was chosen in order to give the optimum image quality as further increase in resolution would cause reduction in signal-to-noise ratio and would result in sub-optimal image quality. Improvements in image quality in infants should be the subject of future studies. It is hoped that, in the future, specific normative coronary dimensions for CMRA are available. The difficulty imaging normal volunteers in this age group has precluded this to date. Hence, until such data becomes available, the utility of coronary measurement below 3 mm lies in serial follow-up rather than for normative scoring. In particular, when reporting MRI coronary dimensions, we should not use published z-score values for echocardiography [3]. In the past, clinicians have merely assumed that dimensions were normal on CMRA if they equated to normal published echocardiographic z-scores. This study shows that this assumption is erroneous. One may argue that this result was to be expected because echocardiography relies on high contrast in the vessel wall and low contrast in the lumen, whereas CMRA is the opposite. Although 'black-blood' coronary MRI exists [13] and contrast-enhanced echocardiography exists, the purpose of this study was to evaluate the commonly used clinical echocardiographic and MRI techniques.

In keeping with previous studies, this study shows an excellent (94 %) success rate for CMRA detection of coronary origins in children [7, 14, 15]. Dual-phase imaging may be advantageous as it has been previously shown that image quality of each proximal coronary segment can vary unpredictably within the same patient according to selection of the systolic or diastolic rest period for imaging [7]. Infants with high heart rates remain challenging [14] and echocardiography remains the modality of choice for this age group. Naturally, echocardiography remains the first choice for cardiac imaging in all children due to the ease of application and the acceptability from a child's perspective. Success rates are difficult to report from literature, as the technique is operator dependent with some operators showing excellent accuracy [16–18]. Success rates are even higher in newborn infants [19]. Nevertheless, there remains an important false negative reporting rate, which is difficult to quantify [20]. Given the operator-dependency, any doubt regarding coronary anomaly with potentially malignant course, should have further imaging [16]. Our study also shows that distal coronary tree imaging in children is superior with CMRA in comparison to echocardiography. This is another useful point of note from this study for clinical follow up of coronary disease in children. Multidetector CT angiography has excellent success rates in determining coronary origins and is becoming routinely used clinically to detect coronary stenosis [21, 22]. However, it does involve potentially harmful radiation use in young children.

Unfortunately, coronary distensibility in children has been largely neglected in the published literature [2, 3, 23]. Although an important recognized variable in adults, [24] this factor has been ignored when generating echocardiographic normal values for coronary dimensions in children [2, 3, 23]. The given reference study [3] was chosen specifically as the details regarding how measurements are to be taken are most precise. Even this study neglects to mention whether values are to be taken in systole or diastole. From clinical experience using echocardiography, it is usually difficult to get clear pictures for each segment in both phases and so it is understandable that this point is not labored. However, our data from the dual-phase CMRA measurements shows that dimensions do indeed vary according to phase. Future normal values for coronary dimensions in children should note this finding and provide phase-specific references.

Conclusions

This study shows that echocardiographic reference values should not be applied to CMRA measurements of coronary dimensions. Looking forward, the development of CMRA-specific reference values would be helpful, although such normative data is difficult to acquire in children. Our study confirms the perception that CMRA remains extremely successful in the identification of coronary origins in children but echocardiography remains superior in small infants. Our study also shows that CMRA is superior to echocardiography in the imaging of the distal coronary tree of children. Finally, the study also demonstrates the need to establish heart phase-specific coronary reference ranges.

Competing interests
The authors declare that they have no competing interests.

Authors' contributions
TH, SM, SP, IV, KB, JS, GG: Planning, data acquisition, data analysis and drafting manuscript. MH, RB: Planning, data analysis and drafting manuscript. All authors read and approved the final manuscript.

Acknowledgements
The authors acknowledge financial support from the Department of Health via the National Institute for Health Research (NIHR) comprehensive Biomedical Research Centre award to Guy's & St Thomas' NHS Foundation Trust in partnership with King's College London and King's College Hospital NHS Foundation Trust".
Dr Gerald Greil's department is part of the Centre of Excellence in Medical Engineering is funded by the Wellcome Trust and EPSRC under grant number WT 088641/Z/09/Z".
King's College London is a British Heart Foundation centre of excellence funded by the British Heart Foundation award RE/08/003.

Author details
[1]Division of Imaging Sciences, King's College London, NIHR Biomedical Research Centre at Guy's & St Thomas' NHS Foundation Trust, London, UK. [2]Department of Paediatric Cardiology, Evelina London Children's Hospital, Guy's & St Thomas' NHS Foundation Trust, Westminster Bridge Road, London, UK. [3]Department of Pediatrics, UT Southwestern Medical Center, Children's Medical Center, 1935 Medical District Drive, Dallas, TX, USA.

References
1. Geva T, Kreutzer J. Diagnostic pathways for evaluation of congenital heart disease. In: Crawford MH, DiMarco JP, editors. Cardiology. London: Mosby International; 2001. p. 7–41.
2. McCrindle BW, Li JS, Minich LL, Colan SD, Atz AM, Takahashi M, et al. Coronary artery involvement in children with Kawasaki disease: risk factors from analysis of serial normalized measurements. Circulation. 2007;116(2):174–9.
3. Olivieri L, Arling B, Friberg M, Sable C. Coronary artery Z score regression equations and calculators derived from a large heterogeneous population of children undergoing echocardiography. J Am Soc Echocardiogr. 2009;22(2):159–64.
4. Greil GF, Stuber M, Botnar RM, Kissinger KV, Geva T, Newburger JW, et al. Coronary magnetic resonance angiography in adolescents and young adults with kawasaki disease. Circulation. 2002;105(8):908–11.
5. Uribe S, Hussain T, Valverde I, Tejos C, Irarrazaval P, Fava M, et al. Congenital Heart Disease in Children: Coronary MR Angiography during Systole and Diastole with Dual Cardiac Phase Whole-Heart Imaging. Radiology. 2011;260(1):232–40.
6. Beerbaum P, Sarikouch S, Laser KT, Greil G, Burchert W, Korperich H. Coronary anomalies assessed by whole-heart isotropic 3D magnetic resonance imaging for cardiac morphology in congenital heart disease. J Magn Reson Imaging. 2009;29(2):320–7.
7. Hussain T, Lossnitzer D, Bellsham-Revell H, Valverde I, Beerbaum P, Razavi R, et al. Three-dimensional dual-phase whole-heart MR imaging: clinical implications for congenital heart disease. Radiology. 2012;263(2):547–554.
8. Uribe S, Tangchaoren T, Parish V, Wolf I, Razavi R, Greil G, et al. Volumetric Cardiac Quantification by Using 3D Dual-Phase Whole-Heart MR Imaging. Radiology. 2008;248(2):606–14.
9. Pruessmann KP, Weiger M, Scheidegger MB, Boesiger P. SENSE: sensitivity encoding for fast MRI. Magn Reson Med. 1999;42(5):952–62.
10. Ustun A, Desai M, Abd-Elmoniem KZ, Schar M, Stuber M. Automated identification of minimal myocardial motion for improved image quality on MR angiography at 3 T. AJR Am J Roentgenol. 2007;188(3):W283–90.
11. Kim WY, Stuber M, Kissinger KV, Andersen NT, Manning WJ, Botnar RM. Impact of bulk cardiac motion on right coronary MR angiography and vessel wall imaging. J Magn Reson Imaging. 2001;14(4):383–90.
12. Newburger JW, Takahashi M, Gerber MA, Gewitz MH, Tani LY, Burns JC, et al. Diagnosis, treatment, and long-term management of Kawasaki disease: a statement for health professionals from the Committee on Rheumatic Fever, Endocarditis and Kawasaki Disease, Council on Cardiovascular Disease in the Young. Am Heart Assoc Circ. 2004;110(17):2747–71.
13. Botnar RM, Kim WY, Bornert P, Stuber M, Spuentrup E, Manning WJ. 3D coronary vessel wall imaging utilizing a local inversion technique with spiral image acquisition. Magn Reson Med. 2001;46(5):848–54.
14. Tangcharoen T, Bell A, Hegde S, Hussain T, Beerbaum P, Schaeffter T, et al. Detection of coronary artery anomalies in infants and young children with congenital heart disease by using MR imaging. Radiology. 2011;259(1):240–7.
15. Su JT, Chung T, Muthupillai R, Pignatelli RH, Kung GC, Diaz LK, et al. Usefulness of real-time navigator magnetic resonance imaging for evaluating coronary artery origins in pediatric patients. Am J Cardiol. 2005;95(5):679–82.
16. Attili A, Hensley AK, Jones FD, Grabham J, DiSessa TG. Echocardiography and coronary CT angiography imaging of variations in coronary anatomy and coronary abnormalities in athletic children: detection of coronary abnormalities that create a risk for sudden death. Echocardiography. 2013;30(2):225–33.
17. Frommelt PC, Berger S, Pelech AN, Bergstrom S, Williamson JG. Prospective identification of anomalous origin of left coronary artery from the right sinus of valsalva using transthoracic echocardiography: importance of color Doppler flow mapping. Pediatr Cardiol. 2001;22(4):327–32.
18. Frommelt PC, Friedberg DZ, Frommelt MA, Williamson JG. Anomalous origin of the right coronary artery from the left sinus of valsalva: transthoracic echocardiographic diagnosis. J Am Soc Echocardiogr. 1999;12(3):221–4.
19. Pasquini L, Sanders SP, Parness IA, Wernovsky G, Mayer Jr JE, Van der Velde ME, et al. Coronary echocardiography in 406 patients with d-loop transposition of the great arteries. J Am Coll Cardiol. 1994;24(3):763–8.
20. Pelliccia A, Spataro A, Maron BJ. Prospective echocardiographic screening for coronary artery anomalies in 1,360 elite competitive athletes. Am J Cardiol. 1993;72(12):978–9.
21. Vanhoenacker PK, Heijenbrok-Kal MH, Van Heste R, Decramer I, Van Hoe LR, Wijns W, et al. Diagnostic performance of multidetector CT angiography for assessment of coronary artery disease: meta-analysis. Radiology. 2007;244(2):419–28.
22. Ghadri JR, Kazakauskaite E, Braunschweig S, Burger IA, Frank M, Fiechter M, et al. Congenital coronary anomalies detected by coronary computed tomography compared to invasive coronary angiography. BMC Cardiovasc Disord. 2014;14:81.
23. Dallaire F, Dahdah N. New equations and a critical appraisal of coronary artery Z scores in healthy children. J Am Soc Echocardiogr. 2011;24(1):60–74.
24. Lin K, Lloyd-Jones DM, Liu Y, Bi X, Li D, Carr JC. Noninvasive Evaluation of Coronary Distensibility in Older Adults: A Feasibility Study with MR Angiography. Radiology. 2011;261(3):771–8.

8

Pelvic retroperitoneal pleomorphic hyalinizing angiectatic tumor (PHAT) of soft tissue

Zhi-gang Chu[1], Meng-qi Liu[1], Zhi-yu Zhu[2], Fa-jin Lv[1] and Yu Ouyang[1*]

Abstract

Background: Pleomorphic hyalinizing angiectatic tumor (PHAT) is a rare soft tissue tumor of low malignant potential, which most often arises in the lower extremities. Lesions occurred in other anatomic locations have been rarely reported. Moreover, their imaging features have not been well discussed. Here we report a case of PHAT arising primarily in the pelvic retroperitoneum. To our knowledge, this is the first radiological description for retroperitoneum PHAT.

Case presentation: A 26-year-old female was referred to our hospital for evaluation of a pelvic mass incidentally noted in routine pre-pregnancy ultrasonography examination. Magnetic resonance imaging (MRI) and computed tomography (CT) scan revealed an irregular mass with clear boundary in the pelvic retroperitoneum. Its signal intensity or density was inhomogeneous. On MRI images, it mainly showed isointense and slight hypointense on T1 weighted image and isointense and hyperintense on T2 weighted image. On contrast-enhanced images, it showed marked but heterogenous enhancement. With the delay time increasing, the enhanced area in the lesion increased but the CT value decreased. Dilated vessels and hemorrhage were detected in the tumor. With patience and careful separation, it was completely excised with great amount of bleeding during operation. Pathological and immunohistochemistry analysis confirmed the diagnosis of PHAT of the soft parts. We found no evidence of recurrence 18 months after operation.

Conclusion: We present an extremely rare case of PHAT arising primarily in the pelvic retroperitoneum. To our knowledge, this is the first radiological description for retroperitoneum PHAT. The provided information is useful for summarizing the characteristics of this kind of tumor. It should be included in the differential diagnosis of a well-defined, inhomogenously enhanced hypervascular soft-tissue mass in pelvic cavity.

Keywords: Pleomorphic hyalinizing angiectatic tumor, Computed tomography, Magnetic resonance imaging

Background

Pleomorphic hyalinizing angiectatic tumor (PHAT) of soft parts is a rare tumor described first in 1996 by Smith et al. [1]. To date, different cases have been reported and which usually located at the lower extremities of adults. Other rarer sites involved were forearm, shoulder, axilla, buttock and buccal mucosa [2]. As this lesion in the present study occurred in an extremely rare location, it is necessary to further enrich the relevant information for diagnosing and managing. In this case,

we introduce a large pathologically confirmed PHAT in pelvic retroperitoneum with focus on describing its imaging features. To our knowledge, this was the first reported case of PHAT which occurred in this site and had comprehensive radiological data.

Case presentation

A 26-year-old female was referred to our hospital for evaluation of a pelvic mass incidentally noted in routine pre-pregnancy ultrasonography examination. The lesion did not cause any discomfort, and the patient did not report any symptom. She and her family members had not experienced such lesion in the past. General examination was unremarkable and laboratory findings were normal.

* Correspondence: cyscitg@163.com
[1]Department of Radiology, The First Affiliated Hospital of Chongqing Medical University, 1# Youyi street, Chongqing 400016, China
Full list of author information is available at the end of the article

Magnetic resonance imaging (MRI) of the pelvic cavity was performed. MRI examination revealed an irregular mass with clear boundary in the pelvic retroperitoneum (Fig. 1). It located in the front of sacrum and behind uterus and rectum. The oppression and displacement of neighbor organs were found. No direct invasion was detected. This mass measured 9.4 cm (anterior-posterior), 9.1 cm (transverse), and 9.5 cm (craniocaudal). The signal intensity of this lesion was inhomogeneous. It mainly showed isointense and slight hypointense on T1 weighted image and isointense and hyperintense on T2 weighted image. On contrast-enhanced images, it showed significant but heterogenous enhancement. The left and lower part of the mass showed some areas with hyperintense on T1 weighted image and hypointense on T2 weighted image. On contrast-enhanced images, it showed no enhancement. This abnormal signal indicated the presence of hemorrhage within the tumor. In addition, flow-void sign was identified at the lesion core and margin. The uterus, bilateral ovaries and rectum had no abnormalities.

Subsequently, computed tomography (CT) examination was performed for further understanding this lesion and its surroundings, especially the adjacent vessels. Pre-contrast CT scan demonstrated a well-defined, irregular soft tissue mass in the same location showed on MRI (Fig. 2). The internal density was slightly inhomogenous, with CT values ranging from 34 to 69 HU. The left and lower parts of the mass demonstrated higher density with CT values ranging from 51 to 69 HU. No calcification was identified. On contrast-enhanced CT images, it showed marked but heterogenous enhancement during arterial phase, with a maximum CT value of 228 HU, which was slightly lower than that of the adjacent vessels (CT value: 284 HU). Dilated feeding arteries and drainage veins showed clearly in the mass core and margin. The enhanced area increased but the CT value decreased in the following phases. However, areas with higher density showed on plain CT scan had no obvious enhancement. This manifestation also indicated there was hemorrhage in the mass. In the peripheral parts around hemorrhage, some irregular areas without obvious enhancement were also detected. No other masses or abnormalities were found in abdomen. No enlarged lymph nodes were detected around the mass.

It could be confirmed this mass with abundant blood supply did not arise in the organs in pelvic cavity according to the imaging examinations. Then, the lesion was radically excised. During surgery, the mass was

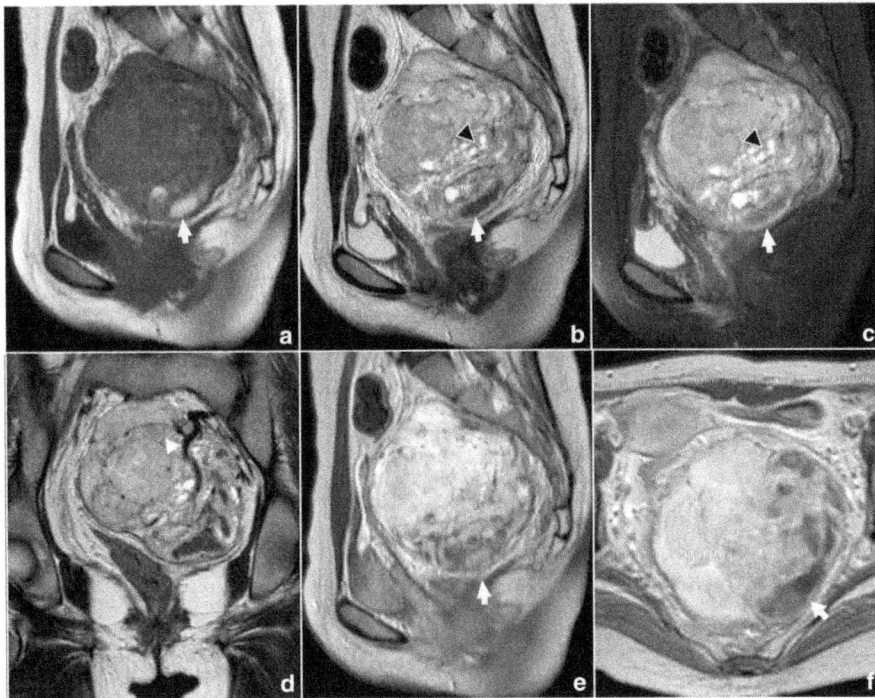

Fig. 1 MRI examination of the pelvic cavity. Sagittal T1-weighted image (**a**) shows a well-defined lobulated mass with isointense and slight hypointense in the pelvic retroperitoneum. The lower part of the mass shows some areas with hyperintense (arrow). Sagittal T2-weighted image (**b**) and T2-weighted image with fat saturation (**c**) show the mass with inhomogeneous isointense and hyperintense. Cystic degeneration could be detected in the inner part (arrowhead). The lower part of the mass showed some areas with hypointense (arrow). Coronal T2-weighted image (**d**) shows large vessels with flow-void sign (arrowhead). Post-contrast T1-weighted images (**e-f**) show the mass with intense heterogeneous enhancement. The lower part with hyperintense on T1-weighted image and hypointense on T2-weighted image shows no significant enhancement (arrow)

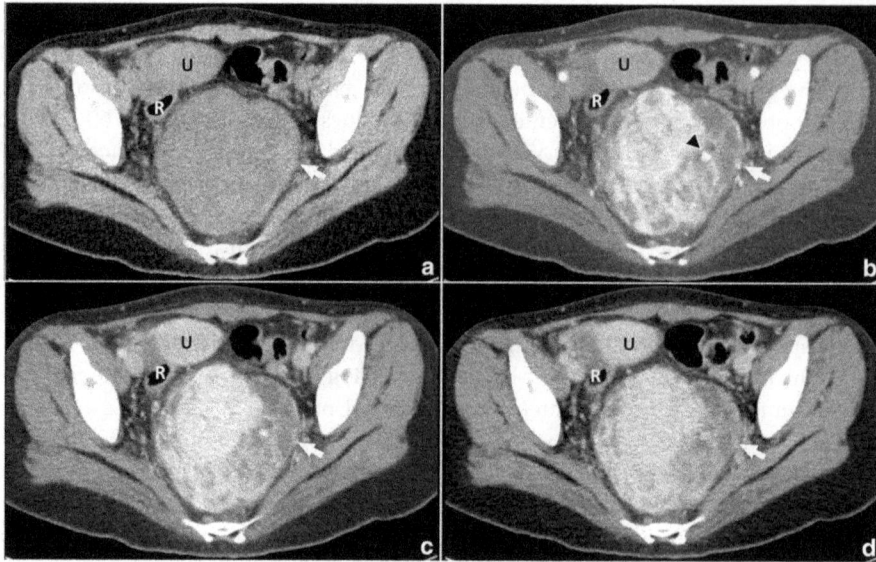

Fig. 2 CT examination of the pelvic cavity. Plain CT scan (**a**) shows a well-defined mass with slightly inhomogenous density in the pelvic retroperitoneum. The left part of the mass has higher density (arrow). On contrast-enhanced CT images (**b**), it shows marked but heterogenous enhancement during arterial phase. Dilated feeding artery shows clearly in the mass (arrow). The enhanced area increases but the CT value decreases in the following phases (**c-d**). Areas with higher density showed on plain CT scan has no obvious enhancement (arrow). Some irregular area without obvious enhancement in the inner part is also detected. U: uterus, R: rectum

found behind the posterior pelvic peritoneum. It is very irregular and tightly adhered to the adjacent tissue. No invasion was detected. There were many vessels in the surface of tumor. With patience and careful separation, it was completely excised with great amount of bleeding during operation. The cut surface was grayish-white in color and necrosis and blood clots were seen in its inner part. It showed solid tissue with a somewhat crisp texture. The histopathology findings showed clusters of dilated thin-walled vessels prominent hyalinization of the vessel walls, and a perivascular and intercellular ground substance. Pleomorphic tumor cells were distributed among these dilated vessels. The mitotic counts was 3/10 HPF. Hemorrhage was also detected. Immunohistochemistry revealed that the tumor cells were positive for vimentin, cluster of differentiation (CD) CD34, CD99, CD117 (focal), and B-cell lymphoma 2 (BCL-2), whereas S-100 protein, CD56, smooth muscle actin (SMA), Desmin, DOG-1, ALK-1 and actin was negative (Fig. 3). The Ki-67 labeling index was 5 %. The final diagnosis was pleomorphic hyalinizing angiectatic tumor (PHAT) of the soft parts.

The postoperative period was uneventful. In the 18 months since the operation, the patient has continued to have no occurrence.

Discussion

Among the reported cases of PHAT in the English language literatures, the patients' sex and age had no significant tendency [3]. A majority of tumors were located in the subcutaneous tissue, mainly in extremities [3–6]. Patients usually had no significant symptoms except showing a local, slowly growing mass. The disease time course and size of tumors varied significantly, which were closely related to their locations [4]. After operation, the local recurrence was relatively common [3, 4], but distal metastasis had not been described. In this study, the mass located in pelvic retroperitoneal space, which is a deep location consisted of loosened tissue. In addition, it did not cause any obvious symptom. Thus, this lesion was very large when it was accidentally discovered.

The CT and MRI manifestations of PHAT arising in neck and extremities have been reported previously [6–8]. However, radiological features of this kind of tumor were still not well understood. It is necessary to enrich the relevant knowledge for its diagnosis and management. We found the image findings of this case reported here had some features. Plain CT and MRI scan showed it was a well-defined mass with inhomogenous dense or signal. Previously reported cases occurred in the neck or renal hilum also had clear boundary [7, 9]. However, some cases arising in extremities were ill-defined [6]. On contrast-enhanced images, this tumor markedly but heterogenously enhanced and many dilated vessels could be detected in it. These manifestations were also illustrated in the previous reported cases [6, 7], which could be seen as the common features of PHAT. Regarding the mass with dilated vessels, preoperative embolization is helpful for reducing intraoperative bleeding and increasing cut rate and safety of

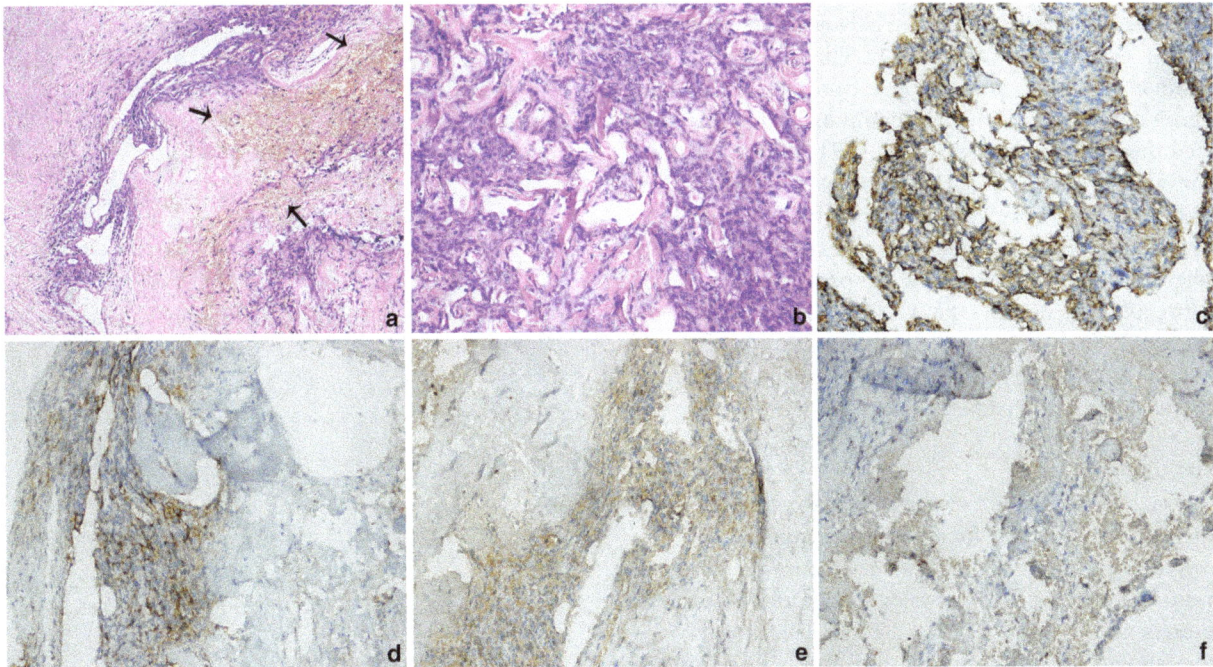

Fig. 3 Hematoxylin and eosin stain (**a-b**) clusters of dilated thin-walled vessels. Pleomorphic tumor cells were distributed among these dilated vessels (A: original magnification, ×100, B: original magnification, ×200). Patchy hemorrhage is detected (arrows). Immunohistochemistry shows positive reactivity for CD34 (**c**), CD99 (**d**), CD117 (**e**) and vimentin (**f**) in the tumor cells (original magnification, ×200)

operation. In addition, hemorrhage in this mass showed on CT and MRI was confirmed by operation and pathological examination. This finding has been reported in previous cases. We suspect it is related to the abundant blood supply and size of the lesion [5, 10]. The larger one might be more prone to have hemorrhage. Beside areas with necrosis and hemorrhage, some irregular areas without obvious enhancement were also detected. Pathologically, it was confirmed to be the prominent hyalinization area of vessel wall and the perivascular ground substance. In summary, the imaging features could well reflect its pathological nature.

Previously reported shapes of masses were usually lobulated, round or oval [3, 4, 11–13]. This large tumor reported here was lobulated. Generally, most of the PHATs were non-encapsulated and incorporated the surrounding normal tissue into the tumor tissue [3, 6]. A few cases had a thin and complete capsule, which manifested smooth and clear boundaries. Though the present case had smooth boundaries, no capsule was detected in operation. In contrast, it tightly adhered to the adjacent tissue. The possible reason was that retroperitoneal fat around the lesion made it showing distinct borders. However, fat space was deficiency among the muscles in the extremities. This tumor has potential for local recurrence. Thus, wide local excision and close follow up are the best approaches for management.

PHAT requires a differential diagnosis with other vascular or hypervascular masses, which includes solitary fibrous tumor (SFT), paraganglioma and gastrointestinal stromal tumor (GIST). SFTs in pelvic cavity appear as well-defined masses with intense heterogeneous enhancement that persists on delayed phase images. Necrosis, hemorrhage, or cystic change may be seen [14]. Paraganglioma appears as a well-defined hypervascular mass in the pelvic retroperitoneum along the course of the common iliac vessels. These tumors may be heterogeneous with foci of calcification. At MR imaging, it appears as areas of low T1 and high T2 signal intensity and shows significant enhancement [15]. Primary pelvic retroperitoneal GIST is extremely rare. They appear as large, hypervascular enhancing masses that frequently harbor areas of necrosis, hemorrhage, or cystic degeneration [16]. The signal of paraganglioma is significantly different from that of PHAT. PHAT usually has intense arterial enhancement and its degree of enhancement is higher than that of SFT and GIST. In addition, hypervascular alveolar soft part sarcoma (ASPS) should also be considered as a differential diagnosis. On contrast-enhanced images, ASPS and PHAT have similar manifestations, while the former usually shows high signal on T1 and T2 weighted images [17–19].

Immunohistochemically, the PHAT is positive for CD34, vimentin, CD99, and VEGF but negative for S-100 protein [1]. The present study showed the similar results. However, these findings are not specific for its diagnosis. Positive findings of CD34 and vimentin only indicate a mesenchymal tumor. The negative S-100 protein excludes a schwannoma from the differential diagnosis, which is the most common lesion that can be confused with this entity [9]. SFT shows a similar immunoprofile to PHAT, both express vimentin, CD34, and CD99 [20]. However, the histopathological findings of PHAT are obviously different from those of SFT [21]. Malignant fibrous histiocytomas can occasionally be CD34 positive but are negative for CD99 [9]. In addition, the negative CD56, SMA, Desmin, DOG-1, ALK-1 and actin in PHAT is distinguishable from neurogenic or myogenic tumors and GIST on pathology.

Conclusion

In conclusion, to the best of our knowledge, this is the first radiological description for retroperitoneum PHAT. This newly recognized, rare neoplasm has some imaging features corresponding to its pathological nature. Although its locations and imaging features are variable, the provided information is useful for summarizing the characteristics of this kind of tumor. It should be included in the differential diagnosis of a well-defined, inhomogeneously enhanced hypervascular soft-tissue mass in the pelvic cavity.

Consent

We pledged to abide by the declaration of Helsinki (2000 EDITION) in accordance with the relevant medical research rules of China in the study. IRB at The Affiliated Hospital of Chongqing Medical University approved this study.

Abbreviations
PHAT: pleomorphic hyalinizing angiectatic tumor; MRI: magnetic resonance imaging; CT: computed tomography; SFT: solitary fibrous tumor; GIST: gastrointestinal stromal tumor; ASPS: alveolar soft part sarcoma.

Competing interests
The authors declare that they have no competing interests.

Authors' contributions
CZG, ZZY, LMQ and LFJ wrote the paper. CZG and OY assessed the imaging study. All authors read and approved the final manuscript.

Authors' information
Ouyang Y and Lv FJ are professors of radiology. Chu ZG, Zhu ZY, and Liu MQ are lecturers.

Acknowledgements
This work was supported by the national key clinical specialist construction programs of China ([2013]544).

Author details
[1]Department of Radiology, The First Affiliated Hospital of Chongqing Medical University, 1# Youyi street, Chongqing 400016, China. [2]Department of Stomatology, The First Affiliated Hospital of Chongqing Medical University, 1# Youyi street, Chongqing 400016, China.

References
1. Smith ME, Fisher C, Weiss SW. Pleomorphic hyaliniz-ing angiectatic tumor of soft parts. A low-grade neoplasm resembling neurilemoma. Am J Surg Pathol. 1996;20(1):21–9.
2. Lee JC, Jiang XY, Karpinski RH, Moore ED. Pleo-morphic hyalinizing angiectatic tumor of soft parts. Surgery. 2005;137(1):119–21.
3. Ke Q, Erbolat, Zhang HY, Bu H, Li S, Shi DN, et al. Clinicopathologic features of pleomorphic hyalinizing angiectatic tumor of soft parts. Chin Med J. 2007; 120(10):876–81.
4. Folpe AL, Weiss SW. Pleomorphic hyalinizing angiectatic tumor analysis of 41 cases supporting evolution from a distinctive precursor lesion. Am J Surg Pathol. 2004;28(11):1417–25.
5. Parameshwarappa S, Rodrigues G, Nagpal N, Rao L. Pleomorphic hyalinizing angiectatic tumor of soft parts involving the upper limb. Indian J Surg. 2010;72(3):263–4.
6. Subhawong TK, Subhawong AP, Montgomery EA, Fayad LM. Pleomorphic hyalinizing angiectatic tumor: imaging findings. Skeletal Radiol. 2012;41(12): 1621–6.
7. Kuang P. CT findings of pleomorphic hyalinizing angiectatic tumor (PHAT) of soft parts of the neck. Jpn J Radiol. 2013;31(3):204–7.
8. Suzuki K, Yasuda T, Hori T, Oya T, Watanabe K, Kanamori M, et al. Pleomorphic hyalinizing angiectatic tumor arising in the thigh: A case report. Oncol Lett. 2014;7(4):1249–52.
9. Idrees MT, Kieffer T, Badve S. Pleomorphic hyalinizing angiectatic tumor of renal hilum. Ann Diagn Pathol. 2012;16(6):489–93.
10. Peng HC, Huang MT, Chen DJ, Leung TK, Chu JS. Pleomorphic hyalinizing angiectatic tumor of soft parts. J Formos Med Assoc. 2010;109(8):616–20.
11. Matsumoto K, Yamamoto T. Pleomorphic hyalinizing angiectatic tumor of soft parts: a case report and literature review. Pathol Int. 2002;52(10):664–8.
12. Fujirawa M, Yuba Y, Wada A, Ozawa T, Tanaka T. Pleomorphic hyalinizing angiectatic tumor of soft parts: report of a case and review of the literature. J Dermatol. 2004;31(5):419–23.
13. Tallarigo F, Squillaci S, Putrino I, Zizzi N, Bisceglia M. Pleomorphic hyalinizing angiectatic tumor of the male breast: a heretofore unreported occurrence. Pathol Res Pract. 2009;205(1):69–73.
14. Shanbhogue AK, Fasih N, Macdonald DB, Sheikh AM, Menias CO, Prasad SR. Uncommon primary pelvic retroperitoneal masses in adults: a pattern-based imaging approach. Radiographics. 2012;32(3):795–817.
15. Qiao HS, Feng XL, Yong L, Yong Z, Lian ZJ, Ling LB. The MRI of extraadrenal pheochromocytoma in the abdominal cavity. Eur J Radiol. 2007;62(3):335–41.
16. Reith JD, Goldblum JR, Lyles RH, Weiss SW. Extragastrointestinal (soft tissue) stromal tumors: an analysis of 48 cases with emphasis on histologic predictors of outcome. Mod Pathol. 2000;13(5):577–85.
17. Suh JS, Cho J, Lee SH, Shin KH, Yang WI, Lee JH, et al. Alveolar soft part sarcoma: MR and angiographic findings. Skeletal Radiol. 2000;29(12):680–9.
18. Castillo M, Lee YY, Yamasaki S. Inframtemporal alveolar soft part sarcoma: CT, MRI and angiographic findings. Neuroradiology. 1992;34(5):367–9.
19. Iwamoto Y, Morimoto N, Chuman H, Shinohara N, Sugioka Y. The role of MR imaging in the diagnosis of alveolar soft part sarcoma: a report of 10 cases. Skeletal Radiol. 1995;24(4):267–70.
20. Shidham VB, Chivukula M, Gupta D, Rao RN, Komorowski R. Immunohistochemical comparison of gastrointestinal stromal tumor and solitary fibrous tumor. Arch Pathol Lab Med. 2002;126(10):1189–92.
21. Cox DP, Daniels T, Jordan RC. Solitary fibrous tumor of the head and neck. Oral Surg Oral Med Oral Pathol Oral Radiol Endod. 2010;110(1):79–84.

9

3D rotational fluoroscopy for intraoperative clip control in patients with intracranial aneurysms – assessment of feasibility and image quality

Thomas Westermaier[1*], Thomas Linsenmann[1], György A. Homola[2], Mario Loehr[1], Christian Stetter[1], Nadine Willner[1], Ralf-Ingo Ernestus[1], Laszlo Solymosi[2] and Giles H. Vince[3]

Abstract

Background: Mobile 3D fluoroscopes have become increasingly available in neurosurgical operating rooms. In this series, the image quality and value of intraoperative 3D fluoroscopy with intravenous contrast agent for the evaluation of aneurysm occlusion and vessel patency after clip placement was assessed in patients who underwent surgery for intracranial aneurysms.

Materials and methods: Twelve patients were included in this retrospective analysis. Prior to surgery, a 360° rotational fluoroscopy scan was performed without contrast agent followed by another scan with 50 ml of intravenous iodine contrast agent. The image files of both scans were transferred to an Apple PowerMac® workstation, subtracted and reconstructed using OsiriX® free software. The procedure was repeated after clip placement. Both image sets were compared for assessment of aneurysm occlusion and vessel patency.

Results: Image acquisition and contrast administration caused no adverse effects. Image quality was sufficient to follow the patency of the vessels distal to the clip. Metal artifacts reduce the assessability of the immediate vicinity of the clip. Precise image subtraction and post-processing can reduce metal artifacts and make the clip-site assessable and depict larger neck-remnants.

Conclusion: This technique quickly supplies images at adequate quality to evaluate distal vessel patency after aneurysm clipping. Significant aneurysm remnants may be depicted as well. As it does not require visual control of all vessels that are supposed to be evaluated intraoperatively, this technique may be complementary to other intraoperative tools like indocyanine green videoangiography and micro-Doppler, especially for the assessment of larger aneurysms. At the momentary state of this technology, it cannot replace postoperative conventional angiography. However, 3D fluoroscopy and image post-processing are young technologies. Further technical developments are likely to result in improved image quality.

Keywords: Aneurysm surgery, Clip control, Intraoperative, Angiography, Vessel patency, 3D fluoroscopy, Contrast, Image quality, Post-processing

* Correspondence: Westermaie_T@ukw.de
[1]Department of Neurosurgery, University of Wuerzburg, Josef-Schneider-Str. 11, 97080 Wuerzburg, Germany
Full list of author information is available at the end of the article

Introduction

Cerebral angiography is the standard procedure for the diagnosis of cerebrovascular lesions [1, 2]. During surgery of intracranial aneurysms micro-Doppler and indocyanin green videoangiography (ICG-VA) are widely used to assess the occlusion of the aneurysm and patency of distal vessels [3, 4]. These techniques are easy and uncomplicated to use. However, a considerable disadvantage of both of these techniques is that for intraoperative assessment the vessels have to be accessible and visible. As a result, the approach and the operative manipulation have to be tailored to visualise the parent vessel, the aneurysm and the departing vessels after placement of a clip. Particularly in large aneurysms, this may result in more manipulation than otherwise necessary to access the aneurysm base and neck. Intraoperative angiography (IA), in turn, does not require this kind of wide exposition. However, it is more time-consuming and requires the positioning of an angiography catheter. We previously reported about the imaging of intracranial aneurysms before placement of an aneurysm clip [5] and the immediate use of this technique in the case of emergency in a patient suffering from intracerebral hemorrhage originating from a ruptured intracranial aneurysm [6]. This series evaluated if image acquisition by intraoperative 3D fluoroscopy with intravenous contrast agent combined with conventional post-processing software is, in principle, possible and supplies appropriate images for clip control after microsurgical clipping.

Materials and methods

This article is the report of a retrospective analysis of intraoperative 3D fluoroscopic angiography in a series of 12 patients with intracranial aneurysms for the assessment of distal vessel patency and clip control after placement of an aneurysm clip. Prior to aneurysm surgery, the patients were offered intraoperative 3D fluoroscopic angiography with the explicit information that the primary target of the procedure was the assessment of distal vessel patency after placement of the clip. They were distinctly informed about the potential risks of the administration of an iodine contrast agent and about the radiation exposure. All patients had given informed consent to the procedure and the possible publication of the results in an anonymized form. The production of data, analysis and publication were approved by the ethics committee of the medical faculty of the Julius-Maximilians-University Wuerzburg, Germany (Reference 268/13).

Inclusion criteria

Patients met the criteria for intraoperative 3D rotational fluoroscopic angiography if they had an intracranial aneurysm, were over 18 years of age, and if microsurgical clipping of the aneurysm was indicated. Exclusion

criteria were a history of hyperthyroidism, an allergy against contrast agent, or serum creatinine concentrations over 100 μmol/l (1.2 mg/100 ml). 12 patients were included in this analysis. Aneurysm details and assessibility before and after clip placement are listed in Table 1.

Patient positioning and image acquisition

All patients were under general anesthesia and had received a central venous catheter in the right jugular vein for infusions of fluid, medication and contrast agent prior to the surgical procedures. Arterial blood pressure was continuously monitored via an arterial line in the left radial artery. All patients of the present series were placed in a supine position with their head fixed in a carbon Mayfield clamp. Prior to surgery, baseline imaging was performed as follows: Positioning of the 3D fluoroscope (O-arm®, Medtronic GmbH, Meerbusch, Germany) was verified by biplanar fluoroscopy. Subsequently, a 360° rotational native fluoroscopy scan was performed. For image acquisition, the "high definition mode" of the O-arm® (digital flat panel detector 40 × 30 cm, camera resolution 2000 × 1500, reconstruction matrix 512 × 512 × 192) was applied requiring an image acquisition time of 24 s for the 360° gantry rotation followed by a reconstruction time of 24 s. Thereafter, a second, contrast-enhanced scan with identical fluoroscopy parameters was performed using 50 ml of iodine contrast agent (Imeron® 350, Bracco Imaging, Konstanz, Germany). During the second scan, 50 ml of contrast agent were injected manually via the central venous line over 25 s. To obtain selective contrast filling of the arterial phase, the 360° fluoroscopy scan was started with a delay of 12 s after the beginning of contrast injection. After placement of the clips, all metallic surgical devices and spatula that were potential causes of artifacts were removed and the imaging procedure was repeated. The image files (DICOM data) were transferred from the O-Arm® to an Apple Power Mac® workstation and post-processed using OsiriX® imaging free software (OsiriX 4.0, 32-bit version).

Post-processing of DICOM data

Native and contrast-enhanced data sets were subtracted using OsiriX® software. From the subtracted data set, a reconstruction was produced (Volume Rendering Mode). Bony structures were virtually removed and brightness and intensity modified in order to selectively demonstrate the contrasted cerebral vessels.

Evaluation of images

The images before and after placement of the clips were assessed for visibility of the aneurysms, accessibility of distal vessel patency, and complete aneurysm occlusion

Table 1 Aneurysm locations and visibility by intraoperative 3D fluoroscopy before and after clipping. Vessel patency was well assessable in the majority of cases after clip placement. Complete aneurysm occlusion, however, was not reliably assessable in most patients. In patient 11, a neck remnant of the MCA aneurysm and clip displacement from the ICA aneurysm were confirmed by DSA. (Acom = anterior communicating artery, Pcom = posterior communicating artery, MCA = middle cerebral artery, ICA = internal carotid artery, A. = artery, SAH = subarachnoid hemorrhage)

Patient number	Aneurysm (size)	Preoperative visibility	Assessment of vessel patentcy	Assessment of aneurysm/neck remnant
1	Acom, coiled (4 mm remnant), SAH	(+) coil artifact	+	(+) no remnant
	Pericallosal A. (3 mm), incidental	+	not treated	not treated
2	Right Pcom (7 mm), incidental	++	++	+ mild carotid stenosis
3	Acom (14 mm), incidental	++	+	-
4	Acom (8 mm), incidental	++	+	+ no remnant
	Left MCA (6 mm), incidental	++	+	+ no remnant
5	Left MCA (8 mm), incidental	++	++	+ no remnant
6	Right MCA (7 mm), incidental	++	++	+ no remnant
7	Left MCA (5 mm), SAH	++	++	++ no remnant
8	Right MCA (9 mm), SAH	++	+	+ no remnant
9	Left ICA bifurcation (5 mm), SAH	++	(+)	-
10	Left MCA (9 mm), incidental	++	++	+ neck remnant
11	Left MCA (9 mm), SAH	++	++	+ neck remnant
	Left ICA (4 mm)	++	++	+ clip displaced
12	left Pcom (11 mm), incidental	++	+	+ no remnant

by two observers (C.S. and N.W.) blinded to the patients' pathology using a four-grade scale: - not visible/assessable; (+) poorly visible/assessable; + sufficiently visible/assessable, details not distinguishable; ++ clearly visible/assessable, details distinguishable. The observers were allowed to use all means of image reconstruction of the OsiriX software for their evaluation including no –subtracted and subtracted images, 2D- and 3D images, maximum intensity projections and volume rendering reconstruction procedures. Examples of images of 2D projections in 3 planes and an Excel file with the observers' ratings can be viewed under https://www.dropbox.com/sh/3qw11d2z7djidwl/AACFxalr1gIPTs7MDjRcspqla?dl=0 and https://www.dropbox.com/s/6db2yzuw0y3ty2m/Aneurysm%20assessment.xls?dl=0.

Results

Patient characteristics
Twelve patients were included in the analysis. As most patients with aneurysms in the posterior circulation are treated by endovascular coiling in our department, all patients included in this analysis had aneurysms in the anterior circulation. Details on patients and aneurysms are shown in Table 1.

Adverse events
We observed no adverse cardiocirculatory or anaphylactic reaction during or after contrast injection. One patient with a middle cerebral artery (MCA) aneurysm suffered an intraoperative seizure during retraction of the temporal lobe, supposedly independent of the administration of contrast agent.

Radiation dose
A "High Definition Mode" with a higher radiation dose was used in order to improve image quality and to slow down the movement of the X-ray generator. 2 rotational fluoroscopy scans to be able to perform an image subtraction to reduce artifacts. The procedure was repeated after occlusion of the aneurysm. Thus 4 rotational scans were performed with a total dose-length product (DLP) of 4×376.82 mGycm. This equals approximately 1–1.5 the DLP of a whole-brain CT [7, 8].

Image quality
The observers' ratings for preoperative visibility of aneurysms by 3D fluoroscopy and post-clip control of distal vessel patency and complete aneurysm occlusion is depicted in Table 1. In case 1, previous endovascular therapy of an aneurysm of the anterior communicating artery made the 4 mm neck remnant invisible to 3D fluoroscopy. Similarly, the occlusion of the aneurysm and the originating proximal anterior cerebral artery (ACA) branches could not be assessed. In contrast, the patency of the distal ACA, including a small (3 mm) aneurysm of the left pericallosal artery could be readily visualized. In all other patients of this series, the aneurysms were well assessable before clipping. It was observed that small vessels,

especially close to the skull base, may not be visualized due to the occurrence of minor beam hardening artifacts and due to the limited image resolution of the original O-arm® images generated by the given image acquisition parameters. (see Fig. 1a-c). The patency of larger-aneurysm-carrying-vessels and their main branches (Fig. 2) was clearly visible after placement of the clip. Subsequently, a slight clip-induced narrowing of the internal carotid artery was visualized by intraoperative 3D fluoroscopy (Fig. 1f) and verified by postoperative digital subtraction angiography (DSA) (Fig. 1d and e). Similarly, the vasospasm-induced narrowing of the distal MCA trunk in case 11 which was most distinct close to the MCA

bifurcation was depicted by DSA (Fig. 3a–c) and by intraoperative 3D fluoroscopy (Fig. 3d). After positioning of the clip, vessel patency distal to the clip was generally verifiable. In general, the exclusion of the aneurysm dome after clipping was also assessable. However, metal artifacts immediately surrounding the clip branches may remain in some cases in spite of image subtraction and made the verification of complete aneurysm occlusion not possible in most cases of this series. The presence of neck remnants may, therefore, remain undetected (Table 1). However, with precise image subtraction and post-processing, it is possible to depict larger aneurysm remnants (Fig. 3d).

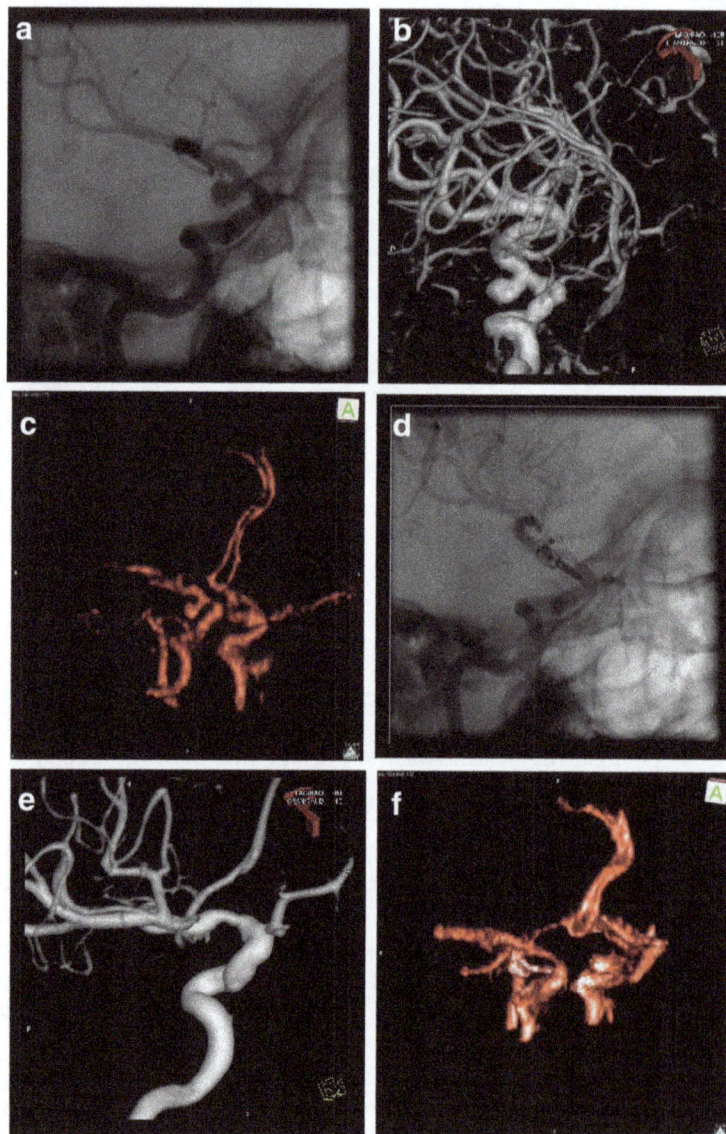

Fig. 1 Preoperative DSA (**a**) with 3D reconstruction (**b**) and intraoperative 3D fluoroscopy after subtraction and reconstruction (**c**) before clip placement in a patient with a carotid artery aneurysm (case 2). **d-f** depict the respective projections after surgery. Postoperative DSA confirms a slight clip-induced narrowing of the ICA depicted by intraoperative 3D fluoroscopy

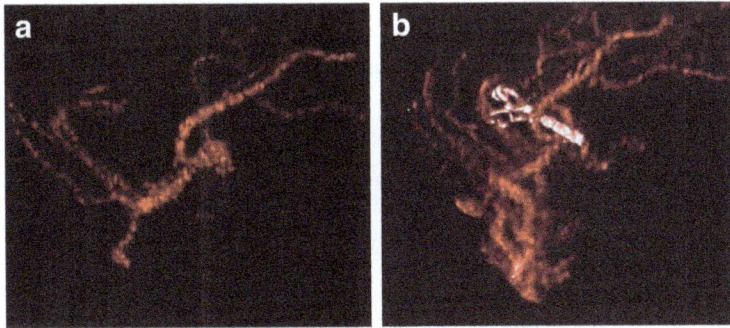

Fig. 2 MCA aneurysm of case 4. MCA bifurcation before (**a**) and after (**b**) placement of the clip

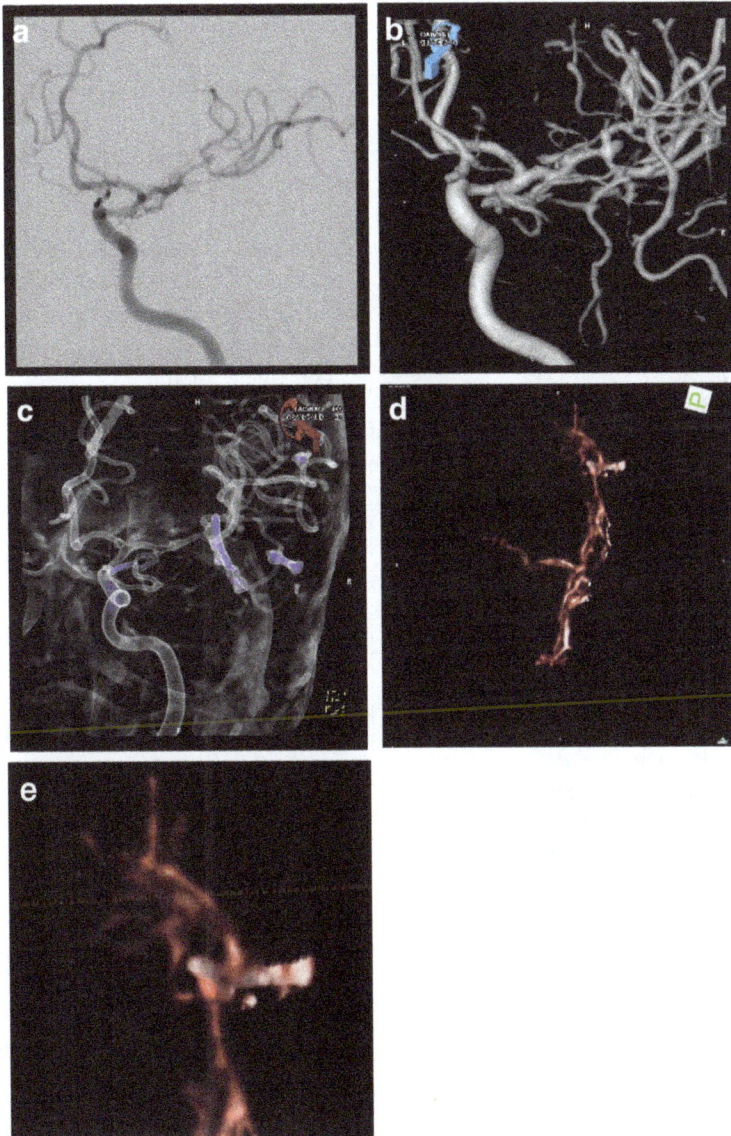

Fig. 3 5 mm neck remnant after clipping of an MCA aneurysm in plain DSA images (**a**), 3D reconstructions (**b** and **c**) and intraoperative 3D fluoroscopy (**d** and **e**)

Discussion

The present case series shows that intraoperative imaging of cerebral vessels and assessment of aneurysm occlusion and vessel patency is possible using 3D rotational fluoroscopy and intravenous contrast agent with appropriate imaging parameters and post-processing software. After a first report on the use of intraoperative 3D rotational fluoroscopy and intraarterial contrast administration for the imaging of cerebral vessels in preparation for electrode implantation in epilepsy surgery [9, 10], we recently demonstrated that cerebral aneurysms can be depicted at adequate image quality using this imaging technology and intravenous contrast administration [5]. Apart from its reported usefulness for the diagnostic imaging of cerebral aneurysms in highly emergent cases [6], evaluating this method for intraoperative evaluation of clip-control and distal vessel patency is a further step in its clinical use. The fundamental advantage of angiographic techniques over "local" techniques like micro-Doppler and ICG-VA is that the vessels do not have to be completely exposed to gain visual control. This is of particular relevance in large aneurysms or after the placement of multiple clips. In both scenarios, the branching vessels may be concealed by the aneurysm or by the clips. In these cases, the application of micro-Doppler or ICG-VA requires a wider exposure which can be avoided by IA.

Intraoperative clip assessment

Washington et al. and Caplan et al. have thoroughly evaluated the sensitivity of catheter-based IA and ICG-VA for the assessment of appropriate clip placement. In both studies, IA showed higher sensitivity than ICG-VA. Consequently, the role of IA as the gold standard for this purpose was underlined by the authors [11, 12]. Micro-Doppler, in turn, is highly sensitive for the assessment of vessel patency but neck remnants cannot be evaluated with this indirect, non-visual technique [3]. These drawbacks can be avoided using IA. Gantry tilts can supply almost any desired perspective. The addition of 3D rotational image acquisition adds a higher degree of image plasticity. Digital image subtraction has further improved image quality. Intraoperative rotational DSA is the ideal technology for this purpose but is limited to hybrid-operating rooms which are only available at a small number of neurosurgical centers. In addition, patients are exposed to a relatively high radiation dose by DSA and its intraoperative use is comparatively time-consuming. It is invasive as it requires the placement of an intraarterial catheter, which necessitates heparinization if placed before surgery or delays surgery if placed after clipping. Intravenous contrast administration, as performed in the present series, can be integrated in the surgical workflow without any further manipulations or invasive procedures.

Using advanced image processing technologies, computed tomography angiography (CTA) has been reported to have a similar diagnostic precision [13] regarding the presence and shape of an aneurysm and the vessel-anatomy for the primary screening for aneurysms [1]. Various series have been published that evaluated 3D fluoroscopic angiography and flat panel detector CT (FD-CT) for the diagnosis of a stenosis of intra- and extracranial vessels and ischemic stroke by intraarterial [14] and intravenous [15] contrast administration and found a good correlation with angiography findings [16]. These studies, however, addressed untreated vessel pathologies and did not have to deal with metal artifacts. Leng et al. used intraoperative FD-CT and intraarterial contrast agent for aneurysm imaging and post clip control in a hybrid operating suite. The authors found good accuracy before and after aneurysm clipping [17]. Intraoperative flat-panel detector 3D rotational angiography with intravenous contrast has, to our knowledge, not been evaluated for the assessment of clip-control after aneurysm surgery. It may be superior in terms of reducing metal artifacts due to the intraprocedural image subtraction. However, an assessment of this technique for its ability to detect aneurysm remnants still has to be conducted. Schnell and coworkers assessed the accuracy of ICG-VA and intraoperative CTA and CT-Perfusion (CTP) for post-clipping assessment. As ICG-VA supplies a good view of the local field, intraoperative CTA/CTP offer conclusive information on the distal vessel patency and tissue perfusion [18].

Mobile 3D-fluoroscopes can be positioned so that they do not interfere with the operative setting and – in contrast to IA and intraoperative CT – can be completely embedded into the surgical workflow. It is evident that this time-frame is important in case of tissue ischemia due to clip-induced vessel occlusion which is exactly the matter of intraoperative assessment. In this case, a significant delay of the intraoperative assessment of vessel patency will favour the development of infarction [19].

Limitations

Our results demonstrate that this procedure can be easily performed and supplies images of acceptable quality concerning the assessment of the parent vessel and the perfusion of the branching vessels. Even smaller vessels are depicted with good quality in locations surrounded by brain tissue. However, quality seems to decrease in the immediate vicinity of the skull-base, most likely due to beam hardening artifacts, similar to CT [20]. The sensitivity of CT angiography to detect cerebral aneurysms has previously investigated and found to be low for aneurysms smaller than 4 mm [21]. Metal artifacts originating from clips and coils can further confine the diagnostic quality [22, 23]. Likewise, the limitations apply for

3D rotational fluoroscopy for intraoperative clip control in patients with intracranial aneurysms – assessment...

79

3D-fluoroscopy. Our images show that is similarly susceptible to metal artifacts as case 1 of our series affirms.

In spite of modern image subtraction techniques, the resolution of the baseline images acquired by the O-Arm® using the afore mentioned settings appears to have arrived at a limit at the present developmental stage of this technology. In unsubtracted images, star-like artifacts are produced by the clip. Similarly, coil artifacts in aneurysms which have previously been occluded by endovascular procedures cause metal artifacts. These can partly be dissolved by image subtraction. However, the immediate vicinity of the clip tends to be surrounded by a slim artifact seam which will conceal a small neck remnant, if present. This might be a problem of the automated image subtraction mode used for post-processing. This mode does not consider e.g. minimal movements of the fluoroscope during the rotational scan which may, however, be relevant in image subtraction and may lead to these artifacts. Using professional post-processing software, a further improvement of image subtraction and reconstruction can be expected. Slight movements of the O-Arm or minor movements of the patient due to mechanical ventilation may be further causes of blurring that will lead to a minor incongruence of image acquisition in spite of identical patient and fluoroscope positions. However, even if the incongruence is only small, it impedes the assessment of complete aneurysm occlusion. Significant movements of the fluoroscope can be prevented by a high definition image acquisition mode in which the image transducer moves at slower motor speed. The latter may be prevented by apnea during the 24 s of image acquisition. One further drawback for intraoperative use is the necessity to remove all metal instruments such as retractors and the need for a carbon head fixation to reduce artifacts.

Higher contrast doses, higher injection speed and a body height dependent injection protocol may further increase image quality. A faster image acquisition time may, combined with optimized injection algorithms, increase the arterial contrast load and selectively enhance the arterial phase of cerebral circulation. Finally, the images obtained by this technique are a summation of X-ray shots gathered during a 360° turn of the transducer and, thus, do not supply information about a possible delay of contrast filling, e.g. caused by a moderate vessel stenosis after placement of the clip. Since 180° image acquisition is sufficient to reconstruct a 3D image, this shortcoming could be solved by the assessment of consecutive 180° sections obtained during the 360° turn. By this way, an evaluation of a contrast delay could be possible.

Rotational fluoroscopy and processing techniques are evolving technologies. Paul and coworkers reported advanced post processing techniques superior to the ones used on this current series to enhance image quality and diagnostic accuracy in liver tumors using ultra-fast cone-beam computed tomography [24, 25]. Further technical advances and improvements of image quality may be expected in the near future.

Conclusion

Intraoperative 3D fluoroscopy with intravenous contrast administration can produce images useful for the assessment of vessel patency after aneurysm clipping. The presence of larger neck remnants can also be detected. Small aneurysm remnants and small vessels, especially those close to the skull-base may not be visible because the image resolution is not high enough with the parameters used for image acquisition in the present series. At the current state, this method of 3D fluoroscopic angiography is technically not mature, but advances can be expected in the near future. 3D rotational fluoroscopy, micro-Doppler and ICG-VA are not rival techniques but may be used complementarily during aneurysm surgery.

Consent for publication

Not applicable.

Abbreviations

ACA: anterior cerebral artery; CTA: computed tomography angiography; CTP: computed tomography perfusion imaging; DICOM: digital imaging and communications in medicine; DLP: dose length product; DSA: digital subtraction angiography; FD-CT: flat panel detector computed tomography; IA: intraoperative angiography; ICA: internal carotid artery; ICG: indocyanin green; ICG-VA: indicyanin green video angiography; MCA: middle cerebral artery; SAH: subarachnoid hemorrhage; VA: video angiography.

Competing interests

The study was not sponsored by public or industrial funding. Dr Westermaier received payments from Johnson&Johnson, Medtronic and Medicon for lectures in spinal neurosurgery. None of the other authors has a conflict of interest to declare.

Authors' contributions

TW – Development of angiography protocol, data acquisition, writing of manuscript. TL – Data acquisition, image post-processing. GAH – Image post-processing. ML – Data acquisition. CS – Image reconstruction and assessment. NW – Image reconstruction and assessment. R-IE – Development of angiography protocol, data acquisition. LS – Development of angiography protocol, image post-processing. GHV – Development of angiography protocol, data acquisition, writing of manuscript. All authors read and approved the final manuscript.

Acknowledgements

The authors cordially thank Mrs. Jennifer Rohmann and Mrs. Nina Menhard for technical assistance in the acquisition of the images. This publication was funded by the German Research Foundation (DFG) and the University of Wuerzburg in the funding program "Open Access Publishing".

Author details
[1]Department of Neurosurgery, University of Wuerzburg, Josef-Schneider-Str. 11, 97080 Wuerzburg, Germany. [2]Department of Neuroradiology, University of Wuerzburg, Josef-Schneider-Str. 11, 97080 Wuerzburg, Germany. [3]Abteilung für Neurochirurgie, Klinikum Klagenfurt, Feschnigstraße 11, 9020 Klagenfurt am Woerthersee, Austria.

References
1. Zhang H1, Hou C, Zhou Z, Zhang H, Zhou G, Zhang G. Evaluating of small intracranial aneurysms by 64-detector CT Angiography: a comparison with 3-dimensional rotation DSA or surgical findings. J Neuroimaging. 2014;24(2):137-43.
2. Fischer G, Stadie A, Oertel JM. Near-infrared indocyanine green videoangiography versus microvascular Doppler sonography in aneurysm surgery. Acta Neurochir (Wien). 2010;152(9):1519–25.
3. Siasios I, Kapsalaki EZ, Fountas KN. The role of intraoperative micro-Doppler ultrasound in verifying proper clip placement in intracranial aneurysm surgery. Neuroradiology. 2012;54(10):1109–18.
4. Raabe A, Beck J, Gerlach R, Zimmermann M, Seifert V. Near-infrared indocyanine green video angiography: a new method for intraoperative assessment of vascular flow. Neurosurgery. 2003;52(1):132–9.
5. Westermaier T, Linsenmann T, Keler AF, Stetter C, Willner N, Solymosi L, Ernestus RI, Vince GH. Intraoperative cerebral angiography by intravenous contrast administration with 3-dimensional rotational fluoroscopy in patients with intracranial aneurysms: a feasibility study. Neurosurgery. 2015;11 Suppl 2:119–26.
6. Westermaier T, Willner N, Vince GH, Linsenmann T, Ernestus RI, Stetter C. Intraoperative 3D rotational angiography: an emergency tool for the diagnosis of intracranial aneurysms. Emerg Radiol. 2015;22(1):97–100.
7. Smith-Bindman R, Moghadassi M, Wilson N, Nelson TR, Boone JM, Cagnon CH, Gould R, Hall DJ, Krishnam M, Lamba R, McNitt-Gray M, Seibert A, Miglioretti DL. Radiation doses in consecutive CT examinations from five university of California Medical Centers. Radiology. 2015;277(1):134–41. doi:10.1148/radiol.2015142728. Epub 2015 May 2015.
8. Geyer LL, Korner M, Harrieder A, Mueck FG, Deak Z, Wirth S, Linsenmaier U. Dose reduction in 64-row whole-body CT in multiple trauma: an optimized CT protocol with iterative image reconstruction on a gemstone-based scintillator. Br J Radiol. 2016:20160003.
9. Cardinale F, Miserocchi A, Moscato A, Cossu M, Castana L, Schiariti MP, Gozzo F, Pero F, Quilici L, Citterio A, Minella M, Torresin A, Lo Russo G. Talairach methodology in the multimodal imaging and robotics era. In: Scarabin JM (ed.), Stereotaxy and Epilepsy Surgery. John Libbey Eurotext. 2012;245-272.
10. Westerlaan HE, Gravendeel J, Fiore D, Metzemaekers JD, Groen RJ, Mooij JJ, Oudkerk M. Multislice CT angiography in the selection of patients with ruptured intracranial aneurysms suitable for clipping or coiling. Neuroradiology. 2007;49(12):997–1007.
11. Caplan JM, Sankey E, Yang W, Radvany MG, Colby GP, Coon AL, Tamargo RJ, Huang J. Impact of indocyanine green videoangiography on rate of clip adjustments following intraoperative angiography. Neurosurgery. 2014;75(4):437–43.
12. Washington CW, Zipfel GJ, Chicoine MR, Derdeyn CP, Rich KM, Moran CJ, Cross DT, Dacey RGJ. Comparing indocyanine green videoangiography to the gold standard of intraoperative digital subtraction angiography used in aneurysm surgery. J Neurosurg. 2013;118(2):420–7.
13. Sun G, Ding J, Lu Y, Li M, Li L, Li GY, Zhang XP. Comparison of standard- and low-tube voltage 320-detector row volume CT angiography in detection of intracranial aneurysms with digital subtraction angiography as gold standard. Acad Radiol. 2012;19(3):281–8.
14. Struffert T, Deuerling-Zheng Y, Kloska S, Engelhorn T, Strother CM, Kalender WA, Kohrmann M, Schwab S, Doerfler A. Flat detector CT in the evaluation of brain parenchyma, intracranial vasculature, and cerebral blood volume: a pilot study in patients with acute symptoms of cerebral ischemia. AJNR Am J Neuroradiol. 2010;31(8):1462–9.
15. Jeon JS, Sheen SH, Hwang GJ, Kim HC, Kwon BJ. Feasibility of intravenous flat panel detector CT angiography for intracranial arterial stenosis. AJNR Am J Neuroradiol. 2013;34(1):129–34.
16. Kamran M, Nagaraja S, Byrne JV. C-arm flat detector computed tomography: the technique and its applications in interventional neuro-radiology. Neuroradiology. 2010;52(4):319–27.
17. Leng LZ, Rubin DG, Patsalides A, Riina HA. Fusion of intraoperative three-dimensional rotational angiography and flat-panel detector computed tomography for cerebrovascular neuronavigation. World Neurosurg. 2013; 79(3-4):504–9.
18. Schnell O, Morhard D, Holtmannspotter M, Reiser M, Tonn JC, Schichor C. Near-infrared indocyanine green videoangiography (ICGVA) and intraoperative computed tomography (iCT): are they complementary or competitive imaging techniques in aneurysm surgery? Acta Neurochir (Wien). 2012;154(10):1861–8.
19. Samson D, Batjer HH, Bowman G, Mootz L, Krippner WJJ, Meyer YJ, Allen BC. A clinical study of the parameters and effects of temporary arterial occlusion in the management of intracranial aneurysms. Neurosurgery. 1994;34(1):22–8.
20. Rozeik C, Kotterer O, Preiss J, Schutz M, Dingler W, Deininger HK. Cranial CT artifacts and gantry angulation. J Comput Assist Tomogr. 1991;15(3):381–6.
21. Anderson GB, Steinke DE, Petruk KC, Ashforth R, Findlay JM. Computed tomographic angiography versus digital subtraction angiography for the diagnosis and early treatment of ruptured intracranial aneurysms. Neurosurgery. 1999;45(6):1315–20.
22. Pechlivanis I, Konig M, Engelhardt M, Scholz M, Heuser L, Harders A, Schmieder K. Evaluation of clip artefacts in three-dimensional computed tomography. Cent Eur Neurosurg. 2009;70(1):9–14.
23. Watanabe Y, Kashiwagi N, Yamada N, Higashi M, Fukuda T, Morikawa S, Onishi Y, Iihara K, Miyamoto S, Naito H. Subtraction 3D CT angiography with the orbital synchronized helical scan technique for the evaluation of postoperative cerebral aneurysms treated with cobalt-alloy clips. AJNR Am J Neuroradiol. 2008;29(6):1071–5.
24. Paul J, Vogl TJ, Chacko A. Detectability of hepatic tumors during 3D post-processed ultrafast cone-beam computed tomography. Phys Med Biol. 2015;60(20):8109–27. doi:10.1088/0031-9155/60/20/8109. Epub 2015 Oct 1 2015.
25. Paul J, Jacobi V, Farhang M, Bazrafshan B, Vogl TJ, Mbalisike EC. Radiation dose and image quality of X-ray volume imaging systems: cone-beam computed tomography, digital subtraction angiography and digital fluoroscopy. Eur Radiol. 2013;23(6):1582–93.

10

Newly recognized cerebral infarctions on postmortem imaging: a report of three cases with systemic infectious disease

Sakon Noriki[1,4]* (iD), Kazuyuki Kinoshita[2,4], Kunihiro Inai[3,4], Toyohiko Sakai[2,4], Hirohiko Kimura[2,4], Takahiro Yamauchi[5], Masayuki Iwano[6] and Hironobu Naiki[3,4]

Abstract

Background: Postmortem imaging (PMI) refers to the imaging of cadavers by computed tomography (CT) and/or magnetic resonance imaging (MRI). Three cases of cerebral infarctions that were not found during life but were newly recognized on PMI and were associated with severe systemic infections are presented.

Case presentations: An 81-year-old woman with a pacemaker and slightly impaired liver function presented with fever. Imaging suggested interstitial pneumonia and an iliopsoas abscess, and blood tests showed liver dysfunction and disseminated intravascular coagulation (DIC). Despite three-agent combined therapy for tuberculosis, she died 32 days after hospitalization. PMI showed multiple fresh cerebral and cerebellar infarctions and diffuse ground-glass shadows in bilateral lungs. On autopsy, the diagnosis of miliary tuberculosis was made, and non-bacterial thrombotic endocarditis that involved the aortic valve may have caused the cerebral infarctions.

A 74-year-old man on steroid therapy for systemic lupus erythematosus presented with severe anemia, melena with no obvious source, and DIC. Imaging suggested intestinal perforation. The patient was treated with antibiotics and drainage of ascites. However, he developed adult respiratory distress syndrome, worsening DIC, and renal dysfunction and died 2 months after admission. PMI showed infiltrative lung shadow, ascites, an abdominal aortic aneurysm, a wide infarction in the right parietal lobe, and multiple new cerebral infarctions. Autopsy examination showed purulent ascites, diffuse peritonitis, invasive bronchopulmonary aspergillosis, and non-bacterial thrombotic endocarditis that likely caused the cerebral infarctions.

A 65-year-old man with an old pontine infarction presented with a fever and neutropenia. Despite appropriate treatment, his fever persisted. CT showed bilateral upper lobe pneumonia, pain appeared in both femoral regions, and intramuscular abscesses of both shoulders developed. His pneumonia worsened, his level of consciousness decreased, right hemiplegia developed, and he died. PMI showed a newly diagnosed cerebral infarction in the left parietal lobe. The autopsy revealed bilateral bronchopneumonia, right-sided pleuritis with effusion, an intramuscular abscess in the right thigh, and fresh multiple organ infarctions. Systemic fibrin thrombosis and DIC were also found. Postmortem cultures showed *E. coli* and *Burkholderia cepacia*.

Conclusion: Cerebral infarction that is newly recognized on PMI might suggest the presence of severe systemic infection.

Keywords: Case report, Postmortem imaging, Cerebral infarction, Infection, Cause of death, Autopsy, Pathology

* Correspondence: noriki@u-fukui.ac.jp
[1]Division of Tumor Pathology, Department of Pathological Sciences, School of Medical Sciences, University of Fukui, 23-3 Shimoaizuki, Matsuoka Eiheiji-cho, Yoshida-gun, 910-1193 Fukui, Japan
[4]Autopsy Imaging Center, School of Medical Sciences, University of Fukui, Fukui, Japan
Full list of author information is available at the end of the article

Background

Cadavers can be evaluated using diagnostic imaging, which comprises one aspect of medical assessment at the time of death. Imaging of cadavers has also been referred to as postmortem imaging (PMI). However, this procedure is variously described as virtopsy in Switzerland [1], virtual autopsy in France [2], radio-autopsy in Germany [3], and autopsy imaging (Ai) in Japan [4]. Although the descriptions and concept of PMI in these countries differ somewhat, all involve analysis of a cadaver by computed tomography (CT) and/or magnetic resonance imaging (MRI) to acquire postmortem medical information.

PMI is a useful diagnostic tool for a forensic case [5] that has no antemortem medical information. However, PMI is often performed in hospital deaths. On the other hand, the rate of the hospital autopsies has been decreasing worldwide in recent years, because the hospital autopsy requires consent in most countries. Furthermore, the brain examination rate of the hospital autopsy is only 20% at our hospital, because another consent is required for the brain examination. Therefore, PMI that can examine the intracerebral state of the cadaver is useful. The findings of PMI are interpreted by taking into consideration the postmortem changes based on the findings of imaging of the living body. Characteristic interpretations of the findings of PMI have yet to be developed.

In this paper, three cases of cerebral infarctions that were not found during life but were newly recognized on PMI are reported. The autopsies revealed severe systemic infectious diseases in all three cases. The aim of this paper is to suggest the possibility of the presence of a severe systemic infection when cerebral infarction is newly recognized on PMI.

Case presentations

Case 1

An 81-year-old woman visited a hospital for a pacemaker check. At that time, slightly impaired liver function was noted. She then developed a fever of 38 °C. Although careful examinations to identify the cause of the fever were performed, the source could not be identified. Various cultures were also negative. Although antibiotic treatment was given, her fever and general status did not improve, and she was admitted to our hospital. On physical examination at admission, her temperature was 38 °C, blood pressure was 140/87 mmHg, and her pulse was 76/min. On blood tests, hemoglobin (Hb) was 11.8 g/dl, C-reactive protein (CRP) was 5.54 mg/dl, soluble interleukin-2 receptor (sIL-2R) was 3732 U/ml (standard 144–518 U/ml), and a tendency to disseminated intravascular coagulation (DIC) (PLT $5.4 \times 10^4/\mu l$, FDP 156 μg/ml, D-dimer 80 μg/ml) was seen. Slightly impaired liver function (aspartate

aminotransferase (AST) 120 IU/l, alanine aminotransferase (ALT) 81 IU/l) was also found.

The chest CT on the second day after hospitalization showed a diffuse ground glass shadow and suspected interstitial pneumonia. On the fifth day after admission, contrast-enhanced CT showed a low-density area (LDA) in the left iliopsoas muscle, suggesting an iliopsoas muscle abscess. *Staphylococcus aureus*, *Escherichia coli (E. coli)*, or tuberculosis was considered as the causative organism of the iliopsoas muscle abscess. Various dysfunctions, such as interstitial pneumonitis, liver damage, and DIC, were also present simultaneously. We assumed that there was a solitary underlying disease that could explain her clinical picture, for example, hematological disease, and treatment was started.

Since intense accumulation of fluoro-deoxy-glucose (FDG) was observed in bilateral lung fields on FDG-positron-emission tomography (PET), an inflammatory disorder, especially tuberculosis was suspected, and three-agent combined therapy was started on the 8th day after admission. However, neither the fever nor her general status improved, and the ground glass appearance had deteriorated further on the chest CT on the 16th day after admission.

On the 22nd day after admission (9 days before death), the patient's respiratory condition deteriorated suddenly, and methylprednisolone pulse therapy resulted in no improvement. She died on the 32nd day after hospitalization. PMI and an autopsy (only thoracoabdominal) were performed 14 h after death (Additional file 1).

PMI findings

Multiple LDAs were recognized in the right middle cerebral artery (MCA) region (Fig. 1), right cerebellum, and left basal ganglia on PMI. They seemed to be infarctions. Since no atrophy was found in the brain, the infarctions seemed to be relatively fresh lesions. There was neither a mass effect nor hemorrhage in the brain. The ground glass shadow was widespread in bilateral lungs, and part of the lungs showed infiltrative shadow and the crazy paving pattern. As the cause of the interstitial shadow, adult respiratory distress syndrome (ARDS), acute interstitial pneumonia, or an infectious disease such as *Pneumocystis jirovecii* pneumonia was considered. No airway obstruction was found. A cardiac pacemaker was confirmed. Neither brain CT nor brain MRI was done during the patient's lifetime.

Pathological findings

On autopsy, white viscous liquid flowed when an incision was made into the left iliopsoas muscle (Fig. 2a). The wall of the abscess was composed of lymphocytes and fibrous tissue, and the contents of the abscess consisted of necrotic material (Fig. 2b). A few neutrophils

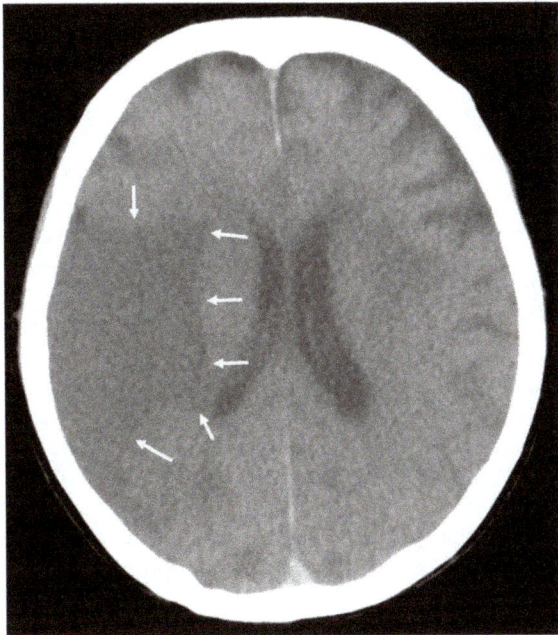

Fig. 1 Brain postmortem CT image 14 h after death (Case 1). An LDA was found in the middle cerebral artery area (*arrows*)

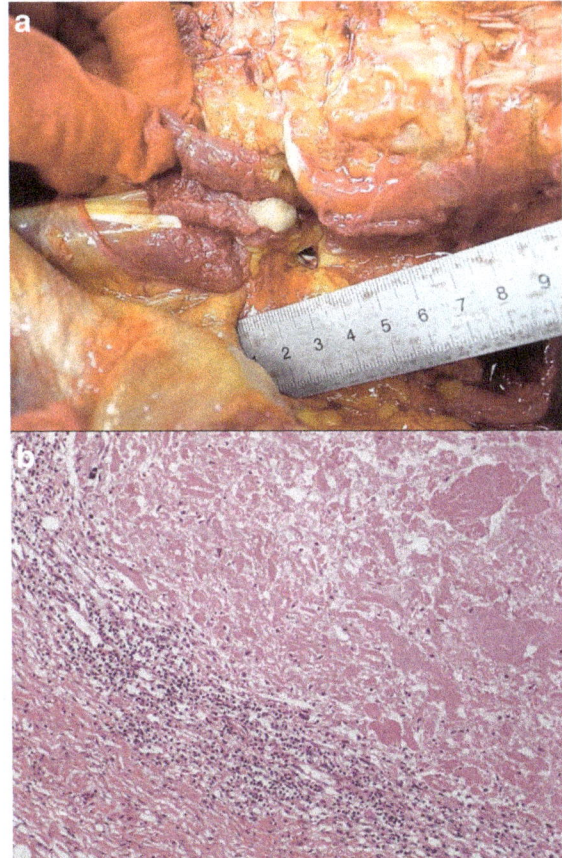

Fig. 2 The cold abscess of the left iliopsoas muscle (Case 1). **a** The left iliopsoas muscle that was cut open at autopsy. White viscous liquid was seen. **b** The micrograph of the iliopsoas abscess. The content of the abscess is necrotic material, and neutrophilic infiltration is not seen (Hematoxylin-Eosin (HE) stain. Original magnification × 4)

infiltrated into the abscess. A few acid fast bacilli were noted in the abscess with Ziehl-Neelsen staining. These histological findings and polymerase chain reaction (PCR) testing showed that the lesion was tuberculous. In addition, tuberculous nodules were found microscopically in bilateral lungs (left 730 g, right 842 g), liver (1118 g), spleen (94 g), left kidney (182 g), bone marrow, and lymph nodes surrounding the pancreas, and miliary tuberculosis was diagnosed. Moreover, vegetations (4 mm and 5 mm in diameter) were noted on the aortic valve (Fig. 3a). The vegetations consisted of fibrin thrombus without bacterial colonies (Fig. 3b), and they were diagnosed as non-bacterial thrombotic endocarditis. This thrombus might have detached from the valve and become the emboli that resulted in the cerebral infarctions.

Case 2

A 74-year-old man was taking a steroid (30 mg/day of predonin) for systemic lupus erythematosus (SLE) and was being followed in the outpatient department. A blood test showed severe anemia (Hb 3.8 g/dl), and he was hospitalized 2 months before death. Melena was found, but no bleeding source was identified even on gastroscopy and colonoscopy. Then, 14 days after admission, free air was found at the subphrenic region on chest X-ray and CT, and intestinal perforation was suspected. The patient was given a course of antibiotic treatment and drainage of ascites because of his general status.

The patient's manifestations were relieved, but the inflammatory response increased again, and his respiratory condition suddenly worsened, requiring intensive care unit (ICU) admission. The onset of ARDS was suspected. He had DIC on admission, and it was exacerbated with progression of the infection. His inflammatory response, renal failure, and respiratory condition deteriorated, and he died 2 months after admission. PMI and an autopsy (only thoracoabdominal) were performed 2 h after death (Additional file 2).

PMI findings

Ascites and an abdominal aortic aneurysm were found on abdominal CT, but the free air had disappeared. On chest CT, infiltrative shadow was found, and ARDS, pneumonia, and interstitial pneumonia were considered. Brain CT showed a wide LDA area in the right parietal lobe, and cerebral infarction was diagnosed (Fig. 4a) [6]. Multiple new cerebral infarctions were seen on PMI. Brain MRI was done 1 year 5 months before death. The

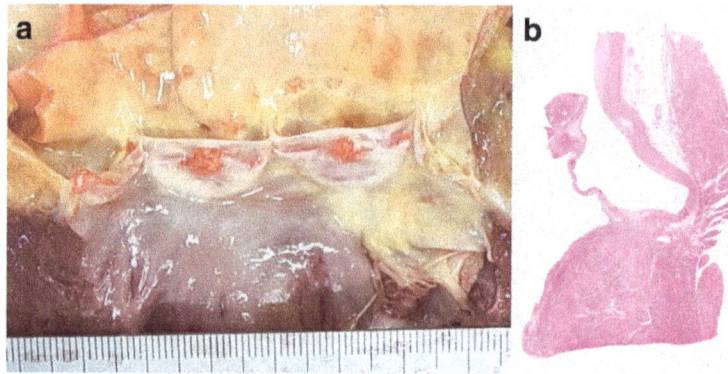

Fig. 3 Vegetations of the aortic valve at autopsy (Case 1). **a** The macroscopic appearance of the aortic valve. The aortic valve has two vegetations of 4 mm and 5 mm in diameter. **b** Loupe image of the aortic valve. Vegetations consist of fibrin without bacterial colonies, and non-bacterial thrombotic endocarditis was diagnosed (HE stain. Original magnification × 1)

T2-weighted image of the MRI corresponding to the CT image is shown (Fig. 4b). At that time, no cerebral infarction was found.

Pathological findings
Yellowish white purulent ascites of 1800 ml was found in the abdominal cavity at autopsy, and it showed diffuse peritonitis. However, the perforation site of the intestine was not confirmed. Moreover, invasive bronchopulmonary aspergillosis was present in the lungs (Fig. 5a,b) [6], and the background lung showed diffuse alveolar damage. Aspergillus species were also found in the peritoneum. There were a few vegetations, up to 10 mm in diameter, on the aortic valve in the heart (Fig. 6a) [6]. Three vegetations, 12 mm, 10 mm, and 7 mm in diameter, were also found on the mitral valve (Fig. 6b) [6]. They were regarded as the cause of the cerebral infarction; these thrombotic vegetations had separated from the valves. In addition, cholesterin crystal embolism was

found in the kidney, heart, liver, spleen, and it was thought that this had caused the progressive renal dysfunction.

Case 3
A 65-year-old man developed a left pontine infarction 2 months before hospitalization. He had a fever of about 39 °C. Blood tests showed white blood cells of 300/μl (3% neutrophils; neutropenia), and he was hospitalized in the Department of Hematology. Drug-induced neutropenia was suspected, and granulocyte colony-stimulating factor and antibiotics were administered with stopping of oral medicine. However, his fever remained, and pneumonia of both upper lobes was diagnosed by CT on the fourth day after admission, and an antifungal drug was added. Pain in both femoral regions then appeared. His pneumonia got worse, and intramuscular abscesses of both shoulders were noted 30 days before death. Though an antimicrobial drug was added, the pneumonia worsened, and an

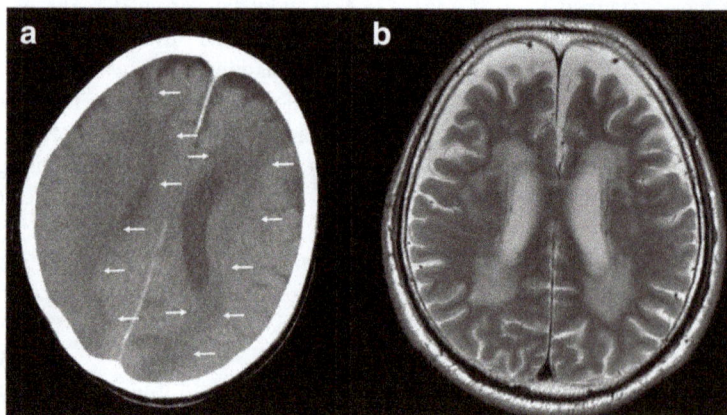

Fig. 4 The postmortem CT and antemortem MRI (Case 2). **a** The postmortem CT image of the brain 2 h after death. LDAs were found widely, resulting in a diagnosis of cerebral infarction (*arrows*). (with permission [6]) **b** Antemortem MRI, T2-weighted image showing no cerebral infarction. The brain MRI was taken 1 year 5 months before death

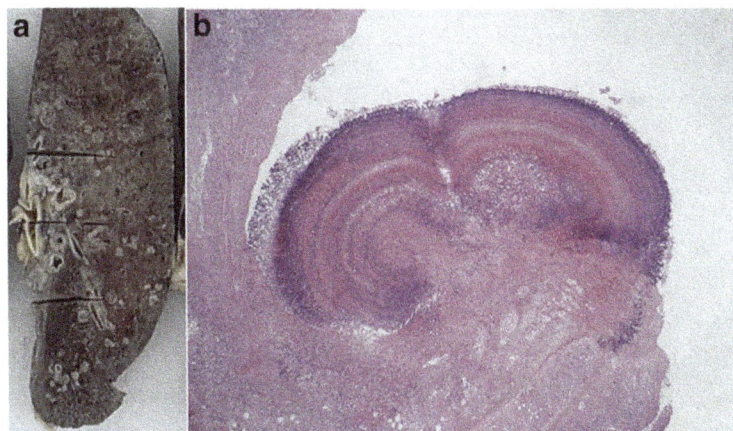

Fig. 5 The aortic valve and mitral valve at autopsy (Case 2). **a** The macroscopic appearance of the aortic valve. The aortic valve has two vegetations of 4 mm and 5 mm. **b** The macroscopic appearance of the mitral valve. The mitral valve has some vegetations diagnosed as non-bacterial thrombotic endocarditis histologically. (with permission [6])

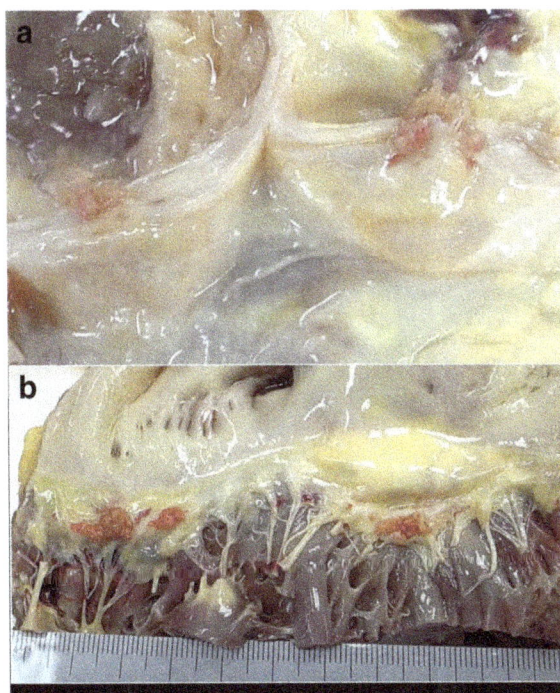

Fig. 6 The lung after fixation (Case 2). **a** The macroscopic appearance of the lung. Diffuse small nodules were noted in the bronchi and parenchyma of the lung. **b** The microscopic appearance of the bronchus. The aspergillus had grown to project into the bronchus in the low-power image of the hilar region. (with permission [6])

inflammatory pleural effusion developed. The patient's level of consciousness decreased, and complete paralysis of the right side arm and leg appeared. He died 3 days after his consciousness level decreased and the right hemiplegia developed. PMI and autopsy were performed 2 h after death (Additional file 3).

PMI findings
An LDA was found in the left parietal lobe, and it was a newly diagnosed cerebral infarction on PMI (Fig. 7a). Brain MRI was done 22 days before death. The T2-weighted image of the MRI corresponding to the CT image is shown (Fig. 7b). At that time, no cerebral infarction was found.

Pathological findings
The autopsy revealed a severe systemic infection: bilateral bronchopneumonia (left 954 g: right 857 g), right-sided pleuritis with effusion, and an intramuscular abscess in the right thigh (Fig. 8). Moreover, systemic fibrin thrombosis and a bleeding tendency due to DIC were seen. The thrombosis resulted in fresh multiple organ infarctions, such as myocardial infarction, left renal infarction, splenic infarction, and cerebral infarctions in the left frontal and parietal lobes. It was also confirmed that the old pontine infarction formed a cyst inside the left pons. The pus of the right thigh abscess was cultured at autopsy, and *E. coli* was detected. *E. coli* and *Burkholderia cepacia* were also detected by blood culture from the right atrium.

Discussion
As described above, both cases 1 and 2 did not show neurological manifestations of the cerebral infarctions during their lifetime, and there were no findings on

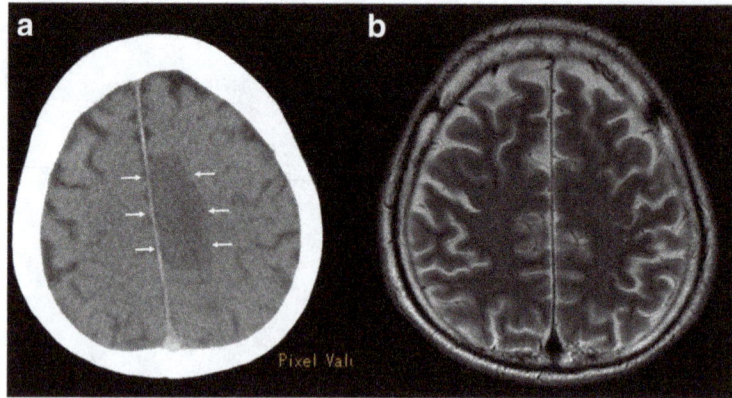

Fig. 7 The postmortem CT and antemortem MRI (Case 3). **a** Brain postmortem CT image 7 h after death. The left parietal lobe has an LDA that was diagnosed as cerebral infarction (*arrows*). **b** Antemortem MRI, T2-weighted showing no cerebral infarction. The brain MRI was taken 22 days before death

brain CT at the final antemortem imaging. However, in both cases, cerebral infarctions were recognized on the postmortem brain CT. In case 3, neurologic symptoms appeared in the agonal stage, and cerebral infarction was newly recognized on postmortem brain CT. The autopsy revealed severe infectious diseases in all three cases.

From October 2010 to January 2014, there were 106 cases that underwent both PMI and autopsy at the University of Fukui Hospital. PMI was performed at the Ai center

of the University of Fukui with an 8-slice multi-detector CT scanner (Hitachi Medico, Tokyo, Japan) used exclusively for autopsies, as described previously [7]. The corpus was placed in the supine position, and a full-body scan from the vertex to the toes was performed. The scanning conditions were 120 kV, 250 mA, 8 × 2.5 collimation, 1.125 pitch, 0.8-s rotation time, 5-mm slice thickness, and 5-mm increments [7, 8]. No contrast reagent was used in these cases.

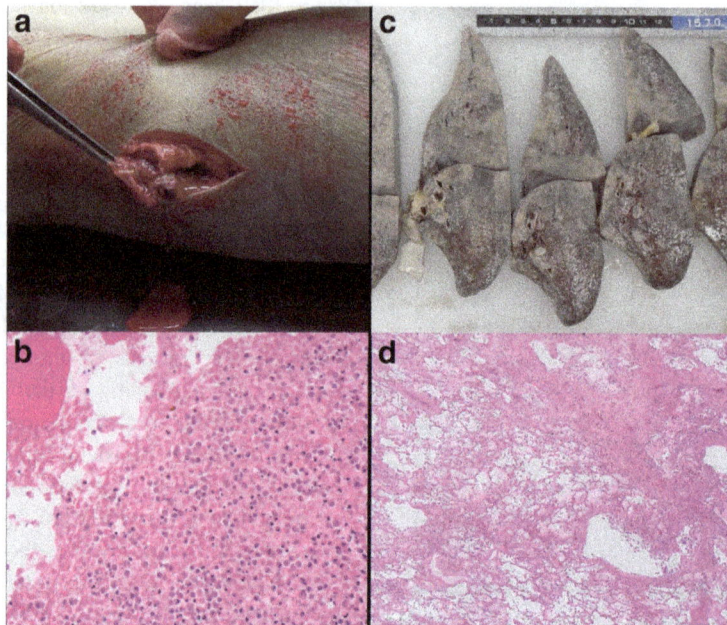

Fig. 8 The left thigh and left lung at autopsy (Case 3). **a** The macroscopic appearance of the thigh. After incision into the abscess of the left thigh, leakage of pus is noted. **b** The microscopic appearance of the abscess. Numerous necrotic cells and neutrophils are noted. The pus was cultured, and *E. coli* was detected (HE stain. Original magnification × 20). **c** The cut surface of the left lung after fixation. The lung was diffusely firm, boggy, and heavy. Whitish lesions were found. **d** The microscopic appearance of the lung. The alveoli were filled with eosinophilic fluid and neutrophils (HE stain. Original magnification × 4)

In three of 106 cases (2.8%), cerebral infarction was newly recognized on PMI, and severe infection was diagnosed on the subsequent autopsy. However, this rate is limited to our hospital, which is a limitation of this report. Many of the autopsied subjects may have had an increased frequency of severe infectious diseases such as ARDS, sepsis, and pneumonia. However, our recent autopsy-based study of histiocytic hyperplasia with hemophagocytosis (polyhemophagocytosis) [9] showed that the incidence of polyhemophagocytosis was equal to that shown in the German, US, and Japanese literature [9–11], suggesting that the characteristics of our autopsied subjects were not biased. Therefore, there might be such cases in other hospitals. However, the exact frequency of cerebral infarction being newly recognized on PMI and severe infection being diagnosed on autopsy is not known.

Some comparison studies of PMI findings and pathological diagnosis by autopsy have been done. In two UK centers in Manchester and Oxford, 182 unselected cases were assessed by radiology (CT and MRI) and autopsy for the cause of death [12]. In Aachen University Hospital, 29 cases were analyzed by CT and autopsy [13], and in the ICUs of Hamburg, 47 cases were analyzed by autopsy and PMI [14]. However, none of these reported cases similar to the ones presented here.

The reported case of a woman in her 40s with familial hypercholesterolemia is similar [15]. She underwent aortic valve replacement and coronary bypass surgery for aortic stenosis and stenosis of the left main coronary artery. However, she developed acute myocardial infarction and died of postoperative mediastinitis and multiple organ failure. PMI and autopsy were done. An LDA was found in the right parietal lobe on PMI. The autopsy revealed that she had disseminated cryptococcosis and developed multiple organ failure due to sepsis.

In the present three cases and the one case in the literature, the systemic infectious disease had already been known before death. However, if the cerebral infarction is newly found on PMI even if infection is not suspected or adequate testing is not possible before the death, systemic infectious diseases might be suspected.

The cause of cerebral infarction in all cases was considered to be a thrombus of thrombotic endocarditis or DIC due to the severe infection. In fact, some studies reported the association of cerebral infarction with prior infection and inflammatory processes [16–20]. However, no article has referred to the relationship between cerebral infarction in PMI and systemic infection. Thus, we would like to emphasize that findings of brain infarctions on PMI might imply systemic infection.

The rate of hospital autopsies has been decreasing worldwide in recent years. For example, autopsies are performed in less than 10% of all U.S. deaths [21]. In the United Kingdom, the mean hospital autopsy rate in 2013 was 0.69% of hospital deaths [22]. In Japan, according to the Japan Council for Quality Health Care, the autopsy rate in 2012 was 4.0%. To make matters worse, another consent is required for the brain examination, so the rate of brain examination at autopsy is still lower; it is only about 20% at our hospital. Therefore, the finding of brain infarction on PMI of the cadaver is important because it suggests the presence of systemic infection.

Systemic infection such as miliary tuberculosis is regarded as a disease for which diagnosis is difficult on PMI at present. However, there is a possibility that systemic infection might become a disease for which a diagnosis can be suspected on PMI based on an accumulation of cases similar to those presented here. Thus, we believe that we can improve the certainty of PMI by comparative examinations between PMI and autopsy findings.

Conclusion

Three cases with systemic infectious disease were presented in this report. All of them showed newly recognized cerebral infarctions on PMI. Cerebral infarction that is newly recognized on PMI might suggest the presence of severe systemic infection.

Abbreviations
Ai: Autopsy imaging; ALT: Alanine aminotransferase; ARDS: Adult respiratory distress syndrome; AST: Aspartate aminotransferase; CRP: C-reactive protein; CT: Computed tomography; DIC: Disseminated intravascular coagulation; *E. coli*: *Escherichia coli*; FDG: Fluoro-deoxy-glucose; Hb: Hemoglobin; HE: Hematoxylin-eosin.; ICU: Intensive-care unit; LDA: Low density area; MCA: Middle cerebral artery; MRI: Magnetic resonance imaging; PET: Positron-emission tomography; PMI: Postmortem imaging; sIL-2R: Soluble interleukin-2 receptor; SLE: Systemic lupus erythematosus

Acknowledgement
None.

Funding
This report was partially supported by Grants-in-Aid from the Ministry of Education, Culture, Sports, Science and Technology of Japan to S. Noriki (MEXT/JSPS KAKENHI Grant Number 26108009 and 26670348).

Authors' contributions
SN was involved in the overall supervision and drafted the manuscript. KK, TS, and HK interpreted the PMI of all patients. SN, KI, and HN autopsied the patients and diagnosed the pathological findings. TY participated in the management of the patients of Cases 1 and 3. MI participated in the

management of the patient of Case 2. All authors read and approved the final manuscript.

Authors' information

SN: MD, PhD, Associate Professor, Division of Tumor Pathology, Department of Pathological Sciences, School of Medical Sciences, University of Fukui, Fukui, Japan 23-3 Shimoaizuki, Matsuoka, Eiheiji, Fukui 910-1193, Japan. KK: MBBS, Junior Associate Professor of Radiology, School of Medical Sciences, University of Fukui. TS: MD, PhD, Associate Professor of Radiology, School of Medical Sciences, University of Fukui. KI: MD, PhD, Junior Associate Professor of Molecular Pathology, School of Medical Sciences, University of Fukui. HK: MD, PhD, Professor of Radiology, School of Medical Sciences, University of Fukui. TY: MD, PhD, Professor of Hematology and Oncology, School of Medical Sciences, University of Fukui. MI: MD, PhD, Professor of Nephrology, School of Medical Sciences, University of Fukui. HN: MD, PhD, Professor of Molecular Pathology, School of Medical Sciences, University of Fukui.

Competing interests

The author(s) declare that they have no competing interests.

Consent for publication

Written, informed consent for publication of this case report and any accompanying images was obtained from the family of each deceased patient prior to autopsy.

Author details

[1]Division of Tumor Pathology, Department of Pathological Sciences, School of Medical Sciences, University of Fukui, 23-3 Shimoaizuki, Matsuoka Eiheiji-cho, Yoshida-gun, 910-1193 Fukui, Japan. [2]Division of Radiology, Department of Radiology and Laboratory Medicine, School of Medical Sciences, University of Fukui, 23-3 Shimoaizuki, Matsuoka Eiheiji-cho, Yoshida-gun, 910-1193 Fukui, Japan. [3]Division of Molecular Pathology, Department of Pathological Sciences, School of Medical Sciences, University of Fukui, Fukui, Japan. [4]Autopsy Imaging Center, School of Medical Sciences, University of Fukui, Fukui, Japan. [5]Division of Hematology and Oncology, Faculty of Medical Sciences, University of Fukui, 23-3 Shimoaizuki, Matsuoka Eiheiji-cho, Yoshida-gun, 910-1193 Fukui, Japan. [6]Division of Nephrology, Department of General Medicine, University of Fukui, 23-3 Shimoaizuki, Matsuoka Eiheiji-cho, Yoshida-gun, 910-1193 Fukui, Japan.

References

1. Thali MJ, Yen K, Schweitzer W, Vock P, Boesch C, Ozdoba C, et al. Virtopsy, a new imaging horizon in forensic pathology: virtual autopsy by postmortem multislice computed tomography (MSCT) and magnetic resonance imaging (MRI)–a feasibility study. J Forensic Sci. 2003;48:386–403.
2. Clarot F, Proust B, Eurin D, Vaz E, Le Dosseur P. Sudden infant death syndrome and virtual autopsy: scalpel or mouse? Arch Pediatr. 2007;14:636–9. Epub 2007 Apr 17. [in French].
3. Oesterhelweg L, Lorenzen M, Braun C, Rohwedder D, Adam G, Püschel K. Radiosektion - computertomographie-assistierte rekonstruktion eines erweiterten suizids. Rechtsmedizin. 2006;17:44–7 [in Germany].
4. Ezawa H, Yoneyama R, Kandatsu S, Yoshikawa K, Tsujii H, Harigaya K. Introduction of autopsy imaging redefines the concept of autopsy: 37 cases of clinical experience. Pathol Int. 2003;53:865–73.
5. Ruder TD, Thali MJ, Hatch GM. Essentials of forensic post-mortem MR imaging in adults. Br J Radiol. 2014;87:20130567.
6. Noriki S, Kinoshita K. New findings on pathological autopsy - comparison studies between Ai and autopsy. Innervision. 2015;7:44–6 [in Japanese].
7. Inai K, Noriki S, Kinoshita K, Nishijima A, Sakai T, Kimura H, et al. Feasibility of liver weight estimation by postmortem computed tomography images: an autopsy study. Pathol Int. 2014;64:315–24.
8. Inai K, Noriki S, Kinoshita K, Sakai T, Kimura H, Nishijima A, et al. Postmortem CT is more accurate than clinical diagnosis for identifying the immediate cause of death in hospitalized patients: a prospective autopsy-based study. Virchow Arch. 2016;[in press]
9. Inai K, Noriki S, Iwasaki H, Naiki H. Risk factor analysis for bone marrow histiocytic hyperplasia with hemophagocytosis: an autopsy study. Virchows Arch. 2014;465:109–18.
10. Strauss R, Neureiter D, Westenburger B, Wehler M, Kirchner T, Hahn EG. Multifactorial risk analysis of bone marrow histiocytic hyperplasia with hemophagocytosis in critically ill medical patients–a postmortem clinicopathologic analysis. Crit Care Med. 2004;32:1316–21.
11. Suster S, Hilsenbeck S, Rywlin AM. Reactive histiocytic hyperplasia with hemophagocytosis in hematopoietic organs: a reevaluation of the benign hemophagocytic proliferations. Hum Pathol. 1988;19:705–12.
12. Roberts IS, Benamore RE, Benbow EW, Lee SH, Harris JN, Jackson A, et al. Post-mortem imaging as an alternative to autopsy in the diagnosis of adult deaths: a validation study. Lancet. 2012;379:136–42.
13. Wichmann D, Heinemann A, Weinberg C, Vogel H, Hoepker WW, Grabherr S, et al. Virtual autopsy with multiphase postmortem computed tomographic angiography versus traditional medical autopsy to investigate unexpected deaths of hospitalized patients: a cohort study. Ann Intern Med. 2014;160:534–41.
14. Westphal SE, Apitzsch J, Penzkofer T, Mahnken AH, Knuchel R. Virtual CT autopsy in clinical pathology: feasibility in clinical autopsies. Virchows Arch. 2012;461(2):211–9.
15. Tanei Z, Takazawa Y, Miura Y, Saitou A, Fukayama M. A case report of familial hypercholesterolemia with right coronary artery obstruction with the artificial valve seat at aortic valve replacement and coronary bypass surgery for aortic stenosis and ischemic heart disease. Pathol Clin Med. 2012;30:993–1000 [in Japanese].
16. Macko RF, Ameriso SF, Barndt R, Clough W, Weiner JM, Fisher M. Precipitants of brain infarction. Roles of preceding infection/inflammation and recent psychological stress. Stroke. 1996;27:1999–2004.
17. Ameriso SF, Wong VL, Quismorio Jr FP, Fisher M. Immunohematologic characteristics of infection-associated cerebral infarction. Stroke. 1991;22:1004–9.
18. Das S, Ghosh KC, Pulai S, Pulai D, Bhar D, Gangopadhyay PK. Systemic infection and inflammation as trigger factors of ischemic stroke. Ann Neurosci. 2011;18:17–20.
19. Grau AJ, Buggle F, Becher H, Zimmermann E, Spiel M, Fent T, et al. Recent bacterial and viral infection is a risk factor for cerebrovascular ischemia: clinical and biochemical studies. Neurology. 1998;50:196–203.
20. Dalager-Pedersen M, Sogaard M, Schonheyder HC, Nielsen H, Thomsen RW. Risk for myocardial infarction and stroke after community-acquired bacteremia: a 20-year population-based cohort study. Circulation. 2014;129:1387–96.
21. Nemetz PN, Tanglos E, Sands LP, Fisher Jr WP, Newman 3rd WP, Burton EC. Attitudes toward the autopsy–an 8-state survey. MedGenMed. 2006;8:80.
22. Turnbull A, Osborn M, Nicholas NJ. Hospital autopsy: endangered or extinct? Clin Pathol. 2015;68:601–14.

11

Case report of hyperglycemic nonketotic chorea with rapid radiological resolution

H.M.M.T.B. Herath[*], S.P. Pahalagamage and Sunethra Senanayake

Abstract

Background: Hemichorea is a rare manifestation of nonketotic hyperglycemia that usually affects elderly Asian women with poor glycemic control. Non-contrast computerized Tomography and T1- weighted Magnetic Resonance Imaging shows characteristic hyperintense basal ganglia lesions.

Case presentation: A Fifty-seven year old Sri Lankan female presented with a two-day history of right upper limb chorea. She had been diagnosed with diabetes mellitus one year ago, but was not on any treatment and did not have any micro vascular or macro vascular complications. Random blood sugar was 420 mg/dl and full blood count, liver function tests, renal function tests, inflammatory markers, thyroid function tests, Urine protein / creatinine ratio, electrocardiogram and 2D Echo were normal. Arterial blood gas did not show acidosis and ketone bodies were not detected in urine. Non-contrast computerized Tomography brain on day 1 showed left side hyperdense lentiform and caudate nuclei and MRI on day 3 showed slightly high signal intensity of left side basal ganglia on T1- weighted images and low signal intensity on T2-weighted and Fluid-attenuated inversion recovery images. She was started on insulin and a low dose of clonazepam and glycemic control was achieved on day 3. Two days later, the chorea completely disappeared. CT brain was repeated 4 days and 10 days following glycemic control, which showed rapid resolution of CT changes. Clonazepam was stopped in 2 weeks and chorea did not recur.

Conclusion: This is a rare manifestation of diabetes in Sri lanka and diagnosing this rare entity will direct clinicians to achieve optimum glycemic control as the treatment which will lead to rapid clinical response without any other medications. In this case report we high light that with the clinical improvement, repeating a CT scan even after a very short period like 2 weeks will show rapid radiological resolution. This repeat imaging can also be useful to confirm the diagnosis, which will minimize unnecessary investigations and treatments. Further cases of hyperglycemic nonketotic chorea with brain imaging performed within short intervals is needed to evaluate the nature of rapid radiological changes, which will be useful to understand the pathology of this condition.

Keywords: Hyperglycemic nonketotic chorea, Rapid radiological resolution

Background

Hemichorea is a rare manifestation of nonketotic hyperglycemia that usually affects elderly Asian women with poor glycemic control. The pathophysiology of hemichorea in hyperglycemia is controversial but these patients display distinct neuroimaging features. Non Contrast Computerized Tomography (NCCT) and T1-weighted Magnetic resonance imaging (MRI) show characteristic hyperintense basal ganglia lesions but the T2-weighted brain MRI findings vary [1–3]. In this case we followed up a patient with nonketotic hyperglycemic chorea with serial CT scans performed in very short intervals which revealed rapid radiological resolution.

Case presentation

A Fifty-seven year old Sri Lankan female presented with a two-day history of acute onset right upper limb chorea. She had been diagnosed with diabetes mellitus one year ago, but was not on any treatment and did not have any micro vascular or macro vascular complications. On examination, right upper limb chorea was evident and the rest of the nervous system examination was normal including fundoscopy. Random blood sugar on admission

* Correspondence: tharukaherath11@gmail.com
National hospital, Colombo, Sri Lanka

was 420 mg/dl. Full blood count, liver function tests, renal function tests, inflammatory markers, thyroid function tests, Anti nuclear antibody, Urine protein / creatinine ratio, electrocardiogram and 2D Echo were normal. Arterial blood gas did not show acidosis and ketone bodies were not detected in urine. NCCT brain on day 1 showed left side hyperdense lentiform and caudate nuclei(Fig. 1). MRI on day 3 showed slightly high signal intensity of left side basal ganglia on T1- weighted images and low signal intensity on T2-weighted and Fluid-attenuated inversion recovery images(Fig. 2). Diffusion weighted imaging and Susceptibility weighted imaging were normal. She was started on insulin and a low dose of clonazepam (0.5 mg nocte) and glycemic control was achieved on day 3. Two days later, the chorea completely disappeared. NCCT was repeated 4 days and 10 days following glycemic control, which showed rapid resolution of CT changes (Fig. 1). Clonazepam was stopped in 2 weeks and chorea did not recur.

Discussion

In this case, the patient had hemichorea, nonketotic hyperglycemia and hyperintense caudate and lentiform nuclei on NCCT and T1-MRI supporting the diagnosis of hyperglycemic nonketotic chorea. Several hypotheses have been put forward to explain the mechanism of chorea including relative dopaminergic hypersensitivity, vascular insufficiency causing transient ischemia to basal ganglia and shifting of cerebral metabolism to the anaerobic pathway causing reduction in both GABA and acetylcholine with metabolic acidosis leading to basal

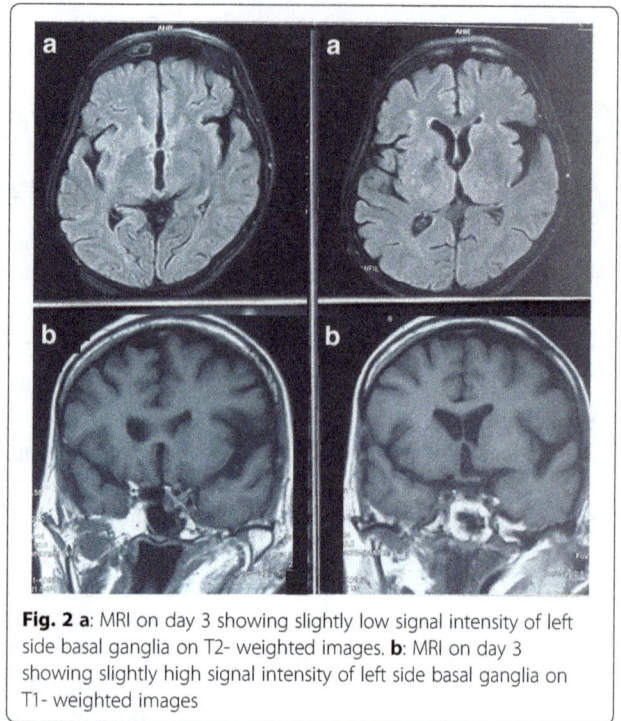

Fig. 2 a: MRI on day 3 showing slightly low signal intensity of left side basal ganglia on T2- weighted images. b: MRI on day 3 showing slightly high signal intensity of left side basal ganglia on T1- weighted images

ganglia dysfunction [1, 2, 4]. As in our case, in most of the cases the chorea ameliorated completely with good glycemic control [1, 5] suggesting a reversible pathology.

Lai, P.H. at el., evaluated neuroimaging of 10 patients with nonketotic hyperglycemic hemichorea in primary diabetes mellitus and CT and T1-weighted MR images showed lesions of the putamen and/or caudate unilaterally or bilaterally. Lin, J.J. and colleagues report 7

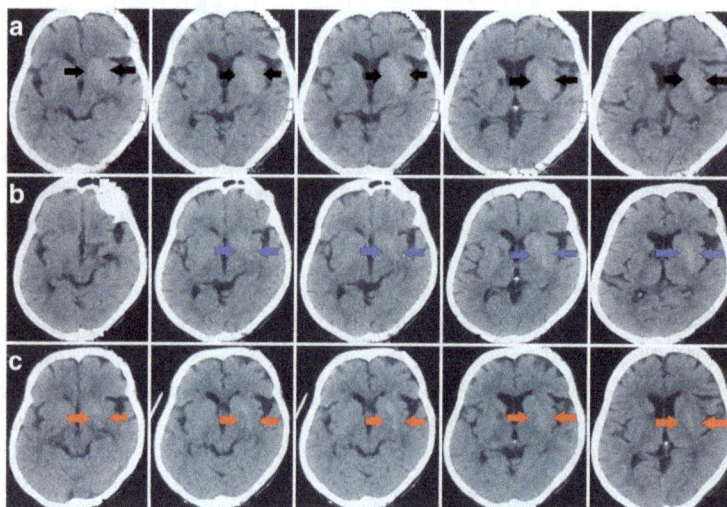

Fig. 1 Serial NCCT brain showing resolution of left side high intensity basal ganglia. a: Day 1 NCCT brain showing left side hyperdense lentiform and caudate nuclei shown by black arrows. b: NCCT brain 4 days after glycemic control showing rapid resolution of left side hyperdense lentiform and caudate nuclei (The hyperdense area is shown by blue arrows). c: NCCT brain 10 days after glycemic control showing rapid resolution of left side hyperdense lentiform and caudate nuclei (The initial hyperdense area is shown by red arrows, which has resolved by day 10)

similar patients with CT showing an increased density in the contralateral putamen and/or caudate and MRI revealing abnormal hyperintensity on T1-weighted and hypointensity on T2-weighted images [5]. The theories for characteristic radiological findings are abnormal deposition of calcium in neurons or glial cells, petechial hemorrhages from small vessels, extravascular hemosiderin deposition and gemistocyte (swollen reactive astrocytes having rich protein content) accumulation following acute injury [4]. Lin, J.J. and colleagues followed up 7 patients and the lesions on CT and MRI showed complete resolution within 3 months and 11 months, respectively [5]. In one literature survey, 19 out of 22 patients who had a follow-up brain MRI after an interval of 2 months – 1.5 years, the high signal intensity basal ganglia lesions resolved along with the improvement in chorea [1]. In another case series, 8 out of 9 patients underwent follow up CT scans within an interval of 1–18 months and the hyperdense striatal lesions had disappeared completely or near-completely [6].

In our patient we did serial CT scans over two weeks, which showed rapid resolution. As mentioned above, we came across on very few case reports in literature where the progression of radiological manifestations was monitored, but in this case we did CT scans in very short intervals. Previous case reports describe rapid clinical improvement but in this case with the resolution of chorea following glycemic control we also noticed the improvement of the CT scan within a very short period of few days. The rapid resolution of radiological changes suggests that the pathological changes in the brain parenchyma in hyperglycemic nonketotic chorea are rapidly reversing.

Conclusion

The patient had poorly controlled diabetes without any complications, suggesting that chorea might not be related to microvascular or macrovascular complications of diabetes. This is a rare manifestation of diabetes in Sri lanka and diagnosing this rare entity will direct clinicians to achieve optimum glycemic control as the treatment which will lead to rapid clinical response without any other medications. In this case report we high light that with the clinical improvement, repeating a CT scan even after a very short period like 2 weeks will show rapid radiological resolution. This repeat imaging can also be useful to confirm the diagnosis, which will minimize unnecessary investigations and treatments. Further case reports and case series of hyperglycemic nonketotic chorea with brain imaging performed within short intervals is needed to evaluate the nature of rapid radiological changes which will be useful to understand the pathology of this condition.

Abbreviations
MRI: Magnetic Resonance Imaging; NCCT: Non-Contrast Computerized Tomography

Acknowledgements
This case report was supported by doctors working in ward 16, national hospital of Sri Lanka, in acquisition, analysis and interpretation of data.

Funding
This case report received no specific grant from any funding agency in the public, commercial, or not-for-profit sectors.

Authors' contributions
Dr. HMMTBH collected data, followed up the patient and did the literature review and designed,drafted the manuscript. Dr. SPP assisted in the literature review, analyzing, and designed, drafted the manuscript. Dr. SS is the consultant managing the patient and collected data, followed up the patient and designed, drafted the manuscript. All authors read and approved the final manuscript.

Consent for publication
Written informed consent was obtained from the patient for publication of this case report and any accompanying images. A copy of the written consent is available for review by the Editor-in-Chief of this journal.

Competing interests
The Authors declare that there they have no competing interest.

References
1. Oh SH, et al. Chorea associated with non-ketotic hyperglycemia and hyperintensity basal ganglia lesion on T1-weighted brain MRI study: a meta-analysis of 53 cases including four present cases. J Neurol Sci. 2002;200(1–2): 57–62.
2. Chang KH, et al. Temporal features of magnetic resonance imaging and spectroscopy in non-ketotic hyperglycemic chorea-ballism patients. Eur J Neurol. 2010;17(4):589–93.
3. Lai PH, et al. Chorea-ballismus with nonketotic hyperglycemia in primary diabetes mellitus. AJNR Am J Neuroradiol. 1996;17(6):1057–64.
4. Cherian A, et al. Concepts and controversies in nonketotic hyperglycemia-induced hemichorea: further evidence from susceptibility-weighted MR imaging. J Magn Reson Imaging. 2009;29(3):699–703.
5. Lin JJ, et al. Presentation of striatal hyperintensity on T1-weighted MRI in patients with hemiballism-hemichorea caused by non-ketotic hyperglycemia: report of seven new cases and a review of literature. J Neurol. 2001;248(9):750–5.
6. *Chromoblastomycosis.* Urol Cutaneous Rev. 1946;50(6):341–3.

12

Radiographic features of Ollier's disease

Jamshid Sadiqi[1,3*], Najibullah Rasouly[1†], Hidayatullah Hamidi[1†] and Salahuddin Siraj[2†]

Abstract

Background: Ollier's disease is a non-hereditary, benign bone tumor which is usually characterized by presence of multiple radiolucent lesions (enchondromas) in the metaphysis of long bones with unilateral predominance. The disease is a rare clinical entity with 1/100000 occurrence in early childhood. Patients mostly present with multiple hard swellings and deformity of the tubular bones specially hands and feet with leg discrepancy and pathologic fractures.

Case presentation: We present two cases of Ollier's disease in a 13 years old female and 8 years old boy which had no specific symptoms. The girl had multiple hard swellings and deformity in the fingers of both hands and left toes with left leg deformity and discrepancy. Her plain radiographs demonstrated multiple expansile enchondromas in the phalanges of hands, left toes and metaphyses of upper humeri as well as left leg bones. The enchondromas were also noted in the left iliac bone and anterior end of ribs. The boy had bowing deformity and shortage of left leg with multiple enchondromas in the metaphyses of left femur, left tibia and fibula as well as left iliac bone in his radiographic images.

Conclusion: Ollier's disease is usually diagnosed by clinical signs and typical location of enchondromas across skeleton in conventional radiography. It usually does not need specific treatment. Well understanding of the clinical manifestation and radiographic features can prevent unnecessary application of other imaging modalities; while other diagnostic imaging modalities like MRI, ultrasound and scintigraphy can be used in complicated and painful conditions.

Keywords: Multiple enchondromatosis, Enchondromas, Tubular bones, Metaphysis, Bone deformity, Conventional radiography

Background

Multiple enchondromatosis is a rare bone disease with six subtypes. Ollier's disease is a non-hereditary subtype of the disease which for the first time was introduced by Ollier in 1899 [1, 2]. It is characterized by presence of at least three enchondromas in the appendicular bones. The disease prevalence is 1/100000 of population with almost equal sex distribution and early manifestation in first decade of life [1–3]. The patients usually present with multiple hard swellings in the fingers and toes associated with asymmetric deformity of the extremities [4]. The plain radiographs of the affected bones demonstrate various number, size and location of enchondromas in the metaphyses of tubular bones with extension into the diaphyseal and epiphyseal regions [2]. Some of these enchondromas may show expansile behavior called enchondromas protuberance. Clusters of enchondromas cause widening of the metaphyseal regions. In the lower extremities the lesions may result in bone deformity and limb discrepancy. Punctate calcifications with light trabeculations are also seen in the metaphysis of long bones [5]. Sometimes Pelvis bone especially the iliac crest is involved but sternum, ribs and skull bones are rarely affected [1]. In one of the present cases, the enchondromas exist in the anterior ribs representing a rare location of the disease.

* Correspondence: jamshid.sadiqi@fmic.org.af
†Equal contributors
[1]Radiology Department of French Medical Institute for Mothers and Children (FMIC), Kabul, Afghanistan
[3]Radiology Department, French Medical Institute for Mothers & Children (FMIC), behind Kabul Medical University Aliabad, P.O. Box: 472, Kabul, Afghanistan
Full list of author information is available at the end of the article

Case presentation

First case

A-13 year old girl was referred to the radiology department of French Medical Institute for Mothers and Children (FMIC) for taking plain radiographs of the axial and appendicular bones. The patient had short left leg with abnormal swelling and deformity of fingers and left toes. The swelling

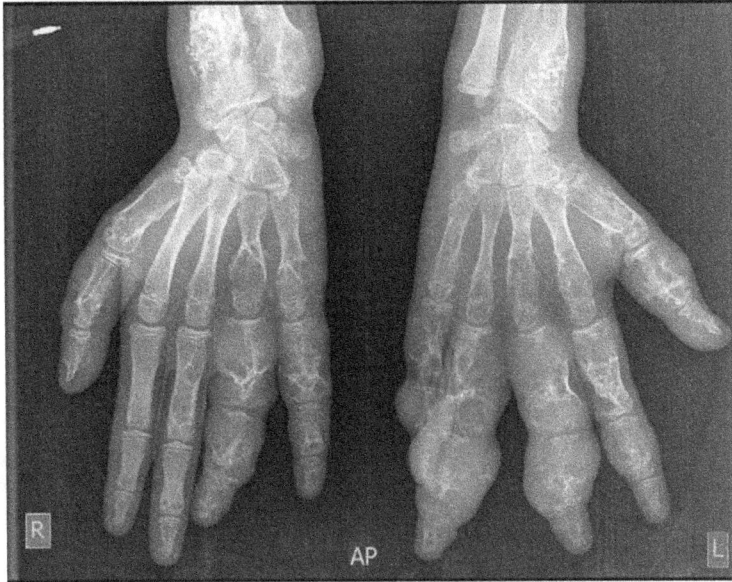

Fig. 1 Multiple expansile lytic lesions in the metacarpi and phalanges of both hands with sparing of right index finger and lytic lesions in the right distal radius and ulna with sparing of the left ulna

were hard in palpation however no pain was noticed. The overlying skin appeared normal. In radiographic images, multiple expansile lytic lesions (enchondromas) were noted in the metacarpi and phalanges of hands with sparing of the index finger of right hand associated with multiple lytic lesions in the distal ulna and radius of both hands with sparing of left distal ulna (Fig. 1). Chest plain image demonstrated multiple enchondromas in the anterior end of the ribs bilaterally as well as proximal metaphyses of both humeri, extending into right humerus diaphysis with multiple punctate like calcifications (Fig. 2). Enchondromas were also noted in the metatarsi and toes of left foot, left distal tibia and fibula in plain image of left foot (Fig. 3). Multiple lytic lesions with punctate

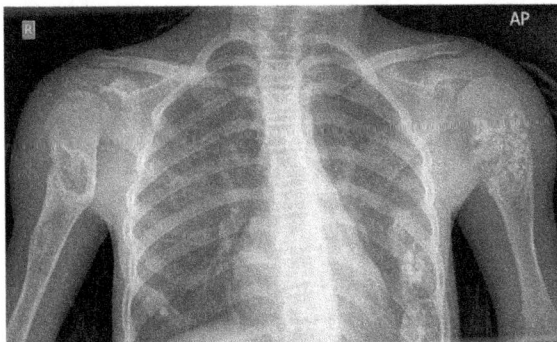

Fig. 2 AP chest x-ray shows multiple lytic lesions with punctate calcifications in the anterior end of ribs and proximal metaphyses of both humeri extending to the diaphysis of right humerus

calcifications were also seen in the left iliac bone and proximal metaphysis of left femur in anterior posterior radiograph of pelvis bone (Fig. 4). Plain image of left calf showed multiple foci of calcifications with lytic lesion in the left distal femur as well as proximal and distal metaphyses of left tibia and fibula (Fig. 5).

Second case

An 8 year-old boy was referred to our radiology department for taking radiographs of left leg and pelvis bones. The patient had left leg discrepancy with bowing deformity without specific pain. The lateral radiograph of the left leg demonstrates bowing deformity with enchondromas in the distal femur as well as proximal and distal ends of left tibia and fibula (Fig. 6). The anterior posterior radiograph of pelvis and both lower extremities showed lytic lesions in the proximal and distal ends of left femur, tibia, fibula and left iliac bone with deformity and significant left leg discrepancy (Fig. 7).

Discussion and conclusion

The etiology of Ollier's disease is not well known however abnormal signaling pathways in the proliferation and differentiation of chondrocytes have been proposed which results in the development of intraosseous cartilaginous foci. Some authors have indicated genetic aberrations like heterozygous mutations of PTHR1, IDH1 and IDH2 genes as the pathogenesis of the disease [3]. The disease has specific radiographic features representing unilateral involvement with presence of multiple lytic lesions in the center of tubular bones of hand, foot

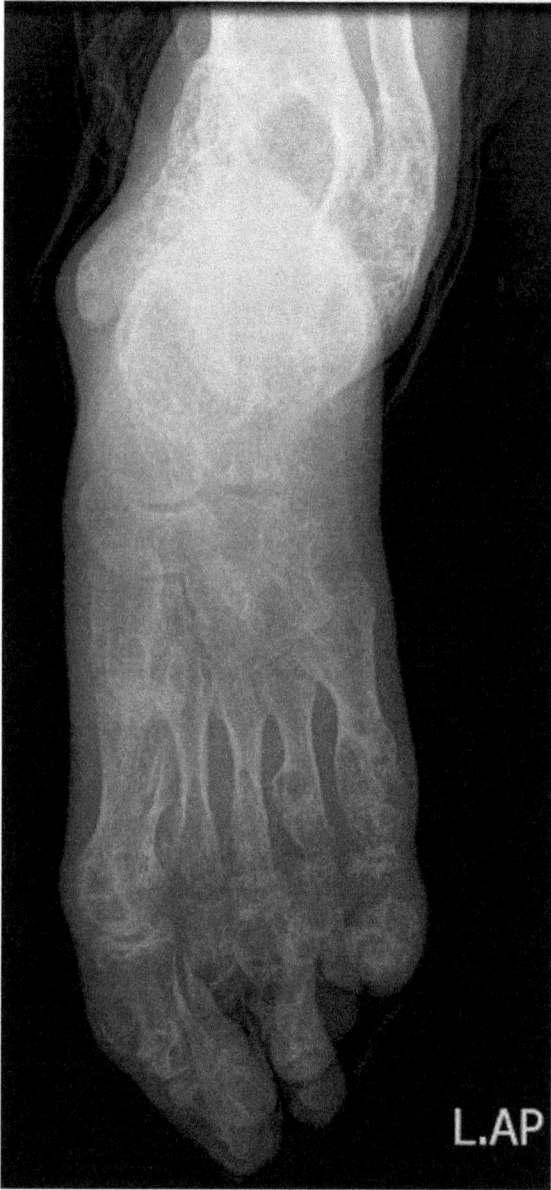

Fig. 3 Anterior posterior x-ray of left foot: Multiple expansile lytic lesions in the metatarsi and toes of left foot with bone deformity and lytic lesions in the metaphysis of distal tibia and fibula

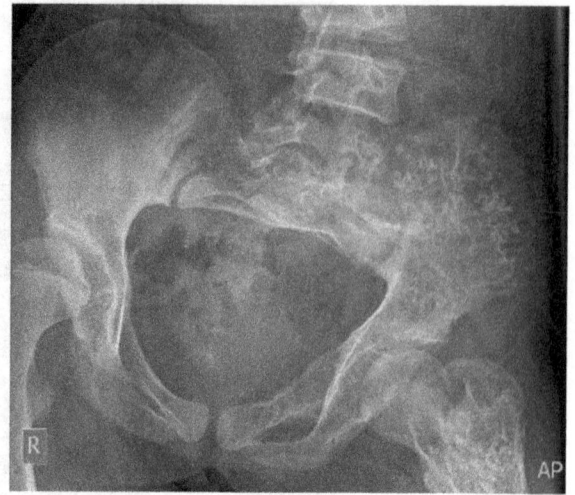

Fig. 4 Multiple lytic lesions with punctate calcifications in the left iliac bone and proximal metaphysis of left femur

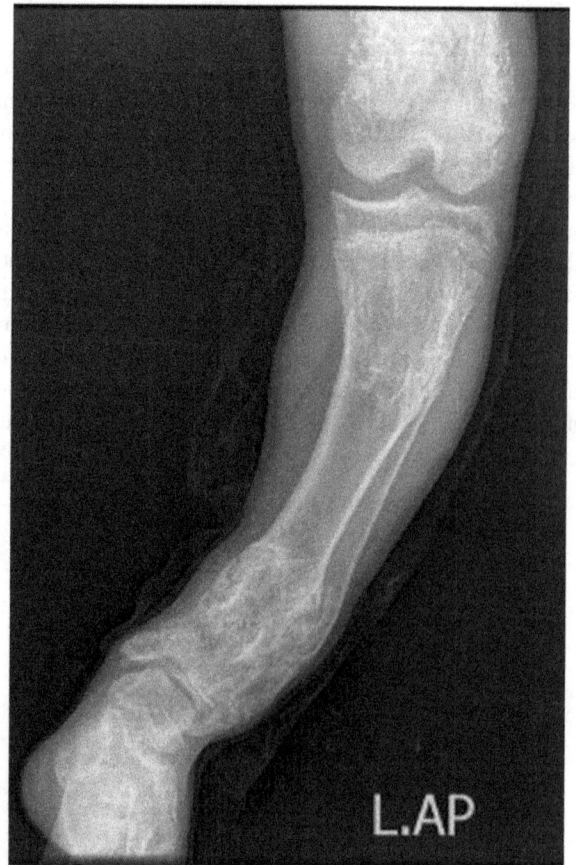

Fig. 5 Anterior posterior x-ray of left leg: lytic lesions in the proximal and distal metaphyses of left tibia and fibula

and long bones particularly in metaphyseal regions. Sometimes there is symmetrical involvement but still with unilateral predominance. Occasionally during the course of the disease pathologic fractures may occur due to the cortical thinning [2]. Ultrasound, Magnetic Resonance Imaging (MRI) and Scintigraphy are used when the lesions increase in size and causing pain. MRI shows lobulated lesions in the affected bones returning intermediate signal intensity in T1 with intermediate to high signal intensity in T2 weighted images [1]. In bone scan multiple foci of radiotracer uptakes are appreciated

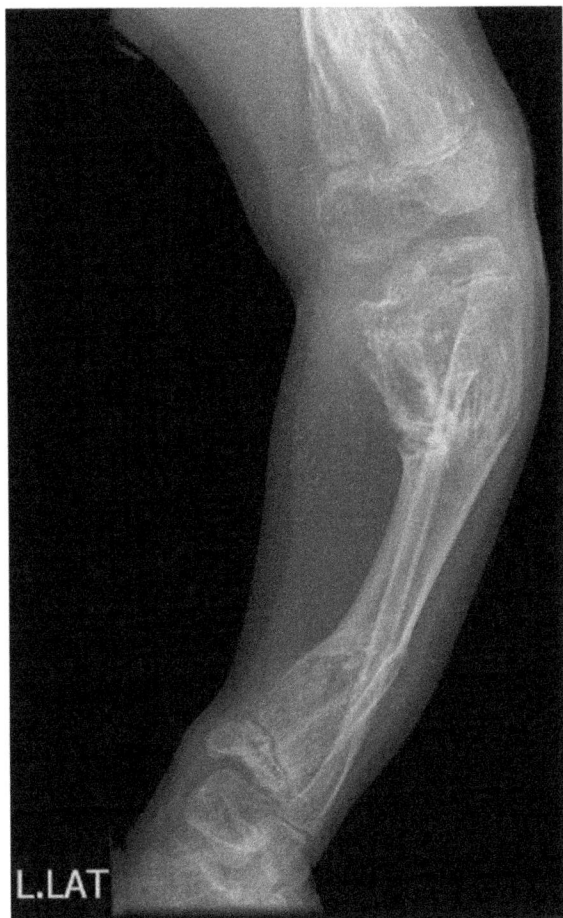

Fig. 6 Lateral radiograph of left lower limb: bone deformity with multiple lytic lesions in the upper and lower metaphyses of tibia and fibula as well as distal end of femur

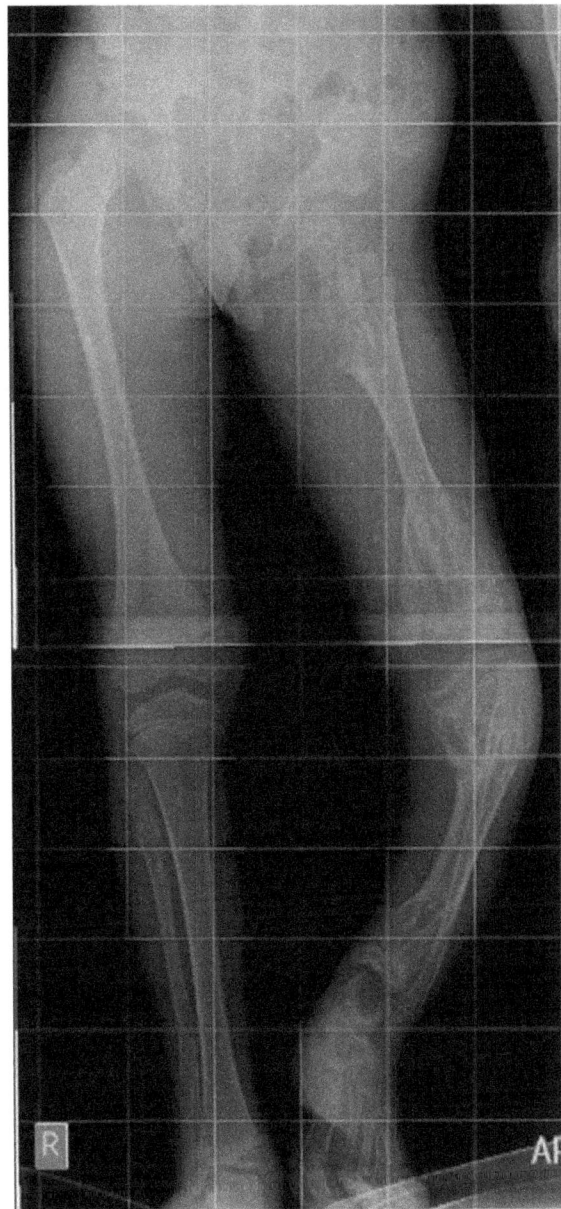

Fig. 7 Anterior-posterior radiograph of pelvis and both lower limbs: enchondromas in the upper and lower ends of left femur, tibia, fibula as well as left iliac crest with left lower limb discrepancy and bowing deformity

mainly in the tubular bones [2].The complication of enchondromatosis is its malignant transformation into the chondrosarcoma which can result in cortical erosion and infiltration into the adjacent soft tissues with indistinguishable and irregular outline of the tumor surface [4]. The differential diagnosis of the Ollier's disease is hereditary multiple exostosis in which the lesions are usually located in the surface of bones rather than in the center (lesions are located in the center of the bones in enchondromatosis) [1]. Another type of multiple enchondromatosis is called Mafucci syndrome which is characterized with presence of multiple enchondromas associated with soft tissue hemangiomas and occasionally lymphangiomas [4]. As the diagnosis of multiple enchondromatosis is based on the clinical features and specific radiographic manifestations therefore the histopathologic examinations are not usually preformed. In cases when malignant transformation is suspected histopathologic exams are necessary. The literature has

indicated a 35% progression into the chondrosarcomas [6, 7]. Asymptomatic patients of multiple enchondromatosis do not need medical or surgical treatments but in cases of growth defects, pathologic fractures and malignant transformation surgical intervention is performed [4]. Radiotherapy and chemotherapy are also advised in cases of malignant transformation [8]. It is concluded that Ollier's disease is a benign bone tumor which is well diagnosed by its unique clinical and radiographic manifestations.

Acknowledgments
We thank Dr. Jamshid Jalal head of pathology department of FMIC for helping us in sending our manuscript for this journal. We also thank the radiographers of FMIC for taking good quality images.

Funding
No financial support was provided for this study.

Authors' contributions
JS reviewed the literature, drafted the manuscript, editing the manuscript according to journal policy and being the corresponding, NS reviewed the manuscript and brought the necessary changes, HH and SS also did the literature review and helped in writing the manuscript and providing the images. All authors read and approved the final manuscript.

Consent for publication
Written informed consent was obtained from the patients' fathers for publication of these case reports and accompanying images. A copy of the written consent will be available for review by the Editor-in-Chief of this journal on request.

Competing interests
The authors declare that they have no competing interests.

Author details
[1]Radiology Department of French Medical Institute for Mothers and Children (FMIC), Kabul, Afghanistan. [2]Orthopedic Department of French Medical Institute for Mothers and Children (FMIC), Kabul, Afghanistan. [3]Radiology Department, French Medical Institute for Mothers & Children (FMIC), behind Kabul Medical University Aliabad, P.O. Box: 472, Kabul, Afghanistan.

References
1. Kumar A, Jain VK, Bharadwaj M, Arya RK. Ollier disease: pathogenesis, diagnosis, and management. Orthopedics. 2015;38(6):e497–506.
2. Fallahi B, Bostani M, Gilani KA, Beiki D, Gholamrezanezhad A. Manifestations of Ollier's disease in a 21-year-old man: a case report. J Med Case Rep. 2009;3(1):7759.
3. Silve C, Jüppner H. Ollier disease. Orphanet J Rare Dis. 2006;1(1):37.
4. George S, Ravi Hoisala V, Cicilet S, Sadashiva S. Multiple Enchondromatosis: Olliers disease-a case report. J Clin Diagn Res. 2016;10(1):TD01.
5. Adam O, Boia E, Mandrusca R, Mejdi R. Enchondroma-tosis-Ollier disease case-report. Jurnalul Pediatrilui. 2009:47-8.
6. Schwartz HERBERTS, Zimmerman NB, Simon MA, Wroble RR, Millar EA, Bonfiglio M. The malignant potential of enchondromatosis. J Bone Joint Surg Am. 1987;69(2):269–74.
7. Pansuriya TC, Oosting J, Krenács T, Taminiau AH, Verdegaal SH, Sangiorgi L, et al. Genome-wide analysis of Ollier disease: Is it all in the genes?. Orphanet J Rare Dis. 2011;6(1):2.
8. Shaheen, Feroze, Nisar Ahmad, Tariq Gojwari, M. Ashraf Teli, Riyaz Resold, and Manjeet Singh. "Multiple Enchondromatosis: Ollier's Disease." (2010).

13

Desmoid-type fibromatosis mimicking cystic retroperitoneal mass

Kyu-Chong Lee[1], Jongmee Lee[1]* 🅓, Baek Hui Kim[2], Kyeong Ah Kim[1] and Cheol Min Park[1]

Abstract

Background: Retroperitoneal desmoid-type fibromatosis (DF) is an uncommon mesenchymal neoplasm presenting as a firm mass with locally aggressive features. It usually manifests as a well-circumscribed or ill-defined, solid mass on cross-sectional imaging. Cystic changes of DF have been described in the literature in association with prolonged medical treatment or abscess formation. However, spontaneous cystic change is rarely reported.

Case presentation: Here we report the case of a 46-year-old patient with a DF mimicked a large cystic tumor in the retroperitoneum. Ultrasonography and computed tomography were performed in order to search for localizations and characteristics of the cystic tumor. Radiological findings showed an oval cystic mass with a relatively thick wall, measuring 18.3 × 12.3 × 21.5 cm in the left upper abdomen. Laparoscopic spleen-preserving distal pancreatectomy was performed and histopathological examination by immunohistochemical study enabled us to diagnose a DF invading the pancreatic parenchyma. The patient remained asymptomatic during an 8-month follow up period.

Conclusions: We report an extremely rare case of retroperitoneal DF with spontaneous cystic change. DF can manifest as a mainly cystic mass with a thick wall, as in our case, which makes the correct diagnosis difficult. DF should be included in the preoperative differential diagnosis of a cystic retroperitoneal mass, regardless of its rarity.

Keywords: Desmoid-type fibromatosis, Desmoid tumor, Retroperitoneum, Ultrasonography, Computed tomography

Background

Desmoid-type fibromatosis (DF), also called desmoid tumor or deep fibromatosis, is an uncommon mesenchymal neoplasm composed of fibrous soft-tissue proliferation. The tumor is characterized by locally aggressive growth and frequent recurrence, although it never metastasizes [1]. DF usually occurs sporadically, but approximately 5% arise in association with familial adenomatous polyposis (FAP) [2]. Retroperitoneal DF is rare and accounts for less than 1% of retroperitoneal masses [3].

DF usually presents as a well-circumscribed solid mass on imaging studies [4]. Cystic changes of DF are rare and a few reports have suggested an association with prolonged medical treatment or abscess formation [5, 6]. Spontaneous cystic degeneration in DF is extremely rare

* Correspondence: jongmee.lee@gmail.com
[1]Department of Radiology, Korea University Guro Hospital, Korea University College of Medicine, 80 Guro-dong, Guro-gu, Seoul 152-703, South Korea
Full list of author information is available at the end of the article

and only a few reports of such masses have been published [7–9]. Most of them were small lesions (less than 10 cm) presenting as pancreatic or mesenteric cystic tumors.

We report here an unusual case of sporadic retroperitoneal DF with spontaneous cystic change mimicking a cystic tumor, including histopathologic correlations.

Case presentation

A 46-year-old man visited the emergency department of our institution due to left lower quadrant pain and a palpable mass in the left upper abdomen. He had no specific relevant past medical history or family history. Physical examination disclosed a large, tender mass in the left abdomen. All laboratory findings were within normal ranges except a slightly increased CRP level (5.82 mg/L). Abdominal plain radiographs showed a large mass-like opacity in the left abdomen (Fig. 1a). Ultrasonography revealed a large, thick-walled cystic mass without evidence of an intracystic

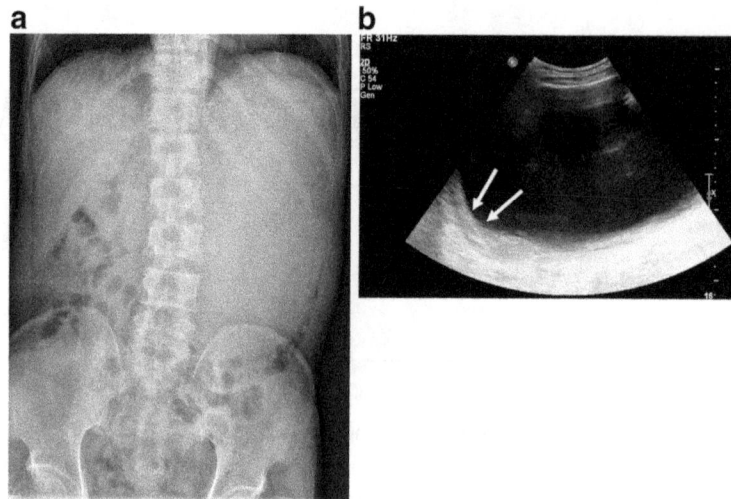

Fig. 1 Retroperitoneal desmoid-type fibromatosis in a 46-year-old man. **a** Abdominal plain radiography shows a large mass-like opacity in the left abdomen. **b** The ultrasonography shows a large anechoic cystic mass with a thick wall (arrows) without an intracystic solid portion or septum in the left abdomen

solid portion or septum (Fig. 1b). The patient underwent computed tomography (CT) scans to evaluate the intra-abdominal mass using a 64-slice multidetector CT scanner. Contrast-enhanced CT images revealed an $18.3 \times 12.3 \times 21.5$ cm sized oval cystic mass with a relatively thick wall in the left upper abdomen (Fig. 2). This lesion caused an extrinsic mass effect on the adjacent stomach and pancreas. The boundary between the mass and adjacent pancreas parenchyma was indistinct. Based on these imaging findings, a neurogenic tumor with cystic changes, a mucinous cystadenoma, and a pseudocyst were considered in the differential diagnoses. The patient underwent laparoscopic

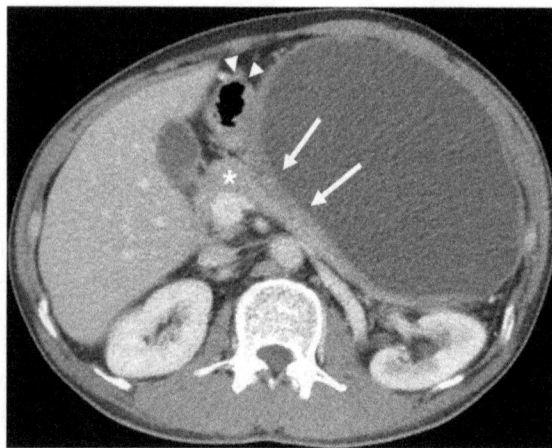

Fig. 2 Retroperitoneal desmoid-type fibromatosis in a 46-year-old man. Axial image of CT shows an $18.3 \times 12.3 \times 21.5$ cm sized oval cystic mass with a thick wall (arrows) that has a mass effect on the stomach (arrowheads) and pancreas (asterisk). There is no evidence of an enhancing septum or a solid portion within the cystic mass

spleen-preserving distal pancreatectomy without preoperative biopsy due to a risk of rupture.

Intra-operatively, the mass was confirmed to have arisen from the retroperitoneum, closely related to the pancreas tail. Surgeons found hemorrhagic fluid within the cystic mass. The surgical specimen was a large round lump of soft tissue measuring $13 \times 10.5 \times 4.3$ cm in size. On gross section, the cut surface revealed a rubbery texture with a whitish to light yellowish color. Almost half of the mass was composed of a cystic space that was filled with clear, light brownish fluid. The mass was diffusely infiltrating the pancreatic parenchyma. Microscopically, the tumor was composed of uniform sheets of elongated, spindle-shaped cells in a collagenous stroma (Fig. 3a). The tumor was intermingled with the pancreatic parenchyma (Fig. 3b). Immunohistochemical study showed the tumor cells were positive for smooth muscle actin (SMA) and beta-catenin (Fig. 3c), but negative for S-100 protein and CD34. The final pathologic diagnosis was DF. The postoperative course was uneventful, and the patient was discharged on postoperative day 20. The patient remained asymptomatic during an 8-month follow up period.

Discussion

The term "fibromatosis" describes a group of conditions that consist of fibroblastic proliferation in a collagenous extracellular matrix. Fibromatosis can be either superficial (fascial) or deep (musculoaponeurotic). In 2002, the World Health Organization (WHO) used the term 'desmoid-type fibromatosis' for deep fibromatosis [10], which is usually called a desmoid tumor. It can be further classified on the basis of its anatomic location, such as abdominal wall, intra-abdominal, or extra-abdominal. In various studies, 28

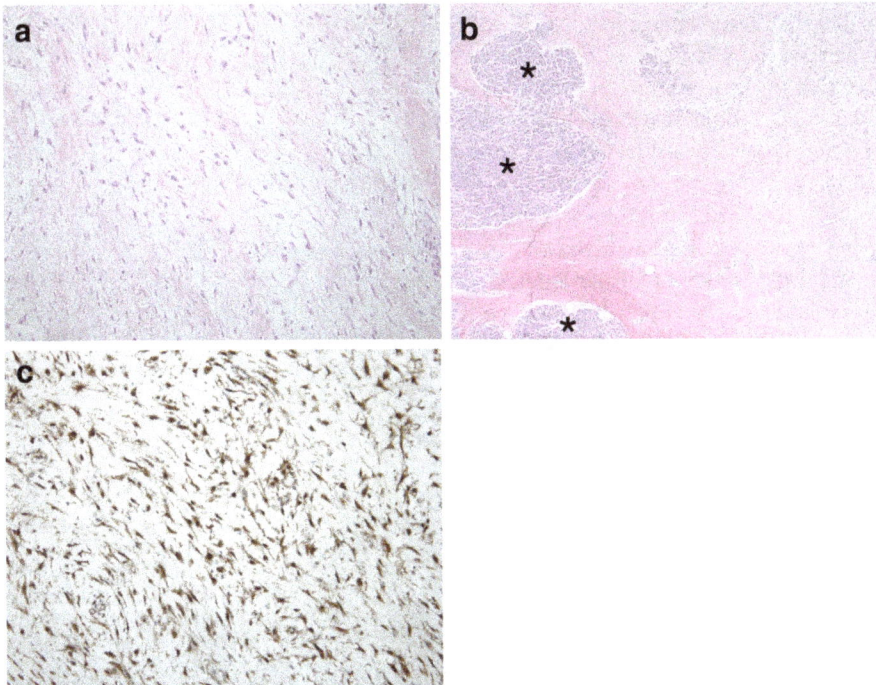

Fig. 3 Retroperitoneal desmoid-type fibromatosis in a 46-year-old man. **a** Microscopically, the tumor is composed of uniform, elongated spindle-shaped cells within a collagenous stroma. Spindle cells show mild nuclear pleomorphism and no mitotic figures (hematoxylin and eosin stain; original magnification ×100). **b** On a lower power view, tumor cells are diffusely infiltrating into the pancreatic parenchyma (asterisks) (hematoxylin and eosin stain; original magnification ×40). **c** Immunohistochemical study of the tumor shows strong nuclear and cytoplasmic positivity for intranuclear β-catenin (β-catenin; original magnification ×100)

to 69% of DF was intra-abdominal (mesenteric or pelvic) or located in the abdominal wall [11]. Retroperitoneal DF accounts for less than 1% of retroperitoneal masses [3]. Multiple risk factors for DF are widely known, including genetic mutations of the adenomatous polyposis coli (APC) gene such as in FAP or the beta-catenin gene (CTNNB1), previous surgery, trauma, pregnancy, and oral contraceptive use [11, 12]. However, the pathogenesis of DF is not completely understood.

DF is more common in young women, from puberty to 40 years of age [1]. However, intra-abdominal fibromatosis shows no gender difference or age predilection [10]. Most patients present with an asymptomatic abdominal mass, but some have mild abdominal pain. Although less common, patients with mesenteric lesions are accompanied by gastrointestinal bleeding or acute abdominal pain secondary to bowel perforation [4].

Histologically, DF is composed of elongated, uniform spindle cells within a collagenous stroma. Although DF appears well-delineated at gross analysis and cross-sectional imaging, at the microscopic level its margins appear to infiltrate the adjacent structures. Immunohistochemically, the tumor cells are negative for CD34, CD117, and S-100 protein [1]. These findings exclude gastrointestinal stromal tumors and neurogenic tumors. Immunoreactivity for β-catenin supports the diagnosis of DF but is not

pathognomonic for this disease because other entities, including superficial fibromatosis, low-grade myofibroblastic sarcomas, and solitary fibrous tumors, may also exhibit nuclear staining for β-catenin [13].

DF usually appears as a well-defined solid mass on imaging studies. The ultrasonographic appearance of DF is a solid, usually well-circumscribed and hypoechoic mass of variable vascularity [4, 11]. On CT, DF appears as a soft tissue mass of variable attenuation and enhancement, which depends on tissue components [3, 4]. DF with a highly collagenous stroma usually displays homogeneous, soft-tissue attenuation on CT scans. DF with a myxoid matrix appears as a hypoattenuating lesion. Some lesions may appear striated or whorled because of the alternating collagenous and myxoid area. Heterogeneous attenuation may be seen due to necrosis or degeneration. The soft-tissue component is such a dominant feature that it often appears similar to solid tumors, such as gastrointestinal stromal tumor, lymphoma, or soft tissue sarcoma [4]. DF has invasive properties and tends to damage blood vessels.

Cystic changes of DF have been rarely reported and an association with prolonged medical treatment or abscess formation has been suggested [5, 6]. However, these causal relationships are irrelevant in this case because our patient was male and there was no evidence of abscess formation in DF on histopathologic examination. Tan et al. [9] postulated that cystic appearance of DF was the result of spontaneous tumor regression. Spontaneous regression of DF is thought to be related to the withdrawal of estrogenic stimulation and could also result from secondary infarction of either superimposed infection or compromised vascular supply to the tumor. DF has an invasive nature and tends to cause vascular compromise. Furthermore, ischemia during rapid tumor growth may be the cause of extensive cystic degeneration of DF. An infarction secondary to a compromised vascular supply may be a possible cause of cystic degeneration in DF in our case. However, it is difficult to explain this extensive cystic change.

In the present case, cystic DF invasion to the pancreas was confirmed by pathology. Only 13 cases have been reported of intra-abdominal DF involving the pancreas [8, 14]. Nine out of 13 cases involved the pancreatic tail, similar to our case. For DF involving the pancreas, which usually appears as a solid mass, only two cases have been considered purely cystic and four cases appeared as mixed cystic and solid masses. DF begins as small scar-like foci of fibrosis in the retroperitoneal fat and, when large, it typically spreads around and between other structures [15]. Therefore, retroperitoneal DF may involve the pancreas and can be interpreted as a pancreas-originating lesion.

A multidisciplinary approach can help patients with DF receive optimal management. Stable, asymptomatic DF can be observed. However, treatment is necessary for symptomatic subjects like our patient. If feasible, surgical excision is regarded as the conventional treatment of choice. However, recurrence is common. The recurrence rate is 15–30% for intra-abdominal DF [11].

Conclusion

We report an extremely rare case of retroperitoneal DF with spontaneous cystic change. It can manifest as a mainly cystic mass with a thick wall, as in our case, that makes it difficult to reach a correct diagnosis. DF should be included in the preoperative differential diagnosis of a cystic retroperitoneal mass, regardless of its rarity.

Abbreviations
APC: Adenomatous polyposis coli; CRP: C-reactive protein; CT: Computed tomography; DF: Desmoid-type fibromatosis; FAP: Familial adenomatous polyposis; SMA: Smooth muscle actin

Funding
This study was supported by a Korea University Grant (K1132871).

Authors' contributions
KL and JL collected and analyzed the patient data and performed the background literature review. KL drafted part of the case presentation and provided manuscript revisions. JL interpreted the data and performed manuscript revisions. KAK participated in the acquisition and interpretation of radiologic images. BHK performed histopathological specimen analysis, prepare the part of the case presentation. KAK and CMP were involved in overall supervision of the case and manuscript. All authors read and approved the final manuscript.

Consent for publication
The patient provided written informed consent for publication of this case report and any accompanying images.

Competing interests
The authors declare that they have no competing interests.

Author details
[1]Department of Radiology, Korea University Guro Hospital, Korea University College of Medicine, 80 Guro-dong, Guro-gu, Seoul 152-703, South Korea. [2]Department of Pathology, Korea University Guro Hospital, Korea University College of Medicine, Seoul, South Korea.

References
1. Goldblum JR, Fletcher JA. Desmoid-type fibromatoses. In: Fletcher CDM, Bridge JA, Hogendoorn PCW, Mertens F, editors. WHO classification of tumors of soft tissue and bone. 4th ed. Lyon: IARC Press; 2013. p. 72–3.
2. Latchford AR, Sturt NJ, Neale K, Rogers PA, Phillips RK. A 10-year review of surgery for desmoid disease associated with familial adenomatous polyposis. Br J Surg. 2006;93:1258–64.
3. Rajiah P, Sinha R, Cuevas C, Dubinsky TJ, Bush WH Jr, Kolokythas O. Imaging of uncommon retroperitoneal masses. Radiographics. 2011;31:949–76.
4. Levy AD, Rimola J, Mehrotra AK, Sobin LH. From the archives of the AFIP: benign fibrous tumors and tumorlike lesions of the mesentery: radiologic-pathologic correlation. Radiographics. 2006;26:245–64.
5. Nakada I, Kawasaki S, Ubukata H, Goto Y, Watanabe Y, Sato S, et al. Transperitoneal drainage for a large cystic degeneration after regression of an intra-abdominal desmoid tumor. Dis Colon Rectum. 2000;43:717–9.
6. Cholongitas E, Koulenti D, Panetsos G, Kafiri G, Tzirakis E, Thalasinou P, et al. Desmoid tumor presenting as intra-abdominal abscess. Dig Dis Sci. 2006;51:68–9.
7. Ko SW, Lee JS. Mesenteric fibromatosis with spontaneous cystic degeneration. J Korean Radiol Soc. 2002;46:179–82.
8. Hsueh C, Lin CY, Huang YC, Ho SY, Lee KW, Liu CK. Desmoid mimicking cystic pancreatic lesion: a case report. J Radiol Sci. 2014;39:91–5.
9. Tan CH, Pua U, Liau KH, Lee HY. Mesenteric desmoid tumour masquerading as a fat-containing cystic mass. Br J Radiol. 2010;83:e200–3.
10. George V, Tammisetti VS, Surabhi VR, Shanbhogue AK. Chronic fibrosing conditions in abdominal imaging. Radiographics. 2013;33:1053–80.
11. Shinagare AB, Ramaiya NH, Jagannathan JP, Krajewski KM, Giardino AA, Butrynski JE, et al. A to Z of desmoid tumors. AJR Am J Roentgenol. 2011; 197:W1008–14.
12. Escobar C, Munker R, Thomas JO, Li BD, Burton GV. Update on desmoid tumors. Ann Oncol. 2012;23:562–9.
13. Braschi-Amirfarzan M, Keraliya AR, Krajewski KM, Tirumani SH, Shinagare AB, Hornick JL, et al. Role of imaging in Management of Desmoid-type Fibromatosis: a primer for radiologists. Radiographics. 2016;36:767–82.
14. Xu B, Zhu LH, Wu JG, Wang XF, Matro E, Ni JJ. Pancreatic solid cystic desmoid tumor: case report and literature review. World J Gastroenterol. 2013;19:8793–8.
15. Giardiello FM, Burt RW, Jarvinen HJ, Offerhaus GJA. Familial adenomatous polyposis. In: Bosman FT, Carneiro F, Hruban RH, Theise ND, editors. WHO classification of Tumours of the digestive system. 4th ed. Lyon: IARC Press; 2010. p. 147–51.

14

Evaluation of magnetic nanoparticle samples made from biocompatible ferucarbotran by time-correlation magnetic particle imaging reconstruction method

Yasutoshi Ishihara[1*†], Takumi Honma[2†], Satoshi Nohara[3] and Yoshio Ito[3]

Abstract

Background: Molecular imaging using magnetic nanoparticles (MNPs)—magnetic particle imaging (MPI)—has attracted interest for the early diagnosis of cancer and cardiovascular disease. However, because a steep local magnetic field distribution is required to obtain a defined image, sophisticated hardware is required. Therefore, it is desirable to realize excellent image quality even with low-performance hardware. In this study, the spatial resolution of MPI was evaluated using an image reconstruction method based on the correlation information of the magnetization signal in a time domain and by applying MNP samples made from biocompatible ferucarbotran that have adjusted particle diameters.

Methods: The magnetization characteristics and particle diameters of four types of MNP samples made from ferucarbotran were evaluated. A numerical analysis based on our proposed method that calculates the image intensity from correlation information between the magnetization signal generated from MNPs and the system function was attempted, and the obtained image quality was compared with that using the prototype in terms of image resolution and image artifacts.

Results: MNP samples obtained by adjusting ferucarbotran showed superior properties to conventional ferucarbotran samples, and numerical analysis showed that the same image quality could be obtained using a gradient magnetic field generator with 0.6 times the performance. However, because image blurring was included theoretically by the proposed method, an algorithm will be required to improve performance.

Conclusions: MNP samples obtained by adjusting ferucarbotran showed magnetizing properties superior to conventional ferucarbotran samples, and by using such samples, comparable image quality (spatial resolution) could be obtained with a lower gradient magnetic field intensity.

Keywords: Magnetic particle Imaging, MPI, Nanoparticle, Ferucarbotran, Resovist, Image reconstruction, Time correlation

* Correspondence: y_ishr@meiji.ac.jp
†Equal contributors
[1]School of Science and Technology, Meiji University, Higashimita Tama, Kawasaki, Kanagawa, Japan
Full list of author information is available at the end of the article

Background

Developments in nanotechnology have been exploited to realize innovative techniques for the diagnosis and treatment of diseases in the field of medicine. In particular, nanotechnology has been applied to drug delivery systems (DDSs) in which a nanoparticle, the surface of which is functionalized with various antibodies, is used to attack cancer cells; furthermore, cellular imaging using the light scattered by a nanoparticle has been actively studied [1]. Cancer treatment has also been attempted using nanoparticles with high sensitivity to light or heat [2,3]. Similarly, the use of magnetic nanoparticles (MNPs) has also been investigated. For example, in the thermal treatment of cancer, MNPs are used as heating elements to selectively heat a cancer cell [4]; in fact, clinical trials of this technique are now underway [5]. Gleich *et al.* reported magnetic particle imaging (MPI), a technique in which MNPs are applied to medical imaging [6,7]. MPI uses the harmonic components of the magnetization signal produced by the interaction between the nonlinear magnetizing properties of an MNP and the alternative magnetic field around the target body. In this technique, MNPs play the role of a contrast medium in blood vessels for the diagnosis of cardiovascular diseases and that of a tracer that images the distribution of MNPs accumulated in the cancer cell. Owing to its various advantages, MPI has attracted considerable research attention as a new diagnostic imaging modality.

The possibility of *in-vivo* real time imaging has already been demonstrated in a mouse [8]. However, a clinical MPI system for humans will require a large magnetic field generator to realize a magnetic field distribution with a steep slope, which is advantageous in identifying the position of an MNP and in obtaining a high-resolution image in MPI. To avoid this problem, the segmentation scanning of the objective region has been proposed as a workaround [9].

In order to realize a feasible clinical system, since 2007, we have focused our attention on developing a high-resolution MPI imaging system that does not require special, high-performance hardware. As a candidate procedure, we have proposed an image reconstruction method to improve the spatial resolution by reducing the interference signal produced around the target region [10]. Through the use of this method, local image artifacts and blurring could be suppressed. Moreover, we reported that the components of image blurring and artifacts could be suppressed based on the difference of the "saturation time" between the ideal magnetization

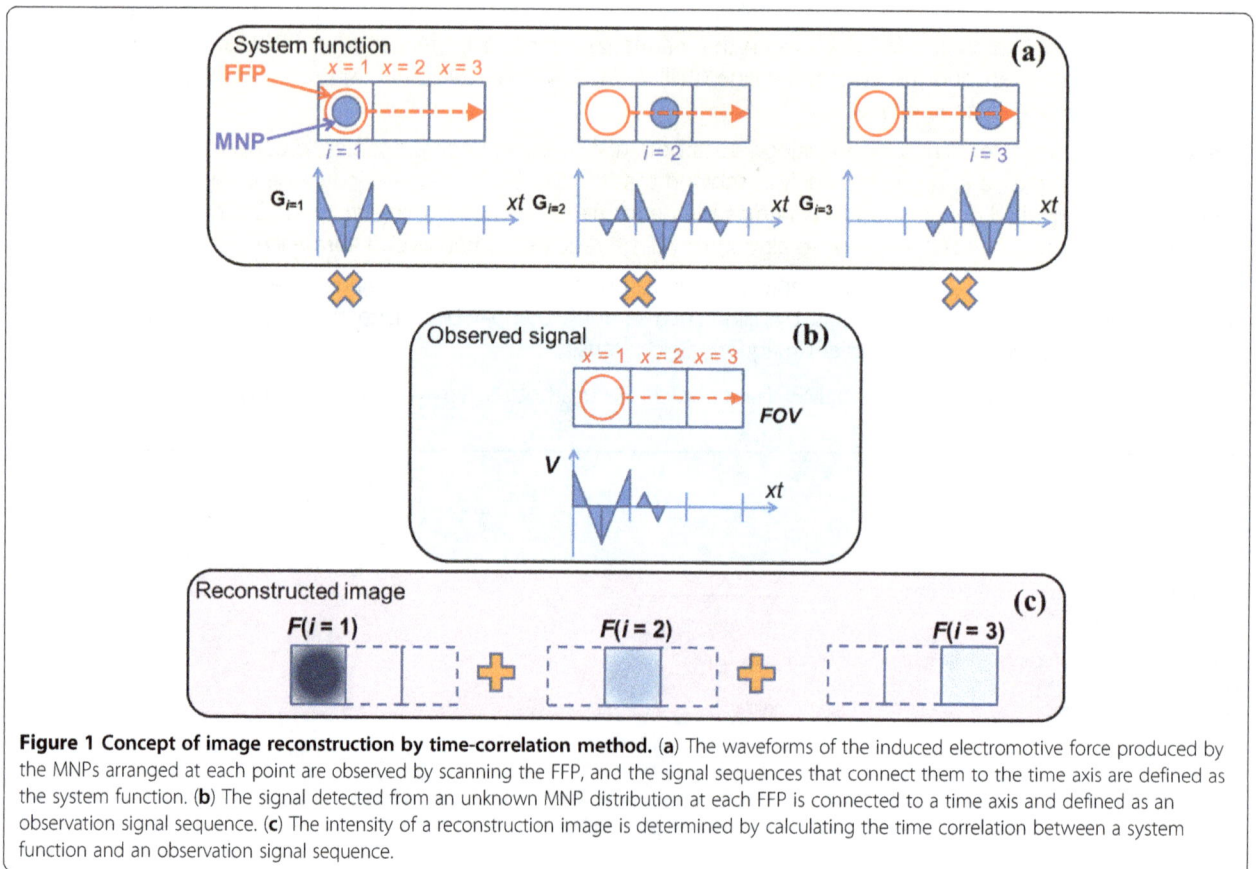

Figure 1 Concept of image reconstruction by time-correlation method. (a) The waveforms of the induced electromotive force produced by the MNPs arranged at each point are observed by scanning the FFP, and the signal sequences that connect them to the time axis are defined as the system function. **(b)** The signal detected from an unknown MNP distribution at each FFP is connected to a time axis and defined as an observation signal sequence. **(c)** The intensity of a reconstruction image is determined by calculating the time correlation between a system function and an observation signal sequence.

signal (corresponding to an impulse response or a point spread function (PSF) of the MPI system), which arises from an isolated MNP and the observed magnetization signal [11]. However, when MNPs are distributed continuously, it becomes difficult to obtain an accurate image of MNPs because of the enhancement of the image edge part, as noted previously. Therefore, we have proposed a new image reconstruction method and evaluated its validity [12]. In this method, the observed magnetization signal produced around a target region is extracted based on the correlation with a system function, and it can be reflected by the intensity of the reconstruction image. However, because the image reconstruction is performed based on a simple correlation, it tends to expand the image blurring theoretically. Therefore, it is necessary to remove the image blurring actively, and we are currently attempting to design an effective algorithm for this purpose [13].

Meanwhile, to improve the image resolution without requiring high-performance hardware, the characteristics of an MNP should be improved in parallel to the image quality improvement by such an image reconstruction method because the spatial broadening of the observed magnetization signal is approximated by the differentiation of the Langevin function [14]. Therefore, high spatial resolution is expected when the particle diameter of an MNP is large because the full width at half maximum (FWHM) of this differentiated waveform narrows with an increase in the particle diameter [15].

Currently, the ferucarbotran (a drug substances of Resovist; supplied only by Meito Sangyo Co., Ltd.) used as a contrast medium for magnetic resonance imaging (MRI) is being used in MPI. However, because the particle diameters of the MNPs contained in ferucarbotran differ, as already pointed out, it is not an optimal contrast medium for demonstrating the performance of MPI. Generally, if the influence of the relaxation time for the magnetization response is ignored, the magnetization properties of an MNP with large particle diameter are advantageous for MPI [16]. Therefore, a trial in which MNPs with large particle diameters are compounded efficiently using an organic solvent is performed [17]. However, sufficient information regarding the biocompatibility of most particles compounded by such processes is not available,

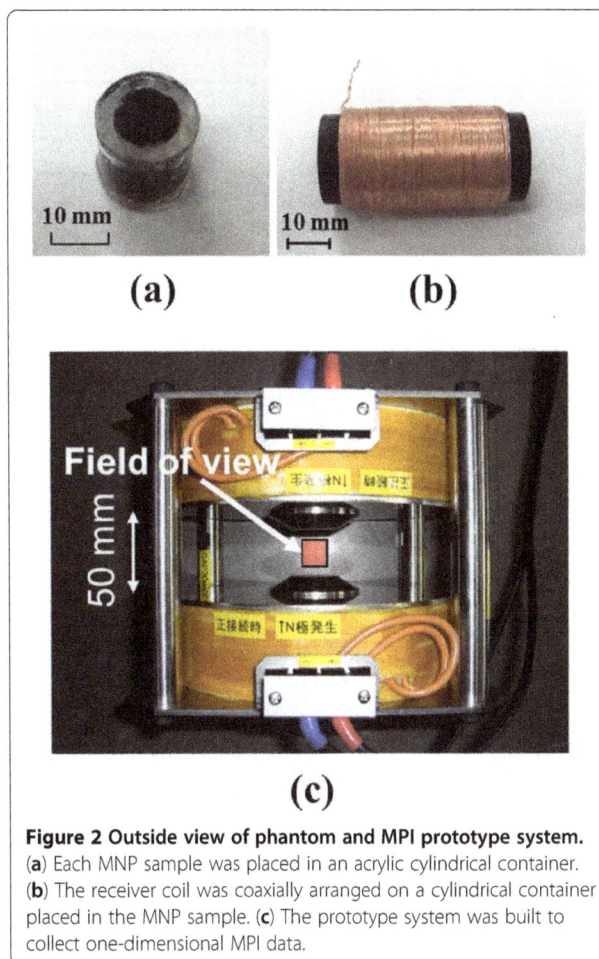

Figure 2 Outside view of phantom and MPI prototype system. (a) Each MNP sample was placed in an acrylic cylindrical container. (b) The receiver coil was coaxially arranged on a cylindrical container placed in the MNP sample. (c) The prototype system was built to collect one-dimensional MPI data.

and it is expected that obtaining such information will require considerable effort and time. On the other hand, some studies have shown that the signal detection sensitivity in magnetic particle spectroscopy (MPS) can be enhanced by using fractionation samples of ferucarbotran [18] or FeraSpin (Miltenyi Biotec GmbH) [19].

In this study, MNP samples adjusted to some particle diameters are prepared by using ferucarbotran, which has already been approved for clinical use, as a base material. In particular, this study aims at estimating the influence of the characteristics of the MNPs based on the difference in particle diameter on the images reconstructed using our proposed method in the

Table 1 Characteristics of each sample based on ferucarbotran

No.	D_a [nm]	PI	D_v [nm]	Magnetic susceptibility [erg · gauss^{-2} · g^{-1}]	T_2 relaxivity [mM^{-1} · s^{-1}]	D [nm]
1	55	0.28	30-110	0.0315	186	15
2	59	0.24	30-120	0.0387	268	18
3	86	0.19	50-200	0.0399	494	20
4	56	0.26	35-110	0.0354	274	17

D_a Average diameter including coating layer.
D_v Particle size distribution of average diameter including coating layer.
D Particle diameter of experimentally evaluated MNP.

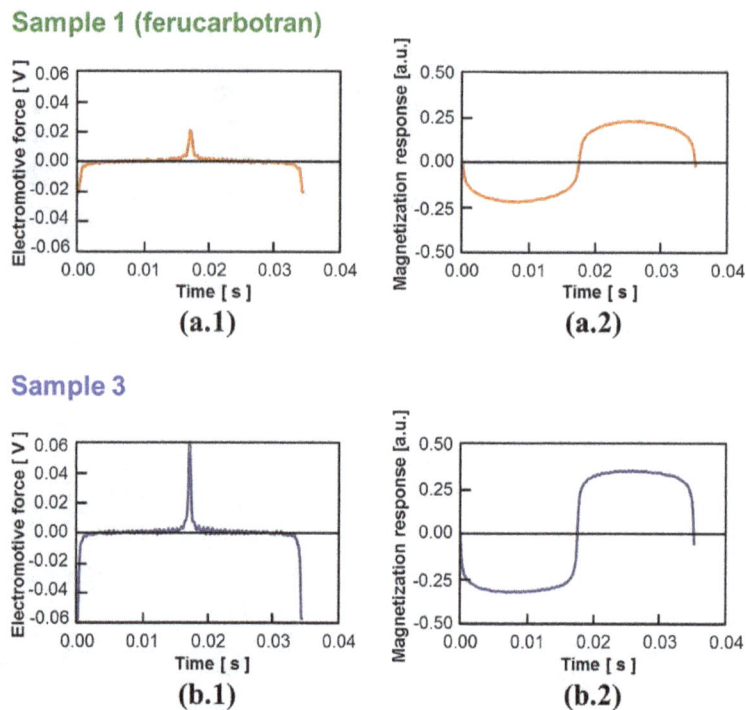

Figure 3 Signal detected with each sample. (a.1), **(b.1)** Waveform of induced electromotive force. **(a.2)**, **(b.2)** Magnetization response waveform.

numerical simulation and the experiments using a prototype. In addition, the relation between the characteristics of the MNP and the hardware ability is discussed based on the results of such reconstructed images.

Principle
Time-correlation MPI reconstruction method
In consideration of the abovementioned problems, we have proposed an image reconstruction method based on the correlation information between an observed signal (induced electromotive force: induced EMF) and a system function without depending on inverse matrix operations [12]. The conceptual diagram of this technique is shown in Figure 1. Here, for simplification, the analyzed matrix is assumed to include three points.

First, a system function is defined. When an MNP is arranged as a delta function at the left end matrix point ($i = 1$), a field free point (FFP) [6,7] where the local magnetic field strength is almost zero is scanned in order ($x = 1, 2, 3$) while applying an alternative magnetic field at each FFP. Here, although such a procedure may be classified under the category of narrow band MPI [20], the FFP scanned by our method is encoded intermittently as in robot position movement [7]. Consequently, a series ($G_{i=1}$) that combines three waveforms of the induced EMF observed at each FFP is created. The system function at each matrix point ($i = 2, 3$) is defined in

a similar manner, with the position of an MNP being changed and the series $G_{i=2}$ and $G_{i=3}$ being created, respectively (Figure 1(a)). Next, the induced EMF generated from the unknown MNPs' distribution is observed at each FFP ($x = 1, 2, 3$), and it is considered as the series V connected to the time-axis as well as the abovementioned system function. Here, the observed signal V shown in Figure 1(b) reflects the outline form of the signal series obtained when the MNP is arranged at the left end matrix as an example. Then, the correlation information of this observed signal and each system function is calculated (Figure 1(c)). It is expected that only the magnetization signal generated from a target region is emphasized and reflected as the image intensity by such correlation processing. In contrast, an interference signal is difficult to reflect as the reconstructed image intensity because the correlation between the observed waveform of the induced EMF and the system function is small. In the case of a general two-dimensional image, the image intensity $F(i, j)$ in the proposed method can be expressed by the following equation:

$$F(i,j) = \int V_{x,z}(t)G_{i,j;x,z}(t)dt \qquad (1)$$

Here, x and z express the scanning position of FFP, $V_{x,z}$ expresses an observed signal, and $G_{x,z}$ expresses the system function as follows [12].

$$G_{i,j;x,z}(t) = G_{i,j}[xt + X(z-1)], \quad \begin{array}{l} x = 1, 2, \cdots, X \\ z = 1, 2, \cdots, Z \end{array} \quad (2)$$

$$V_{x,z}(t) \equiv V[xt + X(z-1)], \quad \begin{array}{l} x = 1, 2, \cdots, X \\ z = 1, 2, \cdots, Z \end{array} \quad (3)$$

Methods

Evaluation of magnetizing properties of MNP

In this study, four types of samples (including ferucarbotran), as listed in Table 1, with ferucarbotran as the base material and adjusted particle diameters were used. These samples were respectively prepared by magnetic separation, centrifugal separation, and gel filtration. The Fe concentration of each sample as well as the Resovist sample was adjusted to 28 [mg/mL]. The average diameter including the coating layer (Da) and the particle size distribution of the average diameter including the coating layer (Dv) were evaluated using a photon correlation spectrometer, the susceptibility was measured using the magnetic balance method, and the T_2 relaxation time was evaluated using 0.47 [T] NMR equipment. The polydispersity index (PI) was evaluated using the light scattering method. A vibrating sample magnetometer (VSM) is commonly used for evaluating the magnetization properties; however, in this case, these properties were evaluated using our MPI prototype because the detection sensitivity in MPI was also evaluated. Each sample was sealed hermetically in 0.7 [cc] cylindrical containers (Ø5 [mm], approximately 12 [mm] in length) made from acrylics, and a solenoid coil of 19 [mm] diameter and with 350 turns was arranged as a receiver coil on the outer circumference (Figure 2). They were installed centered on the gap (50 [mm]) of a customized Maxwell pair coil (Toyojiki Industry Co., Ltd., Niiza, Japan) with an iron core, 180 [mm] diameter, and 285 turns for each coil. An alternative magnetic field with an amplitude of approximately 65 [mT] was generated at the center of those coils by applying an alternative current with an amplitude of 12.0 [A] and frequency of 33.0 [Hz] to each coil in the same direction.

To distinguish between the magnetization components (harmonics) generated from an MNP and the primary magnetic field components applied from the outside, the induced EMF to a coil without a sample was observed previously, and it was defined as the raw flux density applied to an MNP. Then, an induced EMF was generated when an MNP was arranged, and the actual induced EMF generated from the MNP was determined from the difference between this observed signal and the above-described raw flux density. In this case, the absolute value of flux density was corrected using a gauss meter (Model 460; Lakeshore Cryotronics Inc., OH, USA).

The average particle diameter of each sample was computed by approximating the magnetization curve obtained in the abovementioned experiment with a Langevin function.

Evaluation of image reconstruction method by numerical analysis

A gradient magnetic field intensity of 1.5 [T/m] at the center of a Maxwell pair coil and an alternating magnetic field intensity of 32.0 [mT] were used. The FOV was set as 40 [mm] × 40 [mm], and the matrix size was set as 21 × 21. The system function was analytically computed in each matrix point of this FOV based on the Langevin function approximated using the particle diameter of each MNP as evaluated by the abovementioned procedure.

Then, based on equations (1), (2) and (3) and Figure 1, image reconstruction was performed for the signal series that connected the induced EMF observed at the FFP scanned by each matrix point.

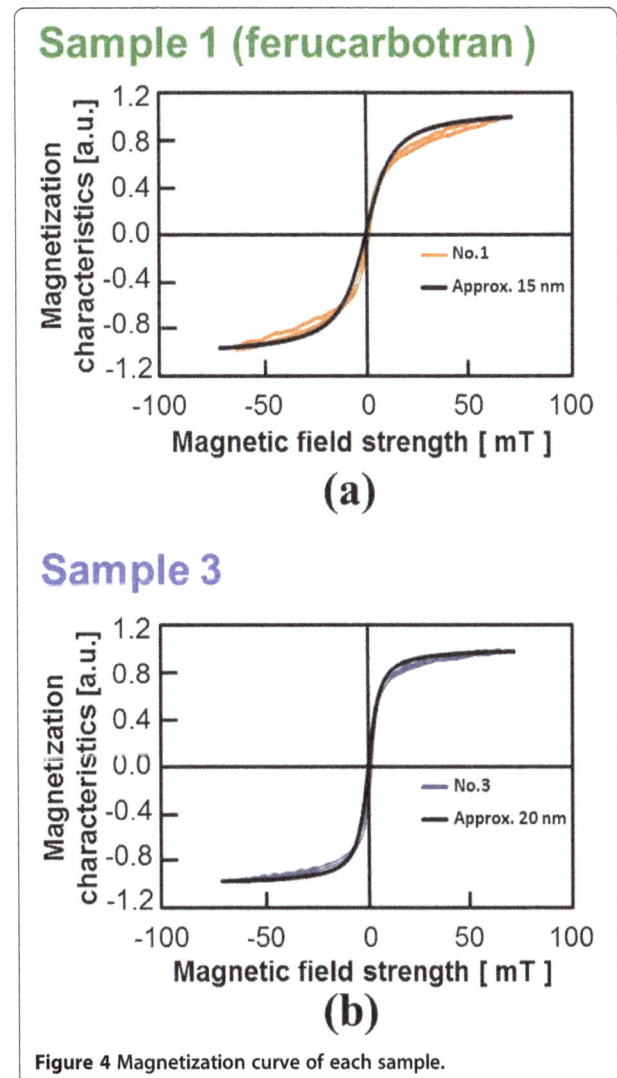

Figure 4 Magnetization curve of each sample.

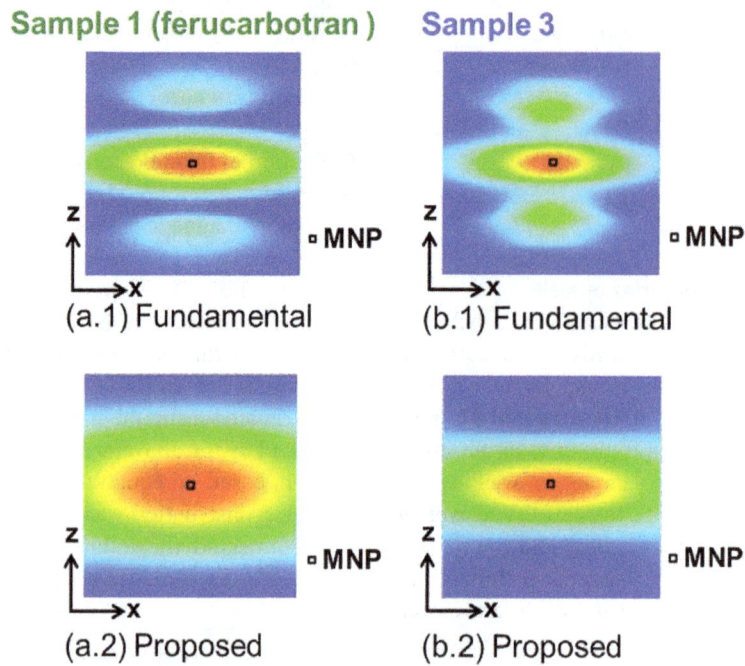

Figure 5 Reconstructed image for each sample by numerical analysis. (a.1), **(a.2)** Images by fundamental and proposed reconstruction methods in the case of sample 1, respectively. **(b.1)**, **(b.2)** Images by fundamental and proposed reconstruction methods in the case of sample 3, respectively.

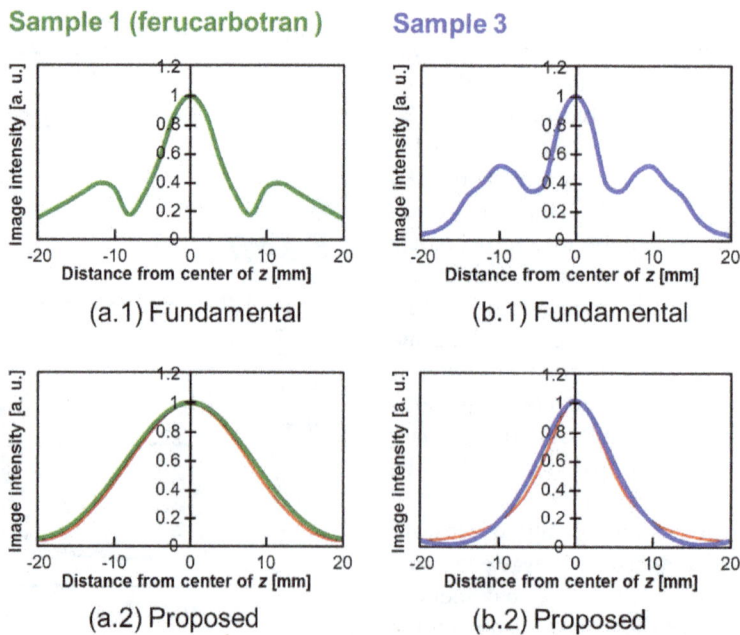

Figure 6 Image profiles of reconstructed images by numerical analysis. (a.1), **(a.2)** Image profiles at $z = 0$ in the case of sample 1, respectively. **(b.1)**, **(b.2)** Image profiles at $z = 0$ in the case of sample 3, respectively. **(a. 2)**, **(b. 2)** Individual theoretical point spread functions indicated by red lines.

Evaluation of one-dimensional reconstructed image using prototype

Both an alternative magnetic field and an FFP were generated using the abovementioned one-axis Maxwell pair coil. The coil current was supplied from a bipolar power supply (BP30-30; Heiwa Electric Co., Ltd., Kashiwa, Japan) in constant current mode, and the current wave for scanning the FFP was controlled by a function generator (AFG3252; Tektronix, Inc., OR, USA). After the induced EMF was detected using the receiver coil (diameter 19 [mm], 350 turns) and passed through the programmable filter (3628, NF Corporation, Yokohama, Japan), it was supplied to a 14-bit AD converter (M2i4031; Spectrum Systementwicklung Microelectronic GmbH, Grosshansdorf, Germany). The detected signal was sampled with a sampling frequency of 20 [kHz] and was sent to a personal computer (dc7800 MT/CT; Hewlett–Packard Co., CA, USA).

As a result of arranging each abovementioned sample at the center of the gap of a Maxwell pair coil and applying the alternative current with an amplitude of 6.0 [A] and frequency of 39.0 [Hz] in the same direction, the MNPs in each sample were subjected to an alternative magnetic field of approximately 30 [mT]. Under such device conditions, a gradient magnetic field of 1.9 [T/m] was generated by applying an offset current of 12.0 [A] simultaneously to the opposite direction of each coil, and an FFP was formed at the center of the Maxwell pair coil.

In a preliminary experiment, the electric current required to move the FFP by a unit length (this corresponds to the spatial resolution) was evaluated; based on this, the scanning of the FFP was controlled by the function generator. In addition, a ±20-mm region from the Maxwell pair coil's center was set as the FOV, and the matrix that divides the inside of this FOV into 21 points was made into each measuring point (FFP).

To detect only the induced EMF generated from an MNP in consideration of the frequency purity of the alternative magnetic field due to the imperfection of the power supply and the coil, difference processing with the induced EMF and without a sample was carried out.

Results and discussion
Magnetization property of each MNP sample

The induced EMF from the samples made with ferucarbotran as the base material to the external alternative magnetic field and the magnetization response obtained from the integration operation of EMF are shown in Figure 3 (in what follows, only the results of sample 1 (ferucarbotran) and sample 3, which show the characteristic tendency, were displayed.). In addition, the average particle diameter of each sample was evaluated by comparing the observed magnetization properties with the magnetization curve of the MNP as indicated by Langevin's approximate expression (Figure 4). These magnetization curves were normalized by the maximum

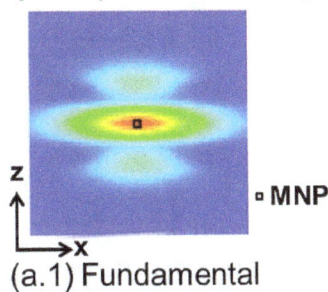

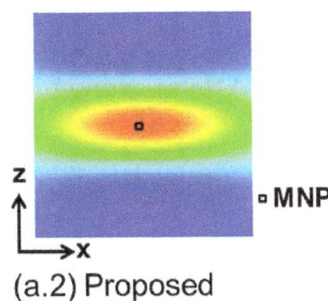

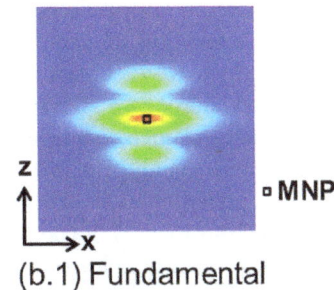

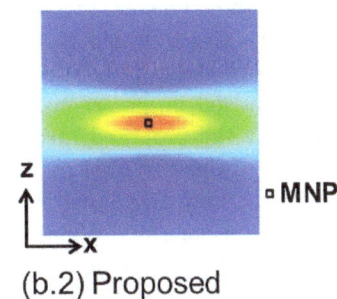

Figure 7 Reconstructed image with numerical analysis for each sample at gradient field of 2.5 T/m. (a.1), (a.2) Images by fundamental and proposed reconstruction methods in the case of sample 1, respectively. **(b.1), (b.2)** Images by fundamental and proposed reconstruction methods in the case of sample 3, respectively.

magnetization of each case. The results are summarized in Table 1.

It was estimated that the average particle diameter D of sample 1 (ferucarbotran), which has been clinically approved, was 15 [nm]. That of sample 3 was 20 [nm], which is the largest among all samples, and it was shown that sample 3 is the most suitable because a sample with large particle diameter is advantageous for MPI. Here, the difference between the obtained magnetization properties and the approximated curve reflected the variation in the particle size distribution of the MNPs in a sample, and it was suggested that the particle diameter of sample 3 was adjusted satisfactorily. This result was also supported by the evaluation results obtained by PI and D_v, shown in Table 1. Because the particle size distribution follows a logarithmic normal distribution [21], it was considered important to adjust the particle diameter in a sample uniformly in order to improve the image resolution in MPI. Moreover, the induced EMF detected from sample 3 was approximately 3 times that from ferucarbotran, indicating that sample 3 also contributes greatly to the improvement of SNR. This is based on the increase in the saturation magnetization of the MNP accompanying the increase in the particle diameter [15].

From the physical properties obtained by this evaluation, as listed in Table 1, it was confirmed that the particle diameter of MNPs was also related to the susceptibility and T_2 relaxation time.

Numerical analysis of time-correlation MPI image reconstruction

Next, the image reconstruction results of the numerical simulation based on the characteristics of sample 1 (ferucarbotran) and sample 3, which were chosen from among all samples as discussed above, are described. The images reconstructed by the fundamental image reconstruction method based on an imaging principle (an alternative magnetic field was applied at each FFP that was scanned for every encoded position [7]) and our proposed time-correlation method for a sample arranged at the center pixel of the FOV are shown in Figure 5. In addition, the profiles at $z = 0$ of these reconstruction images are shown in Figure 6. It was confirmed that the image artifact observed in the upper and lower sides of the actual MNP by the fundamental image reconstruction method was suppressed by the proposed method. However, the image resolution of the proposed method (~12 mm) was slightly degraded compared to that of the fundamental method (~8 mm) using the FWHM for sample 1. Then, it was shown that the image blurring increased. This is because theoretically, the distribution of correlation between the observed signal and the system function at every FFP position (Figure 1) was given as the image intensity with nearly two times the FWHM of

the system function [22]. The PSF of this image reconstruction method was expected as an autocorrelation distribution of the system function, and it was superimposed in Figure 6 for MNPs of each particle diameter. Therefore, it is possible to newly propose the following iterative estimation of the distribution of MNPs in order to improve the image resolution [13].

(1) The position at which the correlation with an observed signal and a system function is the maximum in the FOV is detected.

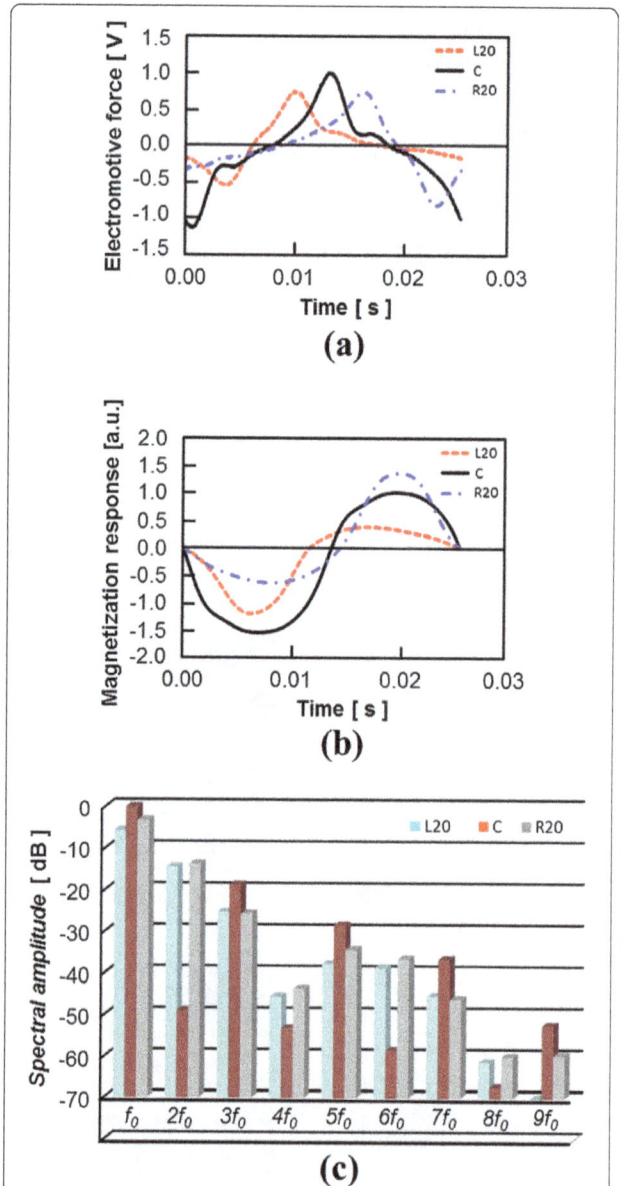

Figure 8 Signal detected using prototype. (a) Waveform of induced electromotive force. (b) Magnetization response waveform. (c) Fourier components of magnetization response waveform. Here, only the waveforms obtained by scanning the FFP at −20 [mm] (L20), 0 [mm] (C), and 20 [mm] (R20) along the z-axis were indicated.

(2) At this position (image matrix), the amount of correlation is given as the reconstructed image intensity.

(3) The distribution of a corresponding system function is subtracted from the observed signal at this position.

Then, the candidate of the processing position is moved to the next FFP and the abovementioned process is repeated until the residual of the subtraction signal at every FFP becomes small. It is considered that a deconvolution with a system function can be carried out equivalently by such processing; therefore, the image blurring can be reduced effectively without inverse matrix operations.

An evaluation of the profile at $z = 0$ (Figure 6) showed that the spatial resolution of sample 3 was approximately 1.3 times better than that of sample 1. This corresponded to the fact that the spatial resolution obtained by a gradient magnetic field strength of 2.5 [T/m] for sample 1 was achieved by a gradient magnetic field strength of approximately 1.5 [T/m] for sample 3 (Figure 7). In other words, it was shown that the dependence on hardware requirements was reduced by 0.6 times under such conditions and that the spatial resolution could be improved by simply adjusting the particle diameter.

One-dimensional imaging experiment using prototype

The waveform of the induced EMF obtained by scanning the FFP, the magnetization response calculated from the integration of the EMF, and the Fourier transform of this magnetization response are shown in Figure 8. Here, when the center coordinate of the FOV was set to 0, only the wave obtained by scanning the FFP at −20 [mm], 0 [mm], and 20 [mm] along the z-axis was indicated in the figure (this corresponds to the sign L20, C, and R20, respectively.). It was confirmed that the difference of the induced EMF's waveform in an experiment appeared depending on the position of the FFP. In other words, because it would reflect that the position of the MNP was indistinguishable when the correlation with an observed signal was evaluated with a system function, the validity of our proposed method based on time-correlation information was also confirmed by experimental data. With regard to sample 1 (ferucarbotran) and sample 3, the one-dimensional images obtained using the fundamental image reconstruction method and the proposed method are shown in Figure 9. In these reconstructed images, although the precise system function should ideally be measured from the signal observed when the MNPs are arranged in a shape like a delta function at each analyzed point in the reconstructed image, the analytically calculated system function corresponding to each particle diameter at every image matrix point was used. This is because considerable time is generally required for the measurement of a system function, and our system's operation might become unstable over such a long time. It was found that sample 3 afforded an image resolution superior to that of sample 1 through both the experimental results as well as the numerical simulation.

Sample 1 (ferucarbotran)   **Sample 3**

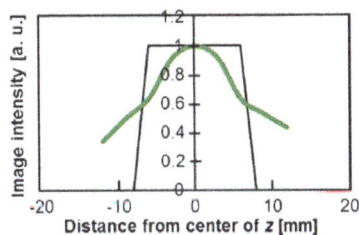

(a.1) Fundamental

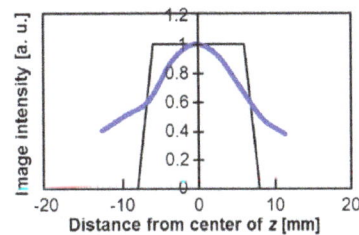

(b.1) Fundamental

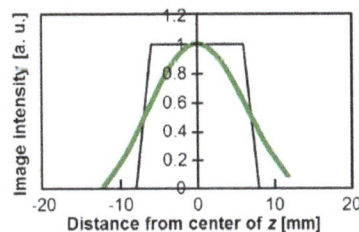

(a.2) Proposed

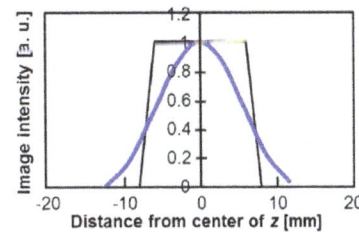

(b.2) Proposed

Figure 9 One-dimensional reconstructed images using prototype. (**a.1**), (**a.2**) Images by fundamental and proposed reconstruction methods in the case of sample 1, respectively. (**b.1**), (**b.2**) Images by fundamental and proposed reconstruction methods in the case of sample 3, respectively. In these cases, the calculated system function corresponding to each particle diameter was used.

Conclusions

In this study, to suppress image artifacts in MPI and improve the spatial resolution without requiring high-performance hardware, an image obtained using an MNP sample made of biocompatible ferucarbotran as the base material and a sample made by our proposed method were compared. It is essential to evaluate the biocompatibility because a large-diameter nanoparticle may behave differently in internal organs compared to Resovist, which is approved for clinical use. Nonetheless, some samples used for MPI were found to have magnetizing properties superior to those of ferucarbotran. Consequently, it was shown that an equivalent image quality (spatial resolution) could be obtained with a smaller gradient magnetic field strength compared to the case in which ferucarbotran was used.

Therefore, if a method for preparing MNP samples consisting of particles with large and equisized diameters made from ferucarbotran as the base material is developed, the MPI image quality can be further improved, and the conditions imposed on hardware ability can be reduced. However, because our study was restricted to the use of an alternating magnetic field with relatively low frequency, evaluations in consideration of the dynamic characteristic of the MNP [19,23] will be required when faster scanning of FFP is used. In addition, because a sufficiently high spatial resolution has not yet been achieved theoretically using the proposed time-correlation MPI reconstruction method, it is necessary to devise an algorithm that can use correlation information more effectively.

Competing interests
The authors have no competing interests to declare.

Authors' contributions
YI conceived the study, built the algorithm, and drafted the manuscript. TH implemented the algorithm in a program, developed the prototype system, performed data collection, and helped to draft the manuscript. SN prepared the experimental MNP samples and helped to draft the manuscript. All authors have read and approved the final manuscript.

Acknowledgements
This study was supported by a Grant-in-Aid for Scientific Research (B), 24300184, 2012, from the Japan Society for the Promotion of Science (JSPS).

Author details
[1]School of Science and Technology, Meiji University, Higashimita Tama, Kawasaki, Kanagawa, Japan. [2]Graduate School of Science and Technology, Meiji University, Higashimita, Tama, Kawasaki, Kanagawa, Japan. [3]The Nagoya Research Laboratory, Meito Sangyo Co., Ltd, Kaechi Nishibiwajima, Kiyosu, Aichi, Japan.

References
1. Huang X, Jain PK, El-Sayed H, El-Sayed MA: Gold nanoparticles: interesting optical properties and recent applications in cancer diagnostics and therapy. *Nanomedicine* 2007, **2**:681–693.
2. Dougherty TJ, Gomer CJ, Henderson BW, Jori G, Kessel D, Korbelik M, Moan J, Peng Q: Photodynamic therapy. *J Natl Cancer Inst* 1998, **90**:889–905.
3. El-Sayed IH, Huang X, El-Sayed MA: Selective laser photo-thermal therapy of epithelial carcinoma using anti-EGFR antibody conjugated gold nanoparticles. *Cancer Lett* 2006, **239**:129–135.
4. Hergt R, Hiergeist R, Zeisberger M, Schüler D, Heyen U, Hilger I, Kaiser WA: Magnetic properties of bacterial magnetosomes as potential diagnostic and therapeutic tools. *Journal of Magnetism and Magnetic Materials* 2005, **293**:80–86.
5. Jordan A, Scholz R, Maier-Hauff K, Johannsen M, Wust P, Nadobny J, Schirra H, Schmidt H, Deger S, Loening S, Lanksch W, Felix R: Presentation of a new magnetic field therapy system for the treatment of human solid tumors with magnetic fluid hyperthermia. *Journal of Magnetism and Magnetic Materials* 2001, **225**:118–126.
6. Gleich B: Method for determining the spatial distribution of magnetic particles. *DE 10151778(A1)05* 2003, **05**:08.
7. Gleich B, Weizenecker J: Tomographic imaging using the nonlinear response of magnetic nanoparticles. *Nature* 2005, **435**:1214–1217.
8. Weizenecker J, Gleich B, Rahmer J, Dahnke H, Borgert J: Three-dimensional real-time *in vivo* magnetic particle imaging. *Phys Med Biol* 2009, **54**:L1–L10.
9. Schmale I, Rahmer J, Gleich B, Kanzenbach J, Schmidt JD, Bontus C, Woywode O, Borgert J: *First phantom and in vivo MPI images with an extended field of view*. Florida: Proc. of SPIE Medical Imaging; 2011:796510.6.
10. Kusayama Y, Ishihara Y: A preliminary study on the molecular imaging device using magnetic nanoparticles. *Technical Report of IEICE. MBE* 2007, **107**:15–18.
11. Kusayama Y, Ishihara Y: High-resolution image reconstruction method on the molecular imaging using magnetic nanoparticles. *IEICE Trans. D* 2009, **J92–D**:1653–1662.
12. Ishihara Y, Kuwabara T, Honma T, Nakagawa Y: Correlation-based image reconstruction methods for magnetic particle imaging. *IEICE Transactions on Information and Systems* 2012, **E95-D**:872–879.
13. Honma T, Shimizu S, Ishihara Y: Correlation-based image reconstruction methods for magnetic particle imaging. In *Proceedings of the Branch Conference of Japanese Society for Medical Biological Engineering 2012*. Edited by Kyoso M. Tokyo; 2012. 2012: C-1-04.
14. Goodwill PW, Conolly SM: The X-space formulation of the magnetic particle imaging process: 1-D signal, resolution, bandwidth, SNR, SAR, and magnetostimulation. *IEEE Trans Med Imaging* 2010, **29**:1851–1859.
15. Chikazumi S: In *Physics of Magnetism*. Edited by Charap SH. New York: John Wiley and Sons; 1964.
16. Ferguson RM, Minard KR, Krishnan KM: Optimization of nanoparticle core size for magnetic particle imaging. *J. Magn. Magn. Mater.* 2009, **321**:1548–1551.
17. Ferguson RM, Minard KR, Khandhar AP, Krishnan KM: Optimizing magnetite nanoparticles for mass sensitivity in magnetic particle imaging. *Med Phys* 2011, **38**:1619–1626.
18. Eberbeck D, Wiekhorst F, Wagner S, Trahms L: How the size distribution of magnetic nanoparticles determines their magnetic particle imaging performance. *Appl Phys Lett* 2011, **98**:182502.1–182502.3.
19. Ludwig F, Wawrzik T, Yoshida T, Gehrke N, Briel A, Eberbeck D, Schilling M: Optimization of magnetic nanoparticles for magnetic particle imaging. *IEEE Transactions on Magnetics* 2012, **48**:3780–3783.
20. Goodwill PW, Scott GC, Stang PP, Conolly SM: Narrowband magnetic particle imaging. *IEEE Trans Med Imaging* 2009, **28**:1231–1237.
21. Chantrell RW, Popplewell J, Charles SW: Measurements of particle size distribution parameters in ferrofluids. *IEEE Transactions on Magnetics* 1978, **14**:975–977.
22. Yarlagadda RKR: *Analog and Digital Signals and Systems*. New York: Springer Science + Business Media; 2010.
23. Yoshida T, Enpuku K, Ludwig F, Dieckhoff J, Wawrzik T, Lak A, Schilling M: Characterization of Resovist® nanoparticles for magnetic particle imaging. *Springer Proceedings in Physics* 2012, **140**:3–7.

15

A workstation-integrated peer review quality assurance program

Margaret M O'Keeffe[1], Todd M Davis[2,3] and Kerry Siminoski[1*]

Abstract

Background: The surrogate indicator of radiological excellence that has become accepted is consistency of assessments between radiologists, and the technique that has become the standard for evaluating concordance is peer review. This study describes the results of a workstation-integrated peer review program in a busy outpatient radiology practice.

Methods: Workstation-based peer review was performed using the software program Intelerad Peer Review. Cases for review were randomly chosen from those being actively reported. If an appropriate prior study was available, and if the reviewing radiologist and the original interpreting radiologist had not exceeded review targets, the case was scored using the modified RADPEER system.

Results: There were 2,241 cases randomly assigned for peer review. Of selected cases, 1,705 (76%) were interpreted. Reviewing radiologists agreed with prior reports in 99.1% of assessments. Positive feedback (score 0) was given in three cases (0.2%) and concordance (scores of 0 to 2) was assigned in 99.4%, similar to reported rates of 97.0% to 99.8%. Clinically significant discrepancies (scores of 3 or 4) were identified in 10 cases (0.6%). Eighty-eight percent of reviewed radiologists found the reviews worthwhile, 79% found scores appropriate, and 65% felt feedback was appropriate. Two-thirds of radiologists found case rounds discussing significant discrepancies to be valuable.

Conclusions: The workstation-based computerized peer review process used in this pilot project was seamlessly incorporated into the normal workday and met most criteria for an ideal peer review system. Clinically significant discrepancies were identified in 0.6% of cases, similar to published outcomes using the RADPEER system. Reviewed radiologists felt the process was worthwhile.

Keywords: Diagnostic errors, Diagnostic imaging, Peer review, Practice performance evaluation, Quality assurance, RADPEER

Background

Even with the recognition that "quality in health care is a complex and rather vague concept" [1], the quality of reporting in diagnostic radiology has become an important issue for radiology professional associations and for regulatory bodies [2-9]. The definitive quality assessment approach in radiology is correlation of radiological findings with the ultimate clinical outcome [1,2,4,10]. Applying this approach across all of diagnostic radiology is cost-prohibitive because of the long timeframes often needed to ascertain the clinical diagnosis and because of the manpower that would be involved [1,4,8,11,12]. In some branches of medicine, including interventional radiology, objective clinical or laboratory parameters are used as markers of quality [1,2,8,10]. This methodology is not applicable to most areas in diagnostic radiology. The surrogate indicator of radiological excellence that has become accepted is consistency of assessments between radiologists, and the technique that has become the standard for evaluating concordance is peer review [1-4,7,8,13]. The underlying intent is that the results of such reviews should act as an impetus for self-learning and other educational activities that ultimately lead to improved radiological performance and better patient outcomes [2,4,7,9,13-16].

There are several peer review approaches in use. One example is 360-degree feedback where radiologists have

* Correspondence: kerrygs@telusplanet.net
[1]Department of Radiology and Diagnostic Imaging, University of Alberta, and Medical Imaging Consultants, 11010-101 Street, Edmonton, AB T5H 4B9, Canada
Full list of author information is available at the end of the article

questionnaires completed by fellow radiologists, referring physicians, other healthcare staff, and patients, assessing a variety of topics including the quality of radiological assessments [6]. A second type of peer review is double reading, in which a random selection of routine cases is chosen for a second read, with any discrepancies between reads adjudicated by a third radiologist [5,7,11]. By far the most-used peer review approach in North America is the RADPEER program of the American College of Radiology (ACR) [3,4]. In this scheme, members of participating radiology groups evaluate prior images and reports of cases currently being reported and rate the quality of the original interpretation [3,4]. A four-point rating scale was originally used, with recent modifications being the addition of score 0 to assign positive feedback, and the incorporation of the option to designate clinical significance [3,4]. The RADPEER evaluation is submitted to the ACR, which provides statistical evaluation of ratings for individual radiologists and for facilities. More than 10,000 radiologists have participated in this program, representing about one-third of radiologists in the United States [3,4,17].

The RADPEER program has several practical drawbacks that have limited participation by the majority of radiologists in the US and that make the implementation of similar national programs in other countries problematic [11]. The first limitation is that case selection is not random [11,18]. The RADPEER program assumes that all active cases with prior studies will be evaluated, but in reality this is generally not the case. When time pressures arise, prior cases are often not evaluated, and it is likely that it is the most complex cases that are not reviewed [4,11,13]. The second problem is that additional time commitments are required to complete either machine-readable cards or internet assessment forms for each evaluated case. Another issue is that participating radiologists and practices are dependent on a third party (the ACR) for statistical compilation and analysis, with an associated time delay [4,19]. Finally, the RADPEER program does not mandate discrepancy case rounds, recognized as a valuable addition to peer review programs [11,13,15,18,20,21].

The concepts involved in performance and evaluation of peer review are evolving, but there is consensus on the characteristics of good peer review [3,4,13,15,18]. We have instituted a pilot peer review program to assess the feasibility of such an approach in a large multifacility radiology practice. The pilot project had the following key characteristics: (1) the review process was workstation-based and integrated into reporting software so that it was seamlessly incorporated into the normal workday; (2) the process was practice-integrated in that the images chosen for review were prior studies related to cases currently being reported, as in the RADPEER system, with the review performed during the reporting process; (3) the cases for review were randomly generated by the software to avoid selection bias; (4) assessment data was immediately locally available and could be used for discrepancy rounds and case-sharing; and (5) discrepancy rounds and case-sharing of discrepant cases were incorporated into the program. In this paper we describe the results of our pilot program and compare them to published results of studies that have also used the RADPEER scoring system.

Methods
Peer review software
This study was performed between September 2009 and March 2010 in community-based outpatient clinic settings. Ethics approval was not required by the Health Research Ethics Board of the University of Alberta as the data was collected as part of a quality control program. Workstation-based peer review was performed using the software Intelerad Peer Review (Intelerad, Montreal, Quebec), which was integrated into the Radiology Information System (RIS; Intelerad). The program used two main steps to determine whether a case underwent review. The first step was determining whether a prior study of a patient whose current images were being evaluated was appropriate for peer review. A case being actively reported was randomly chosen and a paradigm was followed to determine if a prior study was available, was in the same modality as the current study, had either the same fee code or was of the same body area, and had been performed more than four days before the current study for most tests or within nine months of the current study for an obstetrical study.

The adopted terminology used here refers to the physician reporting the current study who is flagged to perform a peer review of prior studies as the reviewing radiologist. The physician who reported the prior study that is undergoing assessment is referred to as the interpreting radiologist [4]. The second step in the computerized selection process involved assessing targets for both the reviewing radiologist and the interpreting radiologist. Reviewing radiologists were each assigned a daily target for the number of peer reviews to perform (four to ten cases per full outpatient clinical reporting day). If the reviewing radiologist had performed fewer reviews than the daily target, the case was designated for possible peer review. If the reviewing radiologist had already met the daily target, or if the prior imaging had been interpreted by the reviewing radiologist, the case was not assessed. Interpreting radiologists were assigned a monthly maximum of 100 peer reviews per modality. If the number of peer reviewed cases for an interpreting radiologist was less than this for the modality of the case under consideration, the case was assigned to the reviewing radiologist for review. If the interpreting radiologist's daily target in that modality had already been met, the case was discarded and not reviewed.

When a case met these criteria, the reviewing radiologist was notified that a relevant prior study had been chosen for peer review. The reviewing radiologist then had the option of reviewing the prior study immediately, reviewing it after dictating the current case, or reviewing it at a later date. To review the case, previous images were viewed in the picture archiving and communication system (PACS: Agfa Impax 6.3.1, Agfa Healthcare Corporation, Greenville, SC, United States) and the prior report was assessed and given a score.

Quality assessment scoring

The reviewing radiologist performing peer review of an identified prior study evaluated the current and prior images and the prior report, then assigned a quality score to the prior report using the modified ACR RADPEER system [3-5,11,19]. A score of 0 indicates positive feedback. A score of 1 was assigned when the reviewer agreed with the original report. Scores 2, 3, and 4 indicated increasing disagreement with the prior report: 2 = error in diagnosis—not usually made; 3 = error in diagnosis – should usually be made; 4 = error in diagnosis – should almost always be made [3,4]. Cases were drawn from the modalities of general radiography, fluoroscopy, mammography, nuclear medicine, and ultrasonography, which encompass 89.1% of the clinic-based caseload of the practice. CT and MRI were not included in this pilot study as in our health region these are primarily hospital-based procedures rather than community-based. For comparison to published data, case scores were grouped as follows based on terminology in the literature: non-discrepant (scores in the range of 0 and 1), concordant (scores of 0 to 2), discrepant (2 to 4), and clinically significant discrepancy (3 and 4) [4,19,22].

Radiologist characteristics and clinical setting

A total of 10 radiologists participated as peer reviewers. The mean amount of time since accreditation in general radiology was 17.5 years (SD, 7.4 years) with a range from 2 to 25 years. Subspecialty accreditation in the imaging modalities relevant to this pilot study included ultrasonography (10/10), mammography (6/10), cardiac echocardiography (6/10), and nuclear medicine (1/10). In subspecialty cases, both the interpreting and reviewing radiologists were accredited in that subspecialty.

Medical Imaging Consultants (MIC) of Edmonton, Alberta is a partnership of approximately 80 general and subspecialty diagnostic radiologists. The mean amount of time since accreditation in general radiology was 15.6 years (SD, 8.9 years) with a range from 1 to 37 years. Subspecialty accreditation in the imaging modalities relevant to this pilot study included ultrasonography (100%), mammography (18.8%), cardiac echocardiography (15%),

and nuclear medicine (12%). Within these subspecialty modalities, reporting was done only by those physicians accredited in the particular modality. Twenty-three radiologists in the practice spent less than one day per month in clinic work, so that 57 radiologists served as the principle interpreting radiologists in this pilot study. A survey was completed by these radiologists at the end of the pilot period.

Approach to discrepant cases

All interpreting radiologists were informed of the results of each of their peer reviewed cases. When a case was scored 2, 3, or 4, the interpreting radiologist was required to reassess the original images and report. The interpreting radiologist also had the option of seeking a subsequent review by another radiologist, but this was not requested for any case during the pilot study. Aggregate peer review statistics were available to all radiologists. A quality assurance (QA) committee reviewed all score 3 and 4 cases. Selected score 3 and 4 cases were presented at discrepancy rounds and made available to the membership as virtual discrepancy rounds on a secure website [11,21].

Statistics

Values are expressed as raw numbers and percentages with 95% confidence intervals (CI). Data was processed using SPSS version 12.0 (SPSS).

Results

A total of 2,241 cases were chosen for review (Table 1). The median number per reviewing physician was 216 cases, with a range from 39 to 529. Reviews were performed on 1,705 of these cases (76%; 95% CI, 74 to 78%). The median proportion of completed reviews per

Table 1 Assigned and reviewed cases for each reviewing radiologist

Reviewing physician	Total assigned cases	Total reviewed cases (%)	Total not reviewed (%)
1	254	254 (100)	0 (0)
2	85	71 (84)	14 (16)
3	133	133 (100)	0 (0)
4	388	315 (81)	73 (19)
5	39	23 (59)	16 (41)
6	529	479 (91)	50 (9)
7	261	220 (84)	41 (16)
8	87	56 (64)	31 (36)
9	177	79 (45)	98 (55)
10	288	75 (26)	213 (74)
Total	2,241	1,705 (76)	535 (24)

Numbers in brackets are percentages of total cases for each reviewing radiologist.

radiologist was 82% with a range from 26% to 100%. The mean non-completion rate was 24% (95% CI, 22 to 26%), while the median non-completion rate was 18%, with a range from 0% to 74%. Four radiologists completed less than two-thirds of assigned cases. Of the reviewed cases, 94% (95% CI, 93 to 95%) were completed within 15 minutes of assignment. Fluoroscopy made up the lowest fraction of the total assigned cases at 3% and general radiography the highest at 34% (Table 2); these comprised approximately similar proportions of the total tests in each modality done by MIC in this time period.

The reviewing radiologist agreed with the prior report (score = 1) in 1,690 cases (99.1%; 95% CI, 98.6 to 99.5%; Table 3). Positive feedback (score = 0) was given in three cases (0.2%; 95% CI, 0.1 to 0.5%). Twelve cases (0.7%; 95% CI, 0.4 to 1.2%) were evaluated as having discrepant opinions in diagnosis (scores of 2, 3, or 4). A score of 2 was assigned in two cases (0.1%; 95% CI, 0.0 to 0.4%), a score of 3 in nine cases (0.5%; 95% CI, 0.3 to 1.0%), and a score of 4 in a single case (0.1%; 95% CI, 0.0 to 0.3%). Of the cases considered to contain discrepant opinions, there were six cases in general radiography (1.0% of general radiography cases; 95% CI, 0.5 to 2.1%), one case in fluoroscopy (2.0%; 95% CI, 0.4 to 10.3%), none in mammography (95% CI, 0.0 to 1.0%), three cases in nuclear medicine (1.4%; 95% CI, 0.5 to 3.9%), and two cases in ultrasonography (0.5%; 95% CI, 0.1 to 1.7%). Clinically significant discrepancies (scores of 3 or 4) were given in four cases in general radiography (0.7% of general radiography cases; 95% CI, 0.3 to 1.7%), one case in fluoroscopy (2.0%; 95% CI, 0.4 to 10.3%), none in mammography (95% CI, 0.0 to 1.0%), three cases in nuclear medicine (1.4%; 95% CI, 0.5 to 3.9%), and two cases in ultrasonography (0.5%; 95% CI, 0.1 to 1.7%). Ten of 12 (83%; 95% CI, 55 to 95%) of the score 3 and 4 cases were false negative findings. These included five in general radiography (calcified pleural plaque, remote thoracic compression fracture, talar osteochondritis dessicans, a stable calcified scapular lesion, and findings indicative of COPD), one in fluoroscopy (radio-opaque gallbladder calculi), three in nuclear medicine (a horseshoe kidney missed on a bone scan, and inferolateral ischemia and dilated left ventricle on MIBI

scans), and one in ultrasound (small pancreatic tail cyst). One discrepant finding was a false positive in ultrasound (a renal pyramid described as a renal cyst). An error was identified in a nuclear medicine study (renal scan) where the dictated history was incorrect but did not adversely affect image interpretation.

An anonymous survey was completed by all 57 interpreting radiologists. Eighty-eight percent considered the peer review process to be worthwhile. Scores received in reviews were considered appropriate by 79%, and 65% considered the feedback to be appropriate. Reviews prompted 26% to review literature or attend relevant continuing medical education activities. The online cases with clinically significant discrepancy (all grade 3 and 4 cases) were found to be valuable by 67% and of no value by 5%, with 28% not having accessed them.

Discussion

The scoring system used in our pilot program was the modified RADPEER system[3,4]. Discrepant reviews (score 2, 3, or 4) were provided in 0.7% (95% CI, 0.4 to 1.2%) of total cases. This was somewhat lower than rates reported in the literature by studies using RADPEER, in which the frequency of scores of 2 to 4 range from 2.9% to 4.4% (Table 4). This difference was primarily due to a lower rate of score 2 in our study. The frequency of scores of 2 have been reported by RADPEER to generally correlate with rates of scores 3 and 4 within a radiology practice (r = 0.83), but our results do not fit that profile [4]. We found a score 2 rate of only 0.1% whereas rates in the literature ranged from 1.4% to 3.6%. There are several possible explanations for this based on analyses presented in the literature. One possibility is simply individual tendencies to assign certain scores. Borgestede et al. gave examples of score 2 rates for individual radiologists ranging from 0% to 7.3% within the same institution [4]. Another explanation may be the mix of imaging modalities in our study compared to published reports. Score 2 occurs less commonly in mammography, ultrasound, and plain film imaging, which comprised a large proportion of our study mix, than in CT and MRI, which were not included in our pilot [4]. Another reason why our study had fewer scores of 2 may relate to the size of our practice, as it has been reported that the rate of interpretation disagreement declines by 0.5% for each additional 10 interpreting radiologists [4]. Another explanatory variable may be that our study took place in a community setting, where score 2 ratings are reported to average 1.5% less than in academic institutions [4]. A final explanation may be a predilection for our radiologists to give certain cases a score of 1 despite minor disagreement that would have justified scores of 2. This is illustrated by one study that examined written comments for score 1 cases and found that some should

Table 2 Assigned and reviewed cases by modality

Modality	Total assigned cases (% of total cases)	Total reviewed cases (% of modality)	Total not reviewed (% of modality)
Radiography	770 (34)	611 (79)	159 (21)
Fluoroscopy	57 (3)	51 (89)	6 (11)
Mammography	499 (22)	385 (77)	114 (23)
Nuclear Medicine	247 (11)	222 (90)	25 (10)
Ultrasound	668 (30)	436 (65)	232 (35)
Total	2,241	1,703 (76)	535 (24)

Table 3 Scoring of reviewed cases

Modality	Score 0	Score 1	Score 2	Score 3	Score 4	Total	Non-discrepant (0–1)	Concordant (0–2)	Discrepant (2–4)	Clinically Significant Discrepancy (3–4)
Radiography (%)	0 (0)	605 (99.0)	2 (0.3)	4 (0.7)	0 (0)	611	605 (99.0)	607 (99.3)	6 (1.0)	4 (0.7)
Fluoroscopy (%)	0 (0)	50 (98.0)	0 (0)	0 (0)	1 (2.0)	51	50 (98.0)	50 (98.0)	1 (2.0)	1 (2.0)
Mammography (%)	0 (0)	385 (100.0)	0 (0)	0 (0)	0 (0)	385	385 (100.0)	385 (100.0)	0 (0)	0 (0)
Nuclear Medicine (%)	1 (0.4)	218 (98.2)	0 (0)	3 (1.4)	0 (0)	222	219 (98.6)	219 (98.6)	3 (1.4)	3 (1.4)
Ultrasound (%)	2 (0.4)	432 (99.1)	0 (0)	2 (0.5)	0 (0)	436	434 (99.5)	434 (99.5)	2 (0.5)	2 (0.5)
Total (%)	3 (0.2)	1690 (99.1)	2 (0.1)	9 (0.5)	1 (0.1)	1705	1693 (99.3)	(1695 (99.4)	12 (0.7)	10 (0.6)

Numbers in brackets are percentages of each modality assigned the corresponding score. Score definitions are: 0 = positive feedback; 1 = agreement with original report. 2 = error in diagnosis- not usually made; 3 = error in diagnosis – should usually be made; 4 = error in diagnosis – should almost always be made.

have been given scores of 2 based on feedback that included minor criticisms of the prior report, indicating there was a tendency to under-score less serious interpretive disagreements [19]. As a result of this tendency, some investigators have chosen to group scores of 1 and 2 as concordant, meaning there is no disagreement of clinical significance [23]. When our concordance rate is determined this way, we had 99.4% of reviews in this category, similar to the literature rates ranging from 98.5% to 99.8%. This result is again consistent with a tendency of our reviewers to rate some score 2 cases as score 1.

In our study, scores indicating errors that should usually or always be made (scores of 3 or 4), considered clinically significant discrepancies, were given in 0.6% (95% CI, 0.3 to 1.1%) of cases. This is consistent with reported values in the literature, which range from 0.2% to 3.0%. Just as with scores of 2, rates in this category have been reported to vary by individual and by institution, to be influenced by the facility type (higher in academic settings compared to community settings), and to vary by imaging modality [4]. The numbers in our pilot study are too low to statistically

differentiate clinically significant feedback rates between modalities, but it is worth noting that no negative feedback was given in any mammography case. Similar low discrepancy results in mammography were described in the ACR RADPEER pilot (0.1% scored 3 or 4) and other studies [4,10,24]. This may reflect the standardized procedures used in assessing and reporting mammograms or the fact that the majority of mammographic studies are screening examinations with no significant abnormal findings [10,24]. Rates of clinically significant discrepancies in our study were similar to results in the literature for ultrasound (0.5%), general radiography (0.7%), and nuclear medicine (1.4%) [4]. Our highest rate was in fluoroscopy at 2.0% (95% CI, 0.4 to 10.3%); this is the first time RADPEER review rating have been described for this modality.

A criticism of the RADPEER program and of similar peer review processes has been that the rates of negative feedback, particularly of clinically significant discrepancies, appears lower than might be expected [3-5,13,25-28]. This has been attributed by some to the reluctance of radiologists to criticize colleagues [4]. The negative feedback rates

Table 4 Comparison of scoring in current study to published data

Author	O'Keeffe	Siegle*	Borgstede	Soffa**	Jackson	Swanson	Bender
Reference	Current	27	4	5	3	19	22
Year	2013	1998	2004	2004	2009	2012	2012
Grades							
0	0.2	NA	NA	NA	NA	NA	NA
1	99.1	95.6	96.3	96.5	97.1	96.2	96.5
2	0.1	1.4	2.9	NA	2.5	3.6	NA
3	0.5	NA	NA	NA	0.3	0.2	NA
4	0.1	NA	NA	NA	0.1	0.0	NA
Non-discrepant (0–1)	99.3	95.6	96.3	96.5	97.1	96.2	96.5
Concordant (0–2)	99.4	97.0	99.2	NA	99.6	99.8	NA
Discrepant (2–4)	0.7	4.4	3.7	3.5	2.9	3.8	3.5
Clinically Significant Discrepancy(3–4)	0.6	3.0	0.8	N/A	0.4	0.2	NA

NA not available.
Values are percentage of cases in each scoring category.
*Siegle et al. used a slightly different scoring system, but it has been accepted by RADPEER; values in the table for this paper are as reported in Borgstede [4].
**Soffa et al. used a 4-point rating system with nominally different definitions of each score, but they are very close to the RADPEER system [4,5].

contrast sharply with the much higher levels of disagreement reported in blinded clinical studies comparing interobserver performance in radiological diagnosis, where disagreement rates up to 30% are more are described [3,5,11,25-28]. In part, this may reflect the fact that the prevalence of abnormal findings is higher in directed research studies while many clinical radiographs are normal. Since most disagreements relate to false negative findings by the interpreting radiologist as judged by the reviewing radiologist, the rate of disagreement will be proportional to the frequency of abnormal findings [27]. In part, the higher disagreements in research studies may also arise from the very nature of the research protocols, where a wider range of findings are systematically evaluated and recorded in contrast to a lesser range in a typical clinical report. There is currently no objective benchmark for an acceptable level of disagreement in clinical practice [5,7,8,14], Given the fact that a number of unexplained variables have been identified to be associated with rates of disagreement, as noted above, there is reluctance to even attempt to define appropriate rates until further information is available [4,13,19,22]. One suggestion to improve the utility of the RADPEER system has been to allow comments in score 1 cases. Given the tendency of radiologists to classify some cases as score 1 when they should have been score 2, the use of comments allows critical input to the interpreting radiologist despite the under-scoring of disagreement [19].

Even though "error" is the terminology used in RADPEER, it is important to note that discrepant reviews simply indicate disagreement between the reviewing radiologist and the initial interpreting radiologist, and does not in itself mean that the interpreting radiologist made a mistake [4]. This points to the potential value of third-party adjudicators to provide consensus, accomplished in our program by review of all score 3 or 4 cases by the QA committee. In our pilot, all of these cases were ultimately considered to be errors. Single adjudicators are probably not sufficient to serve as the gold standard. An evaluation of 25 clinically significant discrepant cases (scores of 3 or 4) found that inter-observer agreement by multiple subspecialty reviewers was only slight to fair (kappa values of 0.11 to 0.20) [22]. Consensus evaluation by a multi-person QA committee will likely produce a more acceptable adjudication [18].

An aspect of the modified RADPEER system is the addition of score 0 to the original regime to allow positive feedback [3,4]. Such feedback can potentially play a role in improving quality by reinforcing performance regarded by a colleague as exemplary. In our study, only three cases (0.2%) received positive feedback. While this is a low proportion, it should be noted that this was greater than the number of cases that received a score of 4 (indicating a missed diagnosis that should almost always be made). In the future, as radiologists become

more familiar with routine peer review, positive feedback may become more common.

In addition to concerns about the low rate of discrepant scoring, another criticism of radiology peer review is the low completion rate by reviewers in RADPEER and other programs. In the RADPEER pilot, less than 10% of participating radiologists completed more than 200 cases despite the fact that participation was voluntary [4]. By way of explanation, it has been stated that radiologists resist time and resource commitments for additional activities outside the normal work activities, even small ones, due to work burden and costs of implementing such programs [4,11]. In our study, we encountered similar issues with completion of reviews, even though our program was designed to be as minimally intrusive and time-consuming as possible, and despite the fact that participation was voluntary, which might be expected to enlist the most enthusiastic partners. Our median noncompletion rate was 18%, with a range from 0% to 74%. Twenty-four % (95% CI, 22 to 26%) of assigned peer reviews were not completed and four of ten radiologists completed less than two-thirds of assigned cases. A recent report of another workstation-based peer review program found an overall one-year average of 53%, much lower than our 76% compliance rate [19]. In our study, the reasons for non-completion were not formally recorded during the pilot period, but some systemic issues were apparent, and may have similarly affected RADPEER or other peer review programs, underscoring the value of undertaking a pilot project for troubleshooting purposes prior to instituting a full peer review program. Some cases selected for random review could not be evaluated as the cases were chosen from the RIS and many of them did not have corresponding images in the PACS, while other cases did not have an accessible prior report in the RIS. The RIS and PACS were implemented two to three years prior to the pilot study so that prior cases predating implementation of these programs were not accessible. Early in the project, procedures that were non-evaluable were presented for review, such as therapeutic joint injections, and these types of procedures were eliminated from subsequent computer selection. In some circumstances, such as gastrointestinal fluoroscopy, the case selected was not a relevant prior as the computer program did not distinguish between upper GI and lower GI examinations. Another contributor to non-completion may have been the option to delay a review. Of the reviewed cases, 94% (95% CI, 93 to 95%) were completed within 15 minutes of assignment, indicating that once a radiologist had committed to a review, it was done during the reporting of the current case. If a review was not done immediately upon presentation, however, the reviewing radiologist was reminded when the current dictation was completed. If the review was delayed further, the case was saved pending completion of the review. The radiologist was then required to sign into the peer review program and manually search for the case in PACS, a less efficient option. The program is being modified so that a second reminder will be issued at the time a radiologist verifies a current report, and so that the reasons for non-completion will be documented. All voluntary peer review programs will suffer from similar variability in commitment, although rates will certainly increase if peer review is made a mandatory part of practice or hospital protocol, or if required for certification or other regulatory reasons. One suggestion that has been made is to institute financial incentives or penalties [19]. Another suggestion for review systems integrated into the workstations has been to block the ability to continue with the daily workload until quality assurance reviews are completed [19]. These approaches have not received acceptance as they place a burden on participating radiologists [14,19]. One mechanism shown to improve compliance, and that will likely be more acceptable to the profession, is monthly compliance reports to individual reviewing radiologists. One study found with this approach that compliance rates rose from 42% to 76% over one year [19].

Many radiologists function in environments with little opportunity to systematically identify errors and thus correct knowledge gaps [2,11], but it has been difficult to achieve such opportunities in routine practice [3,4,11,20]. We have described the results of a pilot peer review program which demonstrates an approach that can be applied in clinical practice, even in a large radiology group with busy outpatient clinics. A key feature of the pilot program was a review process that was workstation-based and integrated into reporting software so that it was seamlessly incorporated into the normal workday [13,29]. In addition, the procedure was practice-integrated in the manner of the RADPEER program in that the images chosen for review were prior studies related to cases currently being reported, and the review was performed during the regular reporting process [3,4,13]. Since relevant prior reports and prior images are routinely evaluated when a current study is being reported, linking the review process to active cases reduces the time and work burden [3,4,13]. Through computerized automation, no work was required in pulling and collating cases, and the cases were randomly selected and representative of the practice [3,7,8,13,18]. The review itself was performed within the reporting software so that there was no need to record paper or online review forms [4,29]. Assessment of data using our approach was done locally, so that interpreting radiologists could be immediately informed of their peer results, individual and aggregate case data could be prepared on an as-needed basis, and cases could be easily identified for discrepancy rounds, case-sharing, and other educational initiatives 11, 13, 19, 20, 21.

In addition to concerns about low discrepancy rates and low review completion rates, a number of other critiques have been leveled at the use of peer review in radiology and some of these remain as limitations of our protocol. One is that this approach does not delve into the ultimate clinical diagnosis so that it can be correlated with radiological findings to provide definitive feedback. The response to this is virtually universal among those involved in quality assessment in radiology: there are no accepted definitions of what constitutes the gold standard for evaluation of most imaging findings and it would be excessively time-consuming and cost-prohibitive to attempt to track cases [1,2,4,8,11,12]. Such an accuracy-assessment program will probably only occur if mandated and funded by external sources. A related criticism is that most peer review systems do not incorporate an evaluation of the clinical significance of radiological discrepancies. For example, among our cases scored 3 or 4 was a stable calcified scapular lesion and inferolateral ventricular ischemia, which would clearly differ in clinical importance. The most recent iteration of RADPEER includes the option for rating clinical significance, but there has been poor uptake [3,4]. The reason is straightforward: it is often difficult to judge the clinical significance of a particular radiological finding in the absence of full clinical information, which is rarely available at the time of reporting. Given the experience of RADPEER, we chose to not include rating of clinical significance in our peer review process.

Our study did not include either CT or MRI studies simply because our pilot program was done in outpatient clinics, and in our health region these modalities are primarily hospital-based. Many published studies have included these modalities, so there is no reason that they should not be included in peer review programs [4,5,19,23,27,30]. By virtue of their increased complexity and the fact that they are often secondary tests done to follow-up an abnormal result or suspected abnormal result on other imaging, a higher disagreement rate is to be expected, and this is what has been found [4,5,19,23,27,30]. We believe that all imaging modalities, including those that are more operator-dependent, such as fluoroscopy and ultrasound, can be incorporated in peer review, although special attention may be needed in choosing and evaluating these cases [4,5,23].

Two-thirds of our interpreting radiologists reported that the review feedback they received was appropriate, 26% reported that the reviews prompted them to review literature or attend educational events, and 67% found the online presentation of score 3 and 4 cases to be valuable. Based on rates of clinically significant discrepancies of 0.2 to 0.8% (Table 4), it requires 125 to 200 peer reviews to find one important disagreement. Is this disruption, with the associated time commitment, expense, and potential exposure to regulatory and legal repercussions, worth the perceived educational benefit? Studies are needed in two areas to better define the appropriate role for peer review in radiology. First, the financial costs of peer review need to be quantified, as they are borne by radiologists or academic departments. Second, the outcomes of the peer review process need to be determined to see whether future practice performance is improved. With such data, cost-effectiveness of peer review can be determined. For now, the approach of the American College of Radiology and of many other groups is that "peer review has become an essential component of a comprehensive radiology department quality assurance program" [19]. Implementing a workstation-based computerized program we have described is one way to effectively incorporate peer review in an active clinical practice.

Conclusions

Peer review should identify opportunities for quality improvement, facilitate improved outcomes, and contribute to increased competence [7,8,13,19]. Review of possible errors made by colleagues is a recognized learning opportunity for the reviewing physician, the interpreting physician, and those participating in discrepancy rounds or related educational activities [18]. Our pilot project has demonstrated one way in which this can be accomplished using a workstation-integrated computerized system that randomly selects prior cases for review based on cases currently being reported. This approach minimizes time and work impact by blending reviews into the normal workday. Cases were drawn fairly equally from different imaging modalities and the selection process is intrinsically random, avoiding bias. Discrepancy rounds or virtual discrepancy rounds that present cases with scores of 3 or 4 facilitate dissemination of information, with the majority of our radiologists feeling such rounds were valuable. Our radiology group has now instituted workstation-integrated peer review with mandatory participation for all radiologists in the clinic-based part of the practice and is actively working towards establishing a similar review system in our hospital departments including all modalities. Peer review should be considered by all radiologists as a means to reduce errors and improve consistency. If widely adopted, this could demonstrate to the public and governments that the radiology profession is committed to the highest standards of clinical care. The cost-effectiveness of peer review needs further study, but for now remains the primary quality assessment tool in radiology.

Abbreviations

ACR: American College of Radiology; CI: Confidence interval; MIC: Medical Imaging Consultants; PACS: Picture archiving and communication system; QA: Quality assurance; RIS: Radiology information system.

Competing interests

Todd Davis is an employee of Intelerad. The other authors have no competing interests.

Authors' contributions

MMO participated in study design, data analysis, and data interpretation, and contributed to drafting the manuscript. TMD participated in study design, collected raw data, and provided critical revision of the manuscript. KS participated in study design, data analysis, and data interpretation, and contributed to drafting the manuscript. All authors have read and approved the manuscript.

Authors' information

MMO and KS are affiliated with the Department of Radiology and Diagnostic Imaging, University of Alberta, and with Medical Imaging Consultants, Edmonton, Alberta, Canada. TMD is an employee of Intelerad, Montreal, Quebec, Canada, and developed the Intelerad Peer Review software.

Author details

[1]Department of Radiology and Diagnostic Imaging, University of Alberta, and Medical Imaging Consultants, 11010-101 Street, Edmonton, AB T5H 4B9, Canada. [2]Intelerad, Montreal, QC, Canada. [3]295 Midpark Way SE, Suite 380, Calgary, AB T2X 2A8, Canada.

References

1. Steele JR, Hovsepian DM, Schomer DF: The Joint Commission practice performance evaluation: a primer for radiologists. *J Am Coll Radiol* 2010, 7:425–430.
2. Johnson CD, Krecke KN, Miranda R, *et al*: Quality initiatives: developing a radiology quality and safety program: a primer. *Radiographics* 2009, 29:951–959.
3. Jackson VP, Cushing T, Abujudeh HH, *et al*: RADPEER scoring white paper. *J Am Coll Radiol* 2009, 6:21–25.
4. Borgestede JP, Lewis RS, Bhargavan M, *et al*: RADPEER quality assurance program: a multifacility study of interpretive disagreement rates. *J Am Coll Radiol* 2004, 1:59–65.
5. Soffa DJ, Lewis RS, Sunshine JH, *et al*: Disagreement in interpretation: a method for the development of benchmarks for quality assurance in imaging. *J Am Coll Radiol* 2004, 1:212–217.
6. Lockyer JM, Violato C, Fidler HM: Assessment of radiologists by a regulatory authority. *Radiol* 2008, 247:771–778.
7. Strife JL, Kun LE, Becker GJ, *et al*: American Board of Radiology perspective on maintenance of certification: part IV-practice quality improvement for diagnostic radiology. *Radiographics* 2007, 27:769–774.
8. Landon BE, Norman ST, Blumenthal D, *et al*: Physician clinical performance assessment. *JAMA* 2003, 290:1183–1189.
9. Munk PL, Forster BB: Accreditation: problem or opportunity? *Can Assoc Radiol J* 2011, 62:88–89.
10. Wadden N: Breast cancer screening in Canada: a review. *Can Assoc Radiol J* 2005, 56:271–275.
11. FitzGerald R: Radiological error: analysis, standard setting, targeted instruction and teamworking. *Eur Radiol* 2005, 15:1760–1767.
12. Steele JR: The role of RADPEER in the Joint Commission Ongoing Practice Performance Evaluation. *J Am Coll Radiol* 2011, 8:6–7.
13. Mahgerefteh S, Kruskal JB, Yam CS, *et al*: Quality initiatives: peer review in diagnostic radiology: current state and a vision for the future. *Radiographics* 2009, 29:1221–1231.
14. Larson DB, Nance JJ: Rethinking peer review: what aviation can teach radiology about performance improvement. *Radiol* 2011, 259:626–672.
15. Halsted MJ: Radiology peer review as an opportunity to reduce errors and improve patient care. *J Am Coll Radiol* 2004, 1:984–987.
16. Ramsey PG, Wenrich MD, Carline JD, *et al*: Use of peer ratings to evaluate physician performance. *JAMA* 1993, 269:1655–1660.
17. American College of Radiologists: *Practice of radiology in the US.* http://www.acr.org/Quality-Safety/RADPEER. Accessed July 5, 2013.
18. The Royal College of Radiologists: *Standards for radiology discrepancy meetings.* London: The Royal College of Radiologists; 2007.
19. Swanson JO, Thapa MM, Iyer RS, Otto RK, Weinberger E: Optimizing peer review: A year of experience after instituting a real-time comment-enhanced program at a Children's Hospital. *Am J Roentgenol* 2012, 198:1121–1125.

20. FitzGerald R: **Performance-based assessment of radiology faculty.** *Am J Roentgenol* 2006, **186**:265.
21. Nakielny R: **Setting up medical discrepancy meetings – the practicalities.** *CME Radiology* 2003, **4**:29–30.
22. Bender LC, Linnau KF, Meier EN, Anzai Y, Gunn ML: **Interrater agreement in the evaluation of discrepant imaging findings with the Radpeer system.** *Am J Roentgenol* 2012, **199**:1320–1327.
23. Ruma J, Klein KA, Chong S, *et al*: **Cross-sectional examination interpretation discrepancies between on-call diagnostic radiology residents and subspecialty faculty radiologists: analysis by imaging modality and subspecialty.** *J Am Coll Radiol* 2011, **199**:1320–1327.
24. Lee JKT: **Quality-a radiology imperative: interpretation accuracy and pertinence.** *J Am Coll Radiol* 2007, **4**:162–165.
25. Yoon LS, Haims AH, Brink JA, *et al*: **Evaluation of an emergency radiology quality assurance program at a level I trauma center: abdominal and pelvic CT studies.** *Radiology* 2002, **224**:42–46.
26. Tilleman EH, Phoa SS, Van Delden OM, *et al*: **Reinterpretation of radiologic imaging in patients referred to a tertiary referral centre with a suspected pancreatic or hepatobiliary malignancy: impact on treatment strategy.** *Eur Radiol* 2003, **13**:1095–1099.
27. Siegle RL, Baram EM, Reuter SR, *et al*: **Rates of disagreement in imaging interpretation in a group of community hospitals.** *Acad Radiol* 1998, **5**:148–154.
28. Rhea JT, Potsaid MS, DeLuca SA: **Errors of interpretation as elicited by a quality audit of an emergency radiology facility.** *Radiology* 1979, **132**:277–280.
29. Prevedello L, Khorasani R: **Enhancing quality assurance and quality control programs: IT tools can help.** *J Am Coll Radiol* 2009, **6**:888–889.
30. Maloney E, Lomasney LM, Schomer L: **Application of the RADPEER scoring language to interpretation discrepancies between diagnostic radiology residents and faculty radiologists.** *J Am Coll Radiol* 2012, **9**:264–269.

16

An evaluation of meniscal collagenous structure using optical projection tomography

Stephen HJ Andrews[1*], Janet L Ronsky[2,3], Jerome B Rattner[4], Nigel G Shrive[2,3] and Heather A Jamniczky[4]

Abstract

Background: The collagenous structure of menisci is a complex network of circumferentially oriented fascicles and interwoven radially oriented tie-fibres. To date, examination of this micro- architecture has been limited to two-dimensional imaging techniques. The purpose of this study was to evaluate the ability of the three-dimensional imaging technique; optical projection tomography (OPT), to visualize the collagenous structure of the meniscus. If successful, this technique would be the first to visualize the macroscopic orientation of collagen fascicles in 3-D in the meniscus and could further refine load bearing mechanisms in the tissue. OPT is an imaging technique capable of imaging samples on the meso-scale (1-10 mm) at a micro-scale resolution. The technique, similar to computed tomography, takes two-dimensional images of objects from incremental angles around the object and reconstructs them using a back projection algorithm to determine three-dimensional structure.

Methods: Bovine meniscal samples were imaged from four locations (outer main body, femoral surface, tibial surface and inner main body) to determine the variation in collagen orientation throughout the tissue. Bovine stifles (n = 2) were obtained from a local abattoir and the menisci carefully dissected. Menisci were fixed in methanol and subsequently cut using a custom cutting jig (n = 4 samples per meniscus). Samples were then mounted in agarose, dehydrated in methanol and subsequently cleared using benzyl alcohol benzyl benzoate (BABB) and imaged using OPT.

Results: Results indicate circumferential, radial and oblique collagenous orientations at the contact surfaces and in the inner third of the main body of the meniscus. Imaging identified fascicles ranging from 80-420 μm in diameter. Transition zones where fascicles were found to have a woven or braided appearance were also identified. The outer-third of the main body was composed of fascicles oriented predominantly in the circumferential direction. Blood vessels were also visualized using this technique, as their elastin content fluoresces more brightly than collagen at the 425 nm wavelength used by the OPT scanner.

Conclusions: OPT was capable of imaging the collagenous structure, as well as blood vessels in the bovine meniscus. Collagenous structure variability, including transition zones between structural regions not previously described in the meniscus, was identified using this novel technique.

Keywords: Meniscus, Optical projection tomography, Collagen structure

Background

The menisci are complex three-dimensional structures with a heterogeneous structure. The semi-lunar, wedge shapes of the menisci increase the contact area between the rounded femoral condyles and the relatively flat tibia plateau, thereby protecting the articular cartilage from excessive stresses [1–3]. Menisci are fibrocartilages, which have been described as having intermediate structural and functional properties between those of dense, fibrous connective tissue (i.e. ligament, tendon) and hyaline cartilage [4].

The composition and structure of the meniscus has been studied extensively since Fairbank discovered the relationship between meniscal removal and the observation of degenerative changes in the knee [5]. An early investigation of the menisci by Bullough et al. in [6], described the structure of human menisci as consisting predominantly of circumferentially oriented fibres [6]. The study

* Correspondence: shjandrews@gmail.com
[1]Department of Biomedical Engineering, Schulich School of Engineering, University of Calgary, Human Performance Lab, 2500 University Drive NW, Calgary, AB T2N 1N4, Canada
Full list of author information is available at the end of the article

also identified the presence of radially oriented tie-fibres that the authors supposed acted to tie the circumferentially oriented fibres together to prevent longitudinal splitting of the tissue. The conceptual model of a predominance of circumferentially oriented fibres has subsequently been supported in numerous studies [7–11].

The major limitation of these previous models is the use of two-dimensional (2D) imaging techniques to evaluate a highly three-dimensional (3D) structure. One can section and image 2D structures sequentially and subsequently reconstruct 3D models, but this technique is time consuming and difficult, and to date has not been completed for the meniscus. Optical sectioning using confocal microscopy can yield 3D structures, but the maximum sample depth of a few hundred microns is a limitation in this technique.

Optical projection tomography (OPT) is a promising technique which could overcome the inherent difficulties in imaging a highly heterogeneous structure [12], as it is an imaging technique capable of imaging samples on the meso-scale (1-10 mm) at a micro-scale resolution. The technique takes two-dimensional images of objects from multiple angles and reconstructs them using a back projection algorithm to determine its three-dimensional structure). It is optically similar to computed tomography (CT), but uses white or fluorescent light rather than x-ray to image the object of interest. The technique requires for the tissue to be cleared to allow light to pass through the object. OPT has primarily been used to evaluate development and gene expression in mouse embryos [12]. To date, no study has attempted to evaluate collagenous structure of connective tissues using OPT. As collagen and elastin both autofluoresce at similar wavelengths (325 nm) [13] in the fluorescent spectrum, this technique may be useful in the evaluation of meniscal tissue structure. The study described here was exploratory in nature. The purpose was to determine the ability of OPT to visualize the collagenous matrix organization of the meniscus.

Methods
Sample preparation
Bovine stifle joints (n = 2) were obtained from a local abattoir within 48 hours of slaughter (18-30 months age) and the medial menisci were carefully dissected. The menisci were fixed in 100% methanol at 4°C for 48 hours. Four specimen (approximately 3-4 mm in each of three dimensions) were dissected from a radial section cut from the anterior portion of the meniscus and prepared for OPT (Figure 1). The scanner is capable of imaging samples up to 10 mm. However, as the scanner resolution is inversely related to the sample size, sample dimensions of 3-4 mm were chosen. The four specimens were prepared from different locations in order to observe site-specific variation

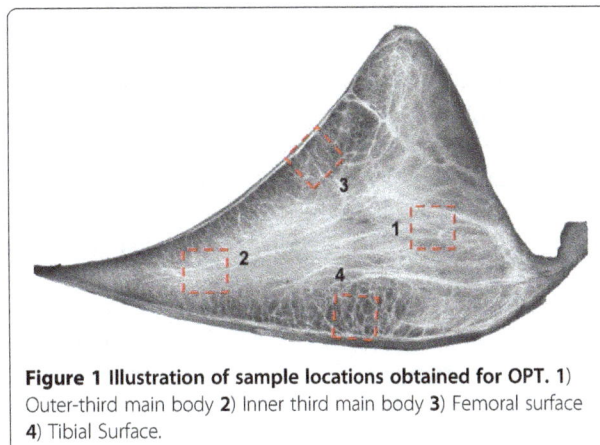

Figure 1 Illustration of sample locations obtained for OPT. 1) Outer-third main body **2)** Inner third main body **3)** Femoral surface **4)** Tibial Surface.

in the structure. The specimens were prepared from: 1) Outer third of the main body 2) Inner third of the main body 3) Femoral surface 4) Tibial Surface. Institutional review board approval was not required for this study.

Optical projection tomography
Specimens were scanned using fluorescence optical projection tomography [12] on a Bioptonics 3001 M OPT scanner (Bioptonics Microscopy, Edinburgh). Each tissue sample was embedded in a block of 1.5% low melting point agarose (Invitrogen). Blocks were trimmed and glued to mounts, and dehydrated through three washes of 100% methanol (Fisher) over 24 hours. Specimens were then cleared for 24 hours in BABB (1 part benzyl alcohol (Fisher): 2 parts benzyl benzoate (Sigma) in a fume hood, allowing any remaining methanol to evaporate.

Native autofluorescence was imaged using the GFP-1 channel (exciter 425 nm/40 nm; emitter LP475 nm) at a resolution of 13.6-20 μm. Raw images were reconstructed into greyscale slices using NRecon (Skyscan NV, Kontich). Each reconstruction results in a stack of 250-500 images, based on the sample size and resolution used. Three dimensional reconstructions were then carried out using ImageJ (NIH open source software) [14]. The stacks of images were imported and visualized using the 3D Viewer plugin and the Volume Viewer plugin. The 3D Viewer renders a 3D surface image of the sample from the slices while the volume viewer allows visualization of sections through the sample in a user defined plane. Images of interest were exported to Adobe Photoshop Elements 9.0 (Adobe Inc.) and filtered with a despeckling filter. Measurements of fascicle diameter were completed using ImageJ pixel information and converting to length using the known resolution of the images.

Results
Optical projection tomography was capable of imaging collagen fascicle orientations in 3D within a specimen. We were also able to identify blood vessels in all

specimens obtained from the outer half of bovine menisci. Specimens imaged with OPT each showed different fascicle orientation patterns. Specimen 1, taken from the outer third of the main body, contained a highly aligned fascicle structure. Sections through the middle, and the extreme ends of the specimen all showed the same predominant fascicle direction (Figure 2). Blood vessels, which fluoresce more brightly than the surrounding collagen, were seen to persist throughout the specimen. Multiple vessels appear to be situated in an area of low collagen density (Figure 2) Blood vessels were observed in samples taken from both the surfaces and outer portion of the menisci (Figure 3). An additional movie file shows this in more detail (see Additional file 1). Specimen 2 was taken in the same orientation as specimen 1, but from the inner third of the tissue. This specimen showed a distinctly different fascicle orientation pattern than specimen 1. The top surface of this sample was composed of a woven pattern with fascicles oriented perpendicular to others within the same plane (Figure 4). Moving through this section in the superior/inferior direction revealed high variability in the fascicle direction. The most superior plane contained aligned fascicles. Moving through the section revealed an intricately woven arrangement with fascicles oriented in multiple directions. The most inferior section through this specimen showed an aligned arrangement, oblique to the arrangement seen in the superior portion of the specimen. The samples from the femoral and tibial surfaces (specimen 3 and 4) demonstrated similar fascicle orientation patterns throughout (Figure 5). The contact surfaces contained fascicles oriented in the direction parallel to the surface in the radial direction. Moving in the direction normal to the contact surfaces, the fascicles changed alignment and in some sections became woven, and in others appeared to be braided. The braided appearance is defined by fascicles running obliquely to

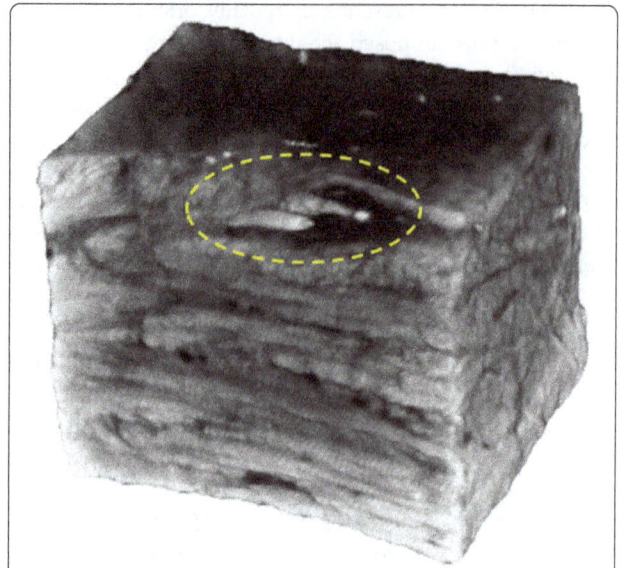

Figure 3 A meniscal specimen taken from the femoral surface of a medial meniscus. Two blood vessels can be seen running parallel inside an area devoid of collagen fascicles.

one another, rather than perpendicular as in the woven arrangement (Figure 6). Surface samples also revealed fluorescence indicative of blood vessels located beneath the lamellar layer. The fascicle size ranged from approximately 80-420 µm. These accuracy of these measurements are limited by manual detection of fascicle borders as well as the resolution of the pixels (14-20 µm based on the sample size).

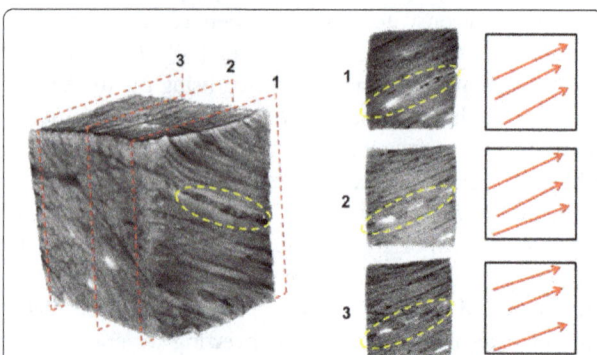

Figure 2 A meniscal sample taken from the outer one-third of the main body of the meniscus. The planes identified by the red dashed lines are shown in the panels **1-3** to the right. Predominant fascicle directions are illustrated by the red arrows. All planes showed similar fascicle orientations. The collagen sparse void space containing blood vessels are indicated by the yellow dashed ellipses.

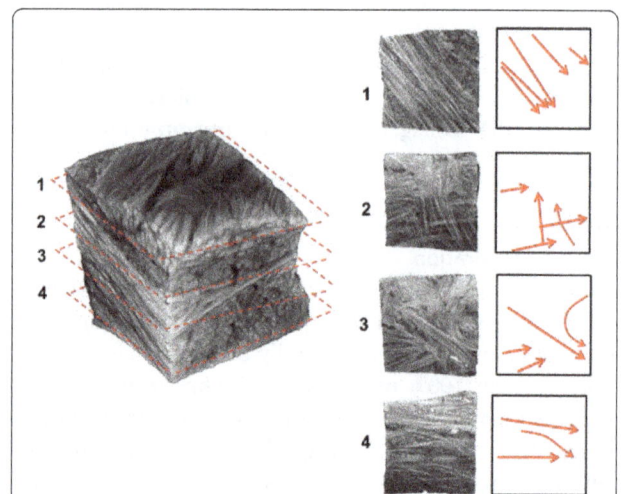

Figure 4 A meniscal sample taken from the inner one-third of the main body of the meniscus. Varying fascicle orientations can be observed in planes **1-4**, moving in the superior to inferior direction. Red arrows to the right indicate the predominant fascicle directions in each breakout section image.

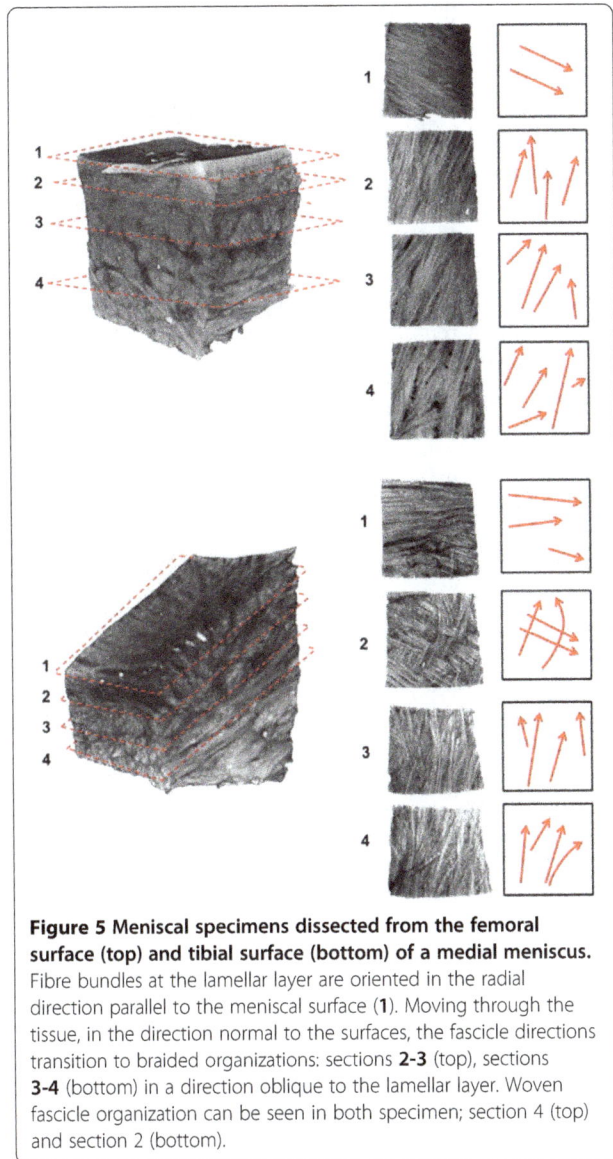

Figure 5 Meniscal specimens dissected from the femoral surface (top) and tibial surface (bottom) of a medial meniscus. Fibre bundles at the lamellar layer are oriented in the radial direction parallel to the meniscal surface (**1**). Moving through the tissue, in the direction normal to the surfaces, the fascicle directions transition to braided organizations: sections **2-3** (top), sections **3-4** (bottom) in a direction oblique to the lamellar layer. Woven fascicle organization can be seen in both specimen; section 4 (top) and section 2 (bottom).

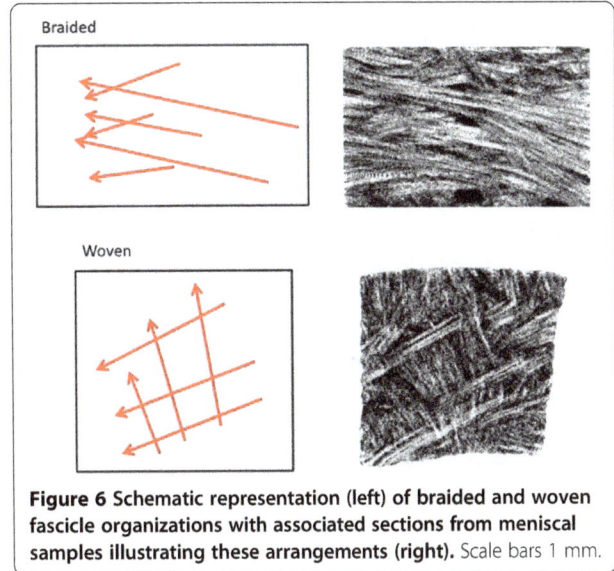

Figure 6 Schematic representation (left) of braided and woven fascicle organizations with associated sections from meniscal samples illustrating these arrangements (right). Scale bars 1 mm.

Discussion

This study has evaluated the ability of optical projection tomography to visualize the collagenous fascicle structure of meniscal specimen. The technique was able to resolve meniscal collagen fascicle orientation, differences between structural layers and blood vessels in three-dimensional space. Specimens dissected from the tibial and femoral surfaces demonstrated a highly aligned lamellar layer near the contact surfaces. This finding agrees with previous findings that showed a distinct layer (150-200 µm thick) with fascicles oriented in the radial direction along the surface of human menisci [10].

The maximum resolution of the system is approximately 5 µm. The resolution of the images obtained here ranged from 13.6-20 µm. Due to the limitation of this resolution, the imaging of individual collagen fibres

(5 µm diameter [11]) is not possible, but collagen fascicles which have a diameters of 80-420 µm could be visualized. These fascicle sizes agree very well with previous scanning electron microscopy studies which found fascicle sizes on the range of 100-400 µm [10]. Further, visualizing the surface layer identified by Peterson and Tillman (10 µm thick) is not practical with samples of this size. This layer may be visible in smaller samples where the system resolution can be maximized.

The specimen from the outer third of the main body demonstrated the aligned circumferential fibre direction described previously [6,9,11]. This specimen also contained multiple blood vessels which were situated within a collagen-sparse void space. Recent unpublished work from our lab has indicated that this void space is likely a proteoglycan rich region which may play a protective role for blood vessels by shielding them from shear stresses. Blood vessels were also seen along the femoral and tibial surfaces. The position of the vasculature within the tissue agree with the findings of Arnoczky and Warren in the human meniscus [15].

We have identified two major types of fascicle organizations, braided and woven (Figure 6), not previously described in the meniscus. These two organizations could play a significant role in the load bearing mechanism and the fracture toughness of the meniscus. The braided fascicle organization is common in various types of rope [16]. This organization results in a non-linear stiffness which increases with increasing deformation. As the fascicles are stretched axially, they compress against adjacent fascicles increasing the friction between them, thereby increasing the stiffness. This is a mechanical behaviour also observed in meniscal samples in tension [17,18]. The woven arrangement is common in fabrics and in structures that withstand compressive loading onto a flat structure (e.g. a basket). This fascicle arrangement allows for the conversion of compressive forces into tensile forces in the weave via attachments to a rigid supporting structure. In the case of the menisci, the ligamentous attachments to the tibial plateau would provide a sufficient supporting structure. These two fascicle organizations could also play a role in increasing the fracture toughness of the menisci. A crack passing through a woven arrangement would encounter fascicles perpendicular to the direction of crack propagation, which would increase the size of deformation zone and divert energy away from the crack tip [19]. The bending of fascicles around one another would also increase the path length and direction a crack would have to follow in order to separate the fascicles. These combined mechanisms may increase the menisci's resistance to failure under physiologic loading conditions. It was observed that many fascicles bifurcate or arborize into multiple smaller fascicles. These arborized fascicles tended to change direction from the path of the branching fascicles. Fascicles were often observed to curve within a plane (Figure 4: Image 3). These findings are also supported by recent findings from our lab [20]. These frequent changes in direction and arborization of fascicles make it difficult to quantify fascicle orientations as well as fascicle size distribution.

Tissue composition varies from the inner cartilage-like tip, to the outer edge of the meniscus [8,21,22]. The results of this study have demonstrated that the structure of the tissue is also transitional. From the outer third of the meniscus to the inner third the fascicle arrangement changes from being highly aligned in the circumferential direction to being a woven, less organized structure at the inner third. The inner tip is similar to hyaline cartilage in both composition and structure. Proteoglycan content is approximately 10% and type II collagen is more abundant than type I collagen [21,23,24]. Taken together, it can be observed that from the inner tip to the outer edge, the bovine meniscus transitions from a hyaline cartilage-like tissue through an intermediate structure in the inner-portion to a highly aligned ligament-like portion at the outer edge. Further, at the contact surfaces there is a transition from the radially oriented lamellar layer at the surface to the woven or braided orientations seen in the sub-lamellar main body. Benjamin and Ralphs previously described fibrocartilage as a transitional tissue, as it is commonly seen in the interface between different tissue types (i.e. at the tendinous junctions with bone) and because of changes in tissue structure throughout development [25]. It has been demonstrated here that the structure within the menisci also fits the paradigm of fibrocartilage as a transitional tissue.

Conclusion

OPT was able to visualize collagen fascicle organization in bovine menisci. This novel technique had not previously been used in the study of connective tissues. We have visualized two fascicle organizations, not previously described in the menisci: braided and woven which may help in further elucidating the load bearing mechanisms within this highly complex tissue. Optical projection tomography is a promising technique in the evaluation of the organization of other connective tissues and changes that occur due to injury or disease processes. For example, changes that occur to tendons after implantation as anterior cruciate ligament (ACL) autografts could be examined to understand remodeling that occurs in soft tissue. This technique also has potential in developmental studies, evaluating collagenous matrix organization of connective tissues throughout the process of growth and maturation.

Abbreviations
BABB: Benzyl alcohol benzyl benzoate; GFP: Green fluorescent protein; OPT: Optical projection tomography.

Competing interests
The authors declare that they have no competing interests.

Authors' contribution
SA was the primary author and responsible for data analysis for this article. JLR was involved in project conception and article revision. NS provided expertise in the mechanical interpretation of the results and article revision. JBR aided in image analysis and article preparation. HJ provided expertise in sample preparation and data collection for OPT as well and article revision and writing. All authors read and approved the final manuscript.

Acknowledgements
Gratitude is due to May Chung for her outstanding technical assistance. The authors gratefully acknowledge funding from NSERC and CIHR.

Author details
[1]Department of Biomedical Engineering, Schulich School of Engineering, University of Calgary, Human Performance Lab, 2500 University Drive NW, Calgary, AB T2N 1N4, Canada. [2]Mechanical and Manufacturing Engineering, Schulich School of Engineering, Faculty of Kinesiology, University of Calgary, Calgary, Canada. [3]McCaig Institute for Bone and Joint Health, University of Calgary, Calgary, Canada. [4]Department of Cell Biology and Anatomy, The McCaig Institute for Bone and Joint Health, Faculty of Medicine, University of Calgary, Calgary, Canada.

References
1. Shrive NG, O'Connor JJ, et al: "Load-bearing in the knee joint". Clin Orthop Relat Res 1978(131):279–287.
2. Baratz ME, Fu FH, et al: Meniscal tears: the effect of meniscectomy and of repair on intraarticular contact areas and stress in the human knee. A preliminary report. Am J Sports Med 1986, 14(4):270–275.
3. Cottrell JM, Scholten P, et al: A new technique to measure the dynamic contact pressures on the Tibial Plateau. J Biomech 2008, 41(10):2324–2329.
4. Benjamin M, Evans EJ: Fibrocartilage. J Anat 1990, 171:1–15.
5. Fairbank TJ: Knee joint changes after meniscectomy. J Bone Joint Surg Br 1948, 30B(4):664–670.
6. Bullough PG, Munuera L, et al: The strength of the menisci of the knee as it relates to their fine structure. J Bone Joint Surg Br 1970, 52(3):564–567.
7. Cameron HU, Macnab I: The structure of the meniscus of the human knee joint. Clin Orthop Relat Res 1972, 89:215–219.
8. McDevitt CA, Webber RJ: "The ultrastructure and biochemistry of meniscal cartilage". Clin Orthop Relat Res 1990(252):8–18.

9. Skaggs DL, Warden WH, *et al*: Radial tie fibers influence the tensile properties of the bovine medial meniscus. *J Orthop Res* 1994, **12**(2):176–185.

10. Petersen W, Tillmann B: Collagenous fibril texture of the human knee joint menisci. *Anat Embryol (Berl)* 1998, **197**(4):317–324.

11. Rattner JB, Matyas JR, *et al*: New understanding of the complex structure of knee menisci: implications for injury risk and repair potential for athletes. *Scand J Med Sci Sports* 2011, **21**(4):543–553.

12. Sharpe J, Ahlgren U, *et al*: Optical projection tomography as a tool for 3D microscopy and gene expression studies. *Science* 2002, **296**(5567):541–545.

13. Richards-Kortum R, Sevick-Muraca E: Quantitative optical spectroscopy for tissue diagnosis. *Annu Rev Phys Chem* 1996, **47**:555–606.

14. Abràmoff MD, Magalhães PJ, *et al*: Image processing with ImageJ. *Biophotonics international* 2004, **11**(7):36–42.

15. Arnoczky SP, Warren RF: Microvasculature of the human meniscus. *Am J Sports Med* 1982, **10**(2):90–95.

16. Leech CM: Theory and numerical-methods for the modeling of synthetic ropes. *Communications in Applied Numerical Methods* 1987, **3**(5):407–413.

17. Fithian DC, Kelly MA, *et al*: "Material properties and structure-function relationships in the menisci". *Clin Orthop Relat Res* 1990(252):19–31.

18. Tissakht M, Ahmed AM: Tensile stress–strain characteristics of the human meniscal material. *J Biomech* 1995, **28**(4):411–422.

19. Briscoe BJ, Court RS, *et al*: The effects of fabric weave and surface texture on the interlaminar fracture toughness of aramid/epoxy laminates. *Compos Sci Technol* 1993, **47**(3):261–270.

20. Andrews SHJ: *Meniscus structure and function.* Calgary, AB, Canada: PhD, University of Calgary; 2013.

21. Nakano T, Dodd CM, *et al*: Glycosaminoglycans and proteoglycans from different zones of the porcine knee meniscus. *J Orthop Res* 1997, **15**(2):213–220.

22. Sanchez-Adams J, Athanasiou KA: "Biomechanics of meniscus cells: regional variation and comparison to articular chondrocytes and ligament cells.". *Biomech Model Mechanobiol* 2012, **11**(7):1047–56. doi:10.1007/s10237-012-0372-0. Epub 2012 Jan 10.

23. Kambic HE, McDevitt CA: Spatial organization of types I and II collagen in the canine meniscus. *J Orthop Res* 2005, **23**(1):142–149.

24. Melrose J, Smith S, *et al*: Comparative spatial and temporal localisation of perlecan, aggrecan and type I, II and IV collagen in the ovine meniscus: an ageing study. *Histochem Cell Biol* 2005, **124**(3–4):225–235.

25. Benjamin M, Ralphs JR: Biology of fibrocartilage cells. *Int Rev Cytol* 2004, **233**:1–45.

17

Diagnostic value of diffusion-weighted MR imaging in thyroid disease: application in differentiating benign from malignant disease

Yingwei Wu[1†], Xiuhui Yue[3†], Weiwen Shen[1], Yushan Du[1], Ying Yuan[2], Xiaofeng Tao[2*] and Cheuk Ying Tang[4]

Abstract

Background: Fine needle aspiration biopsy is usually performed to evaluate thyroid lesions. The purpose of this study was to evaluate the usefulness of diffusion weighted imaging to differentiate malignancy of thyroid lesions.

Methods: The study was approved by ethics committee of Shanghai Changzheng Hospital.Forty-two patients, 10 men and 32 women (range: 20–72 years, mean age 42.4 years) with thyroid lesions were included in the study. Routine neck MR and diffusion-weighted MR imaging was performed using multiple b-values. ADC values were computed for the different b-values. Histological results of the thyroidectomy samples were obtained for all the patients. ADC values of benign and malignant thyroid lesions were compared with the pathology results. Logistic regression analysis was used to detect independent parameters for differentiating benign and malignancy of lesions.

Result: Based on the histology results there were 28 benign and 14 malignant cases. The difference of ADC value between benign and malignant thyroid lesions was significant for ADC values obtained using b-values of 0 and 300 s/mm^2 ($p < 0.001$). The ADC values were significantly higher in benign lesions (benign ADC: $2.37 \pm 0.47 \times 10\text{-}3$ mm^2/s vs. malignant: $1.49 \pm 0.60 \times 10\text{-}3$ mm^2/s). ADC values obtained with b-values of 0 and 300 mm^2/s and max nodular diameter was regarded as the two most discriminative parameters for differentiating malignancy. Using the pathology results as a standard reference, area under ROC curve was found to be 0.876 for an ADC cutoff value of $2.17 \times 10\text{-}3$ mm^2/s that corresponded to an acquisition with b-values of 0 and 300 mm^2/s.

Conclusion: Diffusion-weighted MR imaging is a promising non-invasive method to differentiate malignancy in thyroid lesions.

Keywords: Thyroid lesions, Diffusion weighted imaging, ADC mapping

Background

Incidence and prevalence of thyroid disease has seen a great increase in recent years. An increasing incidence of thyroid cancer has been reported worldwide [1-3]. The reported incidence of thyroid cancer is up to 0.07% over the past 30 years [4]. 44,670 new cases and 1,690 deaths were attributed to thyroid cancer in 2010 [5]. Fine needle aspiration biopsy (FNAB) is regarded as the standard reference for diagnosis, but it has been reported before that FNAB results may mimic some other diseases [6-8].

Ultrasound is the most common non-invasive and sensitive diagnostic imaging modality for diagnosing thyroid lesions, but there are still no reliable criteria for distinguishing benign from malignant lesions. In addition, it is difficult to access the malignancy of the nodule when it is large or multinodular [9]. Despite tremendous improvement in diagnostic techniques such as ultrasound, radionuclide imaging and CT, there is still a big challenge to have a non-invasive and reliable technique to differentiate benign from malignant lesions. Recent developments in MRI may show that some MR protocols are of diagnostic value for these types of lesions [10]. Routine T1- and T2-weighted MR imaging can provide information on the location and size of thyroid lesions. But these protocols still don't have

* Correspondence: cjr.taoxiaofeng@vip.163.com
†Equal contributors
²Radiology Department, Shanghai People's Ninth Hospital, Shanghai Jiaotong University, School of Medicine, Shanghai 200011, China
Full list of author information is available at the end of the article

the specificity for distinguishing benign from malignant nodules or assessing the functional status of these thyroid nodules.

Diffusion-weighted MR imaging (DWI) is an emerging technique for central nervous system (CNS) diseases. DWI is sensitive to changes in the microstructural organization of tissue that may affect water diffusion. It has been used in various forms to evaluate head and neck tumors [11-13]. The Apparent Diffusion Coefficient (ADC) value, a metric obtained from DWI scans, could be a quantitative parameter for distinguishing malignant tumors from benign lesions.

In our current study, we compared ADC values of thyroid lesions with their pathology reports in order to evaluate its usefulness for distinguishing malignancy.

Methods
Patient selection
Between July 2007 and Jan 2011, 42 patients (10 male; 32 female) with palpable or ultrasonography determined thyroid nodules were prospectively enrolled and patient consent was obtained. The study was approved by ethics committee of Shanghai Changzheng Hospital. Mean age of those patients was 42.9 yrs (range 20-72 yrs). Routine neck MR imaging and diffusion-weighted MR imaging was performed for each patient. All patients enrolled for this study have been scheduled to have thyroidectomy within 2 weeks. Thyroidectomy was performed afterwards and pathology results were obtained for each patient. Conventional histology revealed that 28 patients had benign lesions, including thyroid adenoma (N = 20), nodular goiter (N = 5), and Hashimoto's thyroiditis (N = 3) while 14 patients were found to have malignant lesions, including thyroid papillary carcinoma (N = 10), follicular thyroid cancer (N = 3), atypical hyperplasia (N = 1). Thyroid lesions less than 1 cm were excluded because of diagnostic difficulties in evaluation.

MRI protocol
MR scanning was performed on GE Signa HD 1.5 T MR scanner (GE healthcare, USA). Routine MRI examinations were done with the following parameters: fast spin echo FSE scanning for neck, axial T1WI (TR = 520 ms, TE = 14 ms), T2WI (TR = 3500 ms, TE = 95 ms) and coronal T2WI (TR = 3000 ms, TE = 85 ms). Thickness = 4 mm, Spacing = 1 mm. FOV = 14 cm × 14 cm, Matrix = 320 × 256, NEX = 4.

Diffusion Weighted MR Imaging (DWI) was acquired using four different b factors (0, 300, 500, and 800 s/mm^2) in a STIR fat suppressed SE-EPI sequence. All DWI scans were acquired with the same parameters:TR = 3000 ms, TE = 60 ms, Matrix = 96 × 128, thickness - 4 mm and 6 averages were obtained. Total scanning time of about 10 minutes for the DWI scan.

Image post processing
Using the post processing software Functool from GE, ADC maps were automatically generated for each of the b factors. ADC values were extracted from ADC maps. Circular ROIs (regions of interests)with an area of 1 cm^2 were carefully placed on the lesions (areas of necrosis, hemorrhage, calcium and cyst formation were excluded). ROIs were placed on one ADC map and then propagated to the other 2 by two experienced radiologists blinded to each other's delineations. To minimize noise, each radiologist made three measurements for each lesion and the mean ADC value was recorded. Interrater reliability of the ROIs ADC values had ICC > 0.87. Final ADC value was determined by the mean values from two raters.

Analysis
ADC maps were computed for each of the b-values used in the DWI protocol. This was done automatically for the b-factors of 300 s/mm^2, 500 s/mm^2 and 800 s/mm^2. ADC values were extracted from the ADC maps. Statistical analysis was performed using the Statistical Package for the Social Sciences for Windows (SPSS, Chicago, Ill). All ADC data were recorded in Mean ± SD (×10^{-3} mm^2/s) form. Mann–Whitney U-test was performed to compare the quantitative ADC value of benign and malignant thyroid nodules. A value of p < .05 was considered significant. In addition, receiver operating characteristic (ROC) curve was constructed to determine a cutoff value for differentiating benign and malignant thyroid lesions. Receiver operating characteristic (ROC) curves were constructed and areas under the ROC curve (Az) were computed using MedCalc version 10.2.0.0 (http://www.medcalc.com/).

Results
MRI results revealed that among those 42 cases of lesions in the thyroid, 10 were located in the left lobe of thyroid gland, 16 of were in the right lobes, 14 had lesions on both lobes and 2 lesions were in thyroid isthmus. For those with lesions on both lobes, one was randomly chosen (matched with pathology) for ADC measurements. Mean major diameter of the benign and malignant lesions were 3.63 cm and 2.55 cm respectively. Historical findings confirmed there were 28 benign cases and 14 malignant lesions. Independent of malignancy, thyroid lesions occurred more frequently in female than in male (Table 1).

Parameters for differentiating lesion malignancy
Using histology results to group the ADC values we found that the ADC values were significantly different (p < 0.001) between benign and malignant lesions for the ADC values computed for b = 300 s/mm^2. Mean ADC value for benign group (Figure 1) is much higher than that for malignant group (Figure 2), with the values of

Table 1 Historical results and patient characteristics

Histological categories	Number (%)	Mean age (yrs)	Female (%)	Mean maximum diameter (cm)
Benign	28(66.7)	41.7	21(75)	3.63 ± 0.37
Thyroid adenoma	20(47.6)	42.6	15(53.6)	3.53 ± 0.25
Nodular goiter	6(14.3)	39.3	5(17.9)	3.95 ± 0.65
Hashimoto's thyroiditis	2(4.8)	35.6	1(3.6)	3.71 ± 0.11
Malignant	14(33.3)	45.3	11(78.6)	2.55 ± 0.41
Thyroid papillary carcinoma	11(26.2)	41.9	9(64.4)	2.73 ± 0.54
Follicular thyroid cancer	2(4.8)	49.1	1(7.1)	1.7 ± 0.13
Atypical hyperplasia	1(2.4)	45	1(7.1)	2.3

$2.37 \pm 0.47 \times 10^{-3}$ mm^2/s and $1.49 \pm 0.60 \times 10^{-3}$ mm^2/s respectively. However, no significant difference was observed between the two groups for the ADC values obtained using b = 500 s/mm^2 or 800 s/mm^2 (Table 2). Sensitivity, specificity and AUC were also compared among three different b-factors. Highest sensitivity and AUC was observed at b-factor of 300 s/mm^2 (Table 3). We also selected four variables (age, sex, ADC value, max nodular diameter) as independent variables to perform logistic regression analysis. Odds ratios (and 95% CIs) based on the logistic regression model were also calculated. The results obtained from the logistic regression model showed that ADC values obtained with a b factor of 300 s/mm^2 (OR = 4.76, p <0.001) and max nodular diameter (OR = 3.22, p = 0.034) were the two most discriminative independent variables for differentiating between benign and malignant lesions (Table 2).

ROC analysis

Furthermore, a Receiver Operator Characteristic (ROC) curve was computed for the ADC values obtained from DWI scans using b = 300 s/mm^2. We determined a cutoff point from the ROC curve that would differentiate benign from malignant lesions. The area under the ROC curve was 0.876. When we selected a cutoff ADC value of 2.17×10^{-3} mm^2/s, sensitivity and specificity was found to be 76.5% and 100% respectively (Figure 3).

Discussion

To date, only a few studies have focused on the use of DWI in evaluating thyroid disease. Tezuka [14] et al. used both routine T1WI, T2WI and DWI techniques to diagnose thyroid diseases (Graves' disease, sub-acute thyroiditis and Hashimoto's disease). Although no obvious difference using T1WI and T2WI were detected

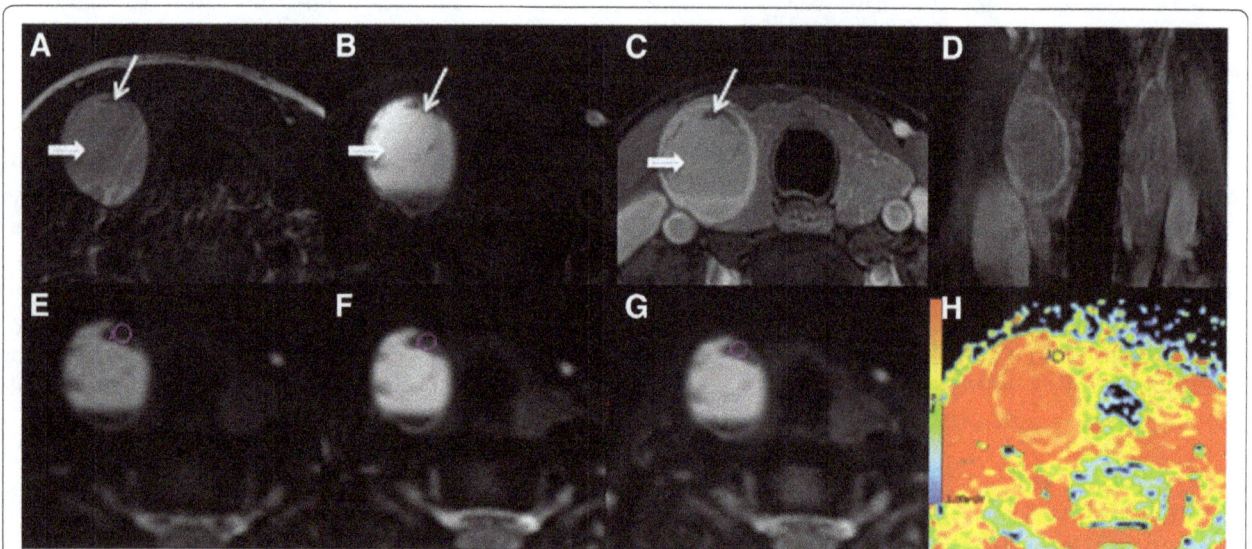

Figure 1 A 44-year-female patient with right lobe thyroid adenoma; (A-C) Non-contrast and contrast transversal images showed a hemorrhage in the right lobe (short thick arrow). Long thin arrow shows the lesion. **(D)** Coronal images showed the well-circumscribed lesion with homogenous enhancement. **(E-G)** showed ADC value obtained from ADC map with b factors of 0, 300, 500 and 800 s/mm^2, respectively. ROIs were placed in the lesion at right upper area to avoid the hemorrhage area. **(H)** ADC map generated at b-factor of 300 s/mm^2.

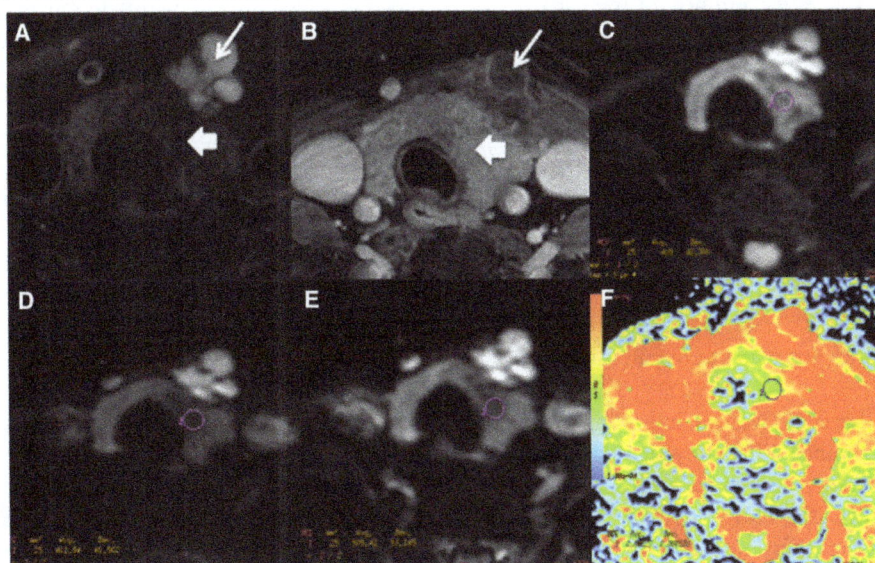

Figure 2 A-36-year-female patient with thyroid papillary carcinoma at left lobe and isthmuses is shown. **(A-B)** Non-contrast and contrast transversal images showed abnormal signal at left lobe and isthmus with multiple cysts (long arrows). **(C-E)** showed ADC value measured from ADC map with b factors of 300, 500 and 800 s/mm², respectively. **(F)** ADC map generated at b-factor of 300 s/mm².

on those thyroid diseases, ADC values of thyroid lesions of Graves' disease was found much higher than that of sub-acute thyroiditis or Hashimoto's disease. An ADC value of 1.82×10^{-3} mm²/s was suggested as the cutoff point to diagnose Graves' disease (Sensitivity 75% and Specificity 80%). DWI has emerged as a potential new noninvasive technique that can provide more quantitative information on thyroid lesions and help make clinical differential diagnosis.

MR technique

Diffusion weighted MR imaging can be done with single shot or multi-shot. Wang and Adel Razek [11,15] applied single-shot multisection echo-planar technique, using b values of 0, 500 and 1000 s/mm² respectively. This sequence is characterized by a train of gradient echoes with a short echo time image and good signal-to-noise ratio

(SNR), but it was associated with more magnetic susceptibility artifacts. Tezuka [14] et al., used a fast spin echo sequence for diffusion-weighted imaging to avoid magnetic susceptibility artifacts, but not only was the imaging time increased but the SNR was also decreased.

In this study, we used a STIR (Short TI Inversion Recovery) fat suppressed SE EPI (Spin-Echo Echo Planar Imaging) sequence. STIR is a very robust fat suppression technique with minimal artifacts. It has low sensitivity to magnetic field inhomogeneities or susceptibility effects and thus improves image quality. It also produces a slight T1-weighted background suppression but does not affect the accuracy of the images. EPI is the fastest acquisition method and it only requires 30 ms ~ 100 ms to collect one image which helps in reducing most physiological movement artifacts [16]. Furthermore, short TE time of 60 ms was used to reduce T2* effect in our study. Thus,

Table 2 Association between parameters and disease property

	Benign group (n = 28)	Malignant group (n = 14)	P value*	OR	95% CI
Age (yrs)	41.7	45.3	0.79	0.62	0.26, 2.59
Sex (Female %)	21(75)	11(78.6)	0.61	0.50	0.16, 1.54
Max nodular diameter (cm)	3.63 ± 0.37	2.55 ± 0.41	0.034	3.22	1.27, 6.76
ADC values [mm²/s]					
b-0,300	2.37 ± 0.47	1.49 ± 0.60	<0.001	4.76	1.56, 9.89
b-0,500	1.87 ± 0.25	1.61 ± 0.45	0.138	1.01	0.3, 1.81
b-0,800	1.68 ± 0.25	1.41 ± 0.34	0.059	0.091	0.03, 0.73

*p value reflected from logistic analysis.

Table 3 Sensitivity, specificity and AUC of the use of mean ADC value as calculated based on 3 different b-values for differentiating benign from malignant thyroid lesions

	b = 0,300	b = 0,500	b = 0,800
AUC	0.88(0.77–0.97)	0.63(0.47–0.77)	0.63(0.46–0.77)
Criterion [10^{-3} mm^2/s]	>2.17	>1.74	>1.65
Sensitivity %	76.5	67.9	53.6
Specificity %	100	64.3	71.4

using this sequence we were able to obtain more accurate tissue ADC values.

The b-factor in the DWI was an important factor for image quality. We obtained diffusion-weighted MR images with different b factors simultaneously to avoid misregistration in computing the different ADC values. Higher b-values produce more diffusion weighting and therefore higher contrast between thyroid lesions and normal tissue. However, higher b value also leads to increased signal attenuation and usually required more averages to compensate for the SNR. Higher b-values also produce more susceptibility distortions and could increase the noise in the DWI images because the distortions are different depending on the gradient directions. In addition, different tumors within different organs or tissues may be more sensitive to different b-values. In this study, we applied an SE EPI diffusion imaging with b-factors of 300, 500 and 800 s/mm^2. Our results showed that a b-factor of 300 s/mm^2 was sufficient to obtain high quality ADC values

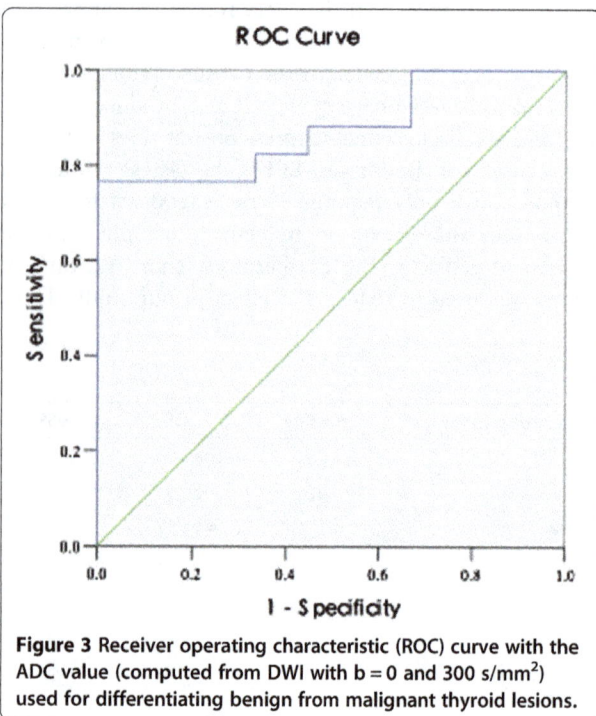

Figure 3 Receiver operating characteristic (ROC) curve with the ADC value (computed from DWI with b = 0 and 300 s/mm^2) used for differentiating benign from malignant thyroid lesions.

and it was also the one with had a high sensitivity and accuracy for differentiating benign and malignancy. These results are consistent with Bozgeyik's [17] results.

Pathological mechanism of ADC values in thyroid lesions

In our study we were able to use the most reliable reference for malignancy which was based on the histopathology of a thyroidectomy. Our results showed a significant difference in the ADC value between benign and malignant thyroid lesions, with ADC values in benign lesions being higher than malignant lesions ($2.37 \pm 0.47 \times 10^{-3}$ mm^2/s vs. $1.49 \pm 0.60 \times 10^{-3}$ mm^2/s) at the b factor of 300 s/mm^2. These results are consistent with other similar studies [17-19]. Diffusion weighted imaging provides more information on the microstructure of tissues and their physiological processes. Changes in the distributions of intracellular organelles and macromolecules in the tissues affect the random motion of water protons. ADC values of tissues vary according to its cellularity and histopathology. Anderson [20]'s study showed that malignant lesions in thyroid glands was characterized by compact cellularity which increased the nucleocyte-cytoplasmic ratio (NCR). These microscopic pathological changes results in the reduction of extracellular space which limits diffusional motion of water protons. Reduced ADC values are presented as high signal on DWI sequences.

Abdel's [21] study demonstrated that when selecting ADC value of 0.98×1.0^{-3} mm^2/s as a cutoff point to differentiate benign and malignant lesions, the sensitivity and specificity was 97.5% and 91.7%, respectively. The accuracy was up to 98.9%. In this study a single pair of b-values (0, 1000 s/mm^2) were studied. Although we also looked at the ADC values obtained using higher b-values (0,800 s/mm^2), we did not detect any useful threshold at the higher b-values. Abdel's study included a variety of cervical lymph nodes whereas our study focused on the thyroid. Lesion heterogeneity might have accounted for the differences in sensitivity. It was also suggested that the ADC values of benign thyroid nodule may vary according to the complex composition within the nodule (colloid, tiny necrosis and cystic change, hemorrhage, fibrosis and calcium). ADC values were highest in thyroid cysts since it contained colloid cyst made of serous or concentrated thyroglobulin. Conversely, increasing NCR and grit-like calcification mainly lead to a decrease of ADC values in papillary thyroid carcinoma.

Bozgeyik [17] also studied thyroid nodules with DWI at lower b-values. Bozgeyik [17] also found that a b-factor of 300 s/mm^2 was the most useful for differentiating benign or malignant lesions. In Bozgeyik's study 3 b-value pairs were used to computed the ADC (0, 100 s/mm^2), (0, 200 s/mm^2) and (0, 300 s/mm^2). We expanded on these results and investigated ADC values obtained using larger b-values. Our sample includes about 33% malignancy rates whereas in Bozgevik's study less than 5% of the nodules were malignant. In their study, malignancy was determined using FNAB whereas in our study we have used pathology results from thyroidectomy, a more accurate reference. Erdem [19] also suggested that tiny calcification was closely correlated with the reduction of ADC values in thyroid malignancy.

However, in Weidekamm's [22,23] study, the opposite result was reported. ADC values were predominantly higher in malignant thyroid nodules than that in benign nodules with values equal or more than 2.25×10^{-3} mm^2/s. The higher ADC values may be due to the over production of thyroprotein follicle in malignant thyroid nodules which do not restrict the diffusion of the water protons.

ADC values has been used as a quantitative parameter for differentiating benign and malignant lesions [24]. The ADC values depend on many factors such as tissue microstructure, necrosis, presence of macromolecules and also perfusion phenomenon. When compared to benign lesions, abnormal blood perfusion is more prevalent in malignant lesions and ADC values will be affected by both blood perfusion and extracellular space. Unlike some other studies [17], in the current study, we chose three different b factors all over 300 s/mm^2 since ADC value would better reflect the true water diffusion in the tissue with larger b factors. However, there was no significant difference in ADC value between benign and malignant lesions when the b factors were 500 s/mm^2 and 800 s/mm^2. Delormere [25] demonstrated that malignant lesions usually do not have a complete basal membrane of blood vessel which enhances the molecular exchange in the capillary bed. ADC values could be influenced by both blood perfusion and extracellular space. In thyroid malignancy, increased blood perfusion increases the apparent speed of the diffusing water protons while narrow extracellular space will restrict its movement. Although at higher b-values the sensitivity to perfusion is reduced, our results show no difference in ADC values between benign and malignant groups with b-values of 500 s/mm^2 or 800 s/mm^2. The ADC values obtained using the lower b-value of 300 s/mm^2 is most likely affected by both perfusion and diffusion effects. It is possible that the discriminatory effect of this lower 300 s/mm^2 reflect a combination of altered vascularity and changes in cellular composition that characterizes malignancy.

Fine-needle aspiration biopsy (FNAB) cytology can give 4 different results: benign, malignant, suspicious and nondiagnostic. No definite diagnosis is possible for the two categories of suspicious and non-diagnostic. Although FNAB is commonly used to screen for malignancy, a unique approach in this study is that we used histological results from thyroidectomy as the standard reference for distinguishing benign and malignant lesions. Based on final histological results, we were able to obtain a definite diagnosis of each lesion. ROC curves and cut off point for b-values are more accurate in this approach.

There are still some limitations in this study. First, the relatively small number (33.3%) of the malignant nodules somehow limits the statistical power. This study needs to be expanded further with a larger number of patients. B-values should be extended to lower values and higher ranges to verify that 300 s/mm^2 is an optimal value. Second, thyroid nodules less than 10 mm were not included in this study. Improvement in the software of diffusion-weighted MR imaging will help in the detection of smaller lesions in future studies. Third, we have not studied the correlation of ADC values with subtypes of thyroid lesions such as cysts from hemorrhagic nodules because of the small number which would reduce its statistical power.

Conclusion

In conclusion, diffusion-weighted MR imaging is a relatively new and non-invasive approach to assess thyroid lesions. ADC values seem to be able to differentiate benign from malignant thyroid disease. Further studies should be performed to expand the utility of DWI in thyroid lesions.

Abbreviations
DWI: Diffusion-weighted imaging; ADC: Apparent diffusion coefficient; T1WI: T1 weighted imaging; T2WI: T2 weighted imaging; FNAB: Fine needle aspiration biopsy; ICC: Intraclass correlation coefficient; ROC: Receiver operating characteristic.

Competing interests
The authors declare that they have no competing interests.

Authors' contributions
YW collect data from patients and drafted the manuscript. XY participated in the sequence alignment. WS participated in the sequence alignment. YD did postprocessing and measurement on images. YY did postprocessing and measurement on images. XT conceived of the study, and participated in its design and coordination. CT participated in the design of the study and performed the statistical analysis. All authors read and approved the final manuscript.

Acknowledgments
The manuscript was supported by grant of National Natural Science Foundation of China (Dr. Xiaofeng Tao No. 81272802) and Key scientific and innovation grant of Education Commission of Shanghai (Dr. Yingwei Wu No. 12ZZ028). Outstanding academic leader of Shanghai Science and Technology Committee of Dr. Xiaofeng Tao (Grant No. 13XD1402400).

Author details
[1]Radiology Department, East Hospital, Tongji University, school of Medicine, Shanghai 200120, China. [2]Radiology Department, Shanghai People's Ninth Hospital, Shanghai Jiaotong University, School of Medicine, Shanghai 200011, China. [3]Radiology Department, Shanghai Changzheng Hospital, Shanghai, China. [4]Radiology Department, Mount Sinai School of Medicine, New York 10029, USA.

References

1. Wong CK, Wheeler MH: **Thyroid nodules: rational management.** *World J Surg* 2000, **24**:934–941.

2. Brander A, Viikinkoski P, Nickels J, Kivisaari L: **Thyroid gland: US screening in a random adult population.** *Radiology* 1991, **181**:683–687.

3. Davies L, Welch HG: **Increasing incidence of thyroid cancer in the United States, 1973–2002.** *JAMA* 2006, **295**:2164–2167.

4. Mazzaferri EL, Harmer C, Mallick UK, Kendall-Taylor P: *Practical management of thyroid cancer: a multidisciplinary approach.* London: Springer; 2006.

5. Jemal A, Siegel R, Xu J, Ward E: **Cancer statistics, 2010.** *CA Cancer J Clin* 2010, **60**:277–300.

6. Bakshi NA, Mansoor I, Jones BA: **Analysis of inconclusive fine-needle aspiration of thyroid follicular lesions.** *Endocr Pathol* 2003, **14**:167–175.

7. Koike E, Yamashita H, Noguchi S, Murakami T, Ohshima A, *et al*: **Effect of combining ultrasonography and ultrasound-guided fine-needle aspiration biopsy findings for the diagnosis of thyroid nodules.** *Eur J Surg* 2001, **167**:656–661.

8. McCoy KL, Jabbour N, Ogilvie JB, Ohori NP, Carty SE, *et al*: **The incidence of cancer and rate of false-negative cytology in thyroid nodules greater than or equal to 4 cm in size.** *Surgery* 2007, **142**:837–844. discussion 844 e831-833.

9. Solbiati L, Osti V, Cova L, Tonolini M: **Ultrasound of thyroid, parathyroid glands and neck lymph nodes.** *Eur Radiol* 2001, **11**:2411–2424.

10. Kiyosue H, Miyake H, Komatsu E, Mori H: **MRI of cervical masses of thymic origin.** *J Comput Assist Tomogr* 1994, **18**:206–208.

11. Wang J, Takashima S, Takayama F, Kawakami S, Saito A, *et al*: **Head and neck lesions: characterization with diffusion-weighted echo-planar MR imaging.** *Radiology* 2001, **220**:621–630.

12. Eida S, Sumi M, Sakihama N, Takahashi H, Nakamura T: **Apparent diffusion coefficient mapping of salivary gland tumors: prediction of the benignancy and malignancy.** *AJNR Am J Neuroradiol* 2007, **28**:116–121.

13. King CH, Higa AT, Culjat MO, Han SH, Bisley JW, *et al*: **A pneumatic haptic feedback actuator array for robotic surgery or simulation.** *Stud Health Technol Inform* 2007, **125**:217–222.

14. Tezuka M, Murata Y, Ishida R, Ohashi I, Hirata Y, *et al*: **MR imaging of the thyroid: correlation between apparent diffusion coefficient and thyroid gland scintigraphy.** *Journal of magnetic resonance imaging: JMRI* 2003, **17**:163–169.

15. Abdel Razek AA, Soliman NY, Elkhamary S, Alsharaway MK, Tawfik A: **Role of diffusion-weighted MR imaging in cervical lymphadenopathy.** *Eur Radiol* 2006, **16**:1468–1477.

16. Murtz P, Krautmacher C, Traber F, Gieseke J, Schild HH, *et al*: **Diffusion-weighted whole-body MR imaging with background body signal suppression: a feasibility study at 3.0 Tesla.** *Eur Radiol* 2007, **17**:3031–3037.

17. Bozgeyik Z, Coskun S, Dagli AF, Ozkan Y, Sahpaz F, *et al*: **Diffusion-weighted MR imaging of thyroid nodules.** *Neuroradiology* 2009, **51**:193–198.

18. Razek AA, Sadek AG, Kombar OR, Elmahdy TE, Nada N: **Role of apparent diffusion coefficient values in differentiation between malignant and benign solitary thyroid nodules.** *AJNR Am J Neuroradiol* 2008, **29**:563–568.

19. Erdem G, Erdem T, Muammer H, Mutlu DY, Firat AK, *et al*: **Diffusion-weighted images differentiate benign from malignant thyroid nodules.** *Journal of magnetic resonance imaging: JMRI* 2010, **31**:94–100.

20. Anderson JR (Ed): *Muir'sTextbook of Pathology.* 13th edition. London: Edward Arnold; 1992.

21. Abdel Razek AA, Soliman NY, Elkhamary S, Alsharaway MK, Tawfik A: **Role of diffusion-weighted MR imaging in cervical lymphadenopathy.** *Eur Radiol* 2006, **16**:1468–1477.

22. Schueller-Weidekamm C, Kaserer K, Schueller G, Scheuba C, Ringl H, *et al*: **Can quantitative diffusion-weighted MR imaging differentiate benign and malignant cold thyroid nodules? Initial results in 25 patients.** *AJNR Am J Neuroradiol* 2009, **30**:417–422.

23. Schueller-Weidekamm C, Schueller G, Kaserer K, Scheuba C, Ringl H, *et al*: **Diagnostic value of sonography, ultrasound-guided fine-needle aspiration cytology, and diffusion-weighted MRI in the characterization of cold thyroid nodules.** *Eur J Radiol* 2010, **73**:538–544.

24. Herneth AM, Guccione S, Bednarski M: **Apparent diffusion coefficient: a quantitative parameter for in vivo tumor characterization.** *Eur J Radiol* 2003, **45**:208–213.

25. Delorme S, Knopp MV: **Non-invasive vascular imaging: assessing tumour vascularity.** *Eur Radiol* 1998, **8**:517–527.

18

Imaging features of primary Sarcomas of the great vessels in CT, MRI and PET/CT

Christian von Falck[1*], Bernhard Meyer[1], Christine Fegbeutel[2], Florian Länger[3], Frank Bengel[4], Frank Wacker[1] and Thomas Rodt[1]

Abstract

Background: To investigate the imaging features of primary sarcomas of the great vessels in CT, MRI and [18] F-FDG PET/CT.

Methods: Thirteen patients with a primary sarcoma of the great vessels were retrospectively evaluated. All available images studies including F-18 FDG PET(/CT) (n = 4), MDCT (n = 12) and MRI (n = 6) were evaluated and indicative image features of this rare tumor entity were identified.

Results: The median interval between the first imaging study and the final diagnosis was 11 weeks (0–12 weeks). The most frequently observed imaging findings suggestive of malignant disease in patients with sarcomas of the pulmonary arteries were a large filling defect with vascular distension, unilaterality and a lack of improvement despite effective anticoagulation. In patients with aortic sarcomas we most frequently observed a pedunculated appearance and an atypical location of the filling defect. The F-18 FDG PET(/CT) examinations demonstrated an unequivocal hypermetabolism of the lesion in all cases (4/4). MRI proved lesion vascularization in 5/6 cases.

Conclusion: Intravascular unilateral or atypically located filling defects of the great vessels with vascular distension, a pedunculated shape and lack of improvement despite effective anticoagulation are suspicious for primary sarcoma on MDCT or MRI. MR perfusion techniques can add information on the nature of the lesion but the findings may be subtle and equivocal. F-18 FDG PET/CT may have a potential role in these patients and may be considered as part of the imaging workup.

Background

Primary malignant sarcomas of the great vessels are exceedingly rare, representing less than 1% of all sarcomas [1,2]. Hence, information on these malignancies is restricted to case reports and small retrospective series. The most frequent sites of origin are the pulmonary arteries and the aorta, followed by venous sarcomas, predominantly of the inferior vena cava [1]. Pulmonary artery sarcomas commonly arise from the pulmonary trunk and the central left or right pulmonary artery. The most dominant histologic subtypes of sarcomas of the great vessels as reported in the literature are undifferentiated intimal sarcoma and leiomyosarcoma. The subtyping of sarcomas has changed in the last decades primarily by the evolvement of modern immunohistological techniques thus making comparisons between published historical and contemporary studies difficult. In both, pulmonary and aortic location, an intraluminal growth pattern is differentiated from a less frequent mural growth type [1-3].

The prognosis of patients with primary malignant sarcomas of the great vessels is poor, mainly due to the late presentation of these patients with locally advanced disease or distant metastases. Clinical features may resemble those of pulmonary or aortic thromboembolic disease [1-3]. The diagnosis may be further delayed by a misinterpretation of imaging studies of this rare disease,

* Correspondence: falck.christian.von@mh-hannover.de
[1]Department of Radiology, Hannover Medical School, Hannover 30625, Germany
Full list of author information is available at the end of the article

e.g. pulmonary artery sarcoma is interpreted as pulmonary embolism [3-5].

The aim of this study was to retrospectively identify typical imaging features suggestive of primary malignancy of intrathoracic vessels in combined F-18-fluorodesoxy-glucose positron emission tomography/computed tomography (F-18 FDG PET/CT), multidetector computed tomography (MDCT) and magnetic resonance imaging (MRI). We therefore analyzed the imaging appearance of primary sarcomas of the great vessels in F-18 FDG PET/CT, MDCT and MRI as seen in 13 consecutive patients who were treated in a single tertiary care university center.

Methods
Study population
This retrospective study was conducted in accordance with the guidelines of the Declaration of Helsinki and according to standards of the local ethics committees. The ethical committee of Hannover Medical School waived the need for written informed consent because routine diagnostic data was analyzed anonymously.

Between 2002 and 2011 a total of 13 patients (m = 7, f = 6) with histologically proven primary sarcoma of the great vessels were treated in a single tertiary care university hospital. The mean patient age was 57.5 (±12.2) years, ranging from 46 to 81 years. All available imaging studies of these patients including F-18 FDG PET/CT ($n = 3$), F-18 FDG PET ($n = 1$), MDCT ($n = 12$) and MRI ($n = 6$) were evaluated by two experienced readers in consensus and typical imaging features of this rare tumor entity were identified.

Imaging studies
The PET/CT scans were acquired 90 minutes after the intravenous application of 5 MBq/Kg body weight of F-18-2-fluoro-2-desoxyglucose (F-18 FDG) on a dedicated dual-slice hybrid imaging system (Siemens biograph 2, Forchheim, Germany) in three patients and on a PET-only scanner in one case (Siemens ECAT Exact, Knox-ville, TN, USA). The acquisition time was five minutes per bed position. A total of 7 – 8 bed positions were scanned to cover a region from the vertex to the upper thigh. A co-registered low-dose CT was used for attenuation correction and anatomical localization (tube voltage = 130 kVp, tube current = $20mAs_{eff}$ (modulated), slice collimation = 2 x 5 mm, pitch = 1.5, reconstruction increment = 2.5 mm, reconstruction kernel = B30s). Neither oral nor intravenous contrast agents were administered for the combined PET/CT scan.

All CT scans were acquired on MDCT scanners with 4 – 64 simultaneously acquired sections (Siemens Somatom Volume Zoom/Sensation 16/Emotion 16/Sensation 64, Forchheim, Germany; General Electric VCT, Chalfont St. Giles, UK; Toshiba Aquillion, Otawara, Japan). The

section thickness was in the range from 0.625 mm to 5 mm and the reconstruction increment in the range from 0.5 mm to 4 mm. The tube voltage was 120 kVp for all examinations. Dose modulation was used with all scanners. The MDCT scans were performed after the power injection of 80-100 ml of an anionic iodinated contrast agent at a flow of 3-4 ml/s followed by a saline chaser. The scan timing was adjusted to maximize the contrast in the region of interest, i.e. the pulmonary arteries or the thoracic and abdominal aorta. The images were reconstructed with standard abdomen kernels, supplemented by an additional high-resolution reconstruction kernel for chest scans. Multiplanar reformations (MPR) in the coronal and sagittal orientation were available in all cases.

The MRI scans were acquired on scanners from three different manufacturers with a field strength of 1.5 T (Siemens Avanto, Erlangen, Germany; Philips Intera, Best, The Netherlands; General Electric CV/i, Chalfont St. Giles, UK). All examinations included T1- and T2-weighted sequences before and T1-weighted sequences with spectral fat suppression after the injection of a gadolinium-based contrast agent as well as a dynamic contrast-enhanced ultra-fast gradient echo acquisition or an MR-angiography (MRA) sequence. Three examinations were supplemented with an additional inversion-recovery (IR) sequence for the detection of late enhancement (LE) and three scans included ECG-gated cine-sequences (FIESTA/Cine Trufi).

Histopathologic diagnosis
The surgically derived specimens were embedded into paraffin and sectioned according to standard histopathologic procedures. Routine staining included hematoxylin and eosin (H&E), Elastica van Gieson (EvG) and periodic acid-schiff (PAS). The diagnosis was supplement by additional immunohistochemical stains. The tumors were classified according to the current WHO classification of soft tissue tumors [6].

Results
Patient demographics and histopathologic diagnosis
A total of 13 patients were included in this retrospective study (m = 7, f = 6). The mean age was 57 (±12) years. With respect to primary *pre-operative* imaging studies MDCT scans were available in 12, MR scans in 6, F-18 FDG PET/CT scans in 3 cases and an F-18 FDG PET scan in one case. The primary tumors were located at the right ($n = 5$), left ($n = 1$) or central ($n = 3$) pulmonary artery ($n = 9$ in total), the right inferior pulmonary vein ($n = 1$), the aortic arch ($n = 1$), the descending aorta ($n = 1$) and the abdominal aorta ($n = 1$). Tumor histology was undifferentiated intimal sarcoma ($n = 8$), angiosarcoma

($n = 2$), leimyosarcoma ($n = 2$) and myxofibrosarcoma ($n = 1$). This information is summarized in Table 1.

We observed a median interval between the first imaging study and the final diagnosis of 11 weeks, ranging from 0 to 12 weeks. However, the interval between the first contact to a physician due to clinical symptoms that could retrospectively attributed to the final diagnosis was much longer in three cases with 30 weeks (dyspnea), 52 weeks (congestive heart failure) and 30 weeks (dyspnea), respectively. The primary tentative diagnoses were pulmonary embolic disease ($n = 8$) and idiopathic pulmonary hypertension ($n = 1$) in the patients with a tumor in the pulmonary arteries. In cases with the tumor being located in the aorta, the tentative diagnoses were atheromatous disease and chronic dissection in two cases. The patient with the sarcoma of the right inferior pulmonary vein was primarily treated for pneumonia as the venous infarction as seen on a chest x-ray was interpreted as a consolidation. One patient underwent an MDCT scan because of B-symptoms including fever, malaise and unintended weight-loss. The MDCT-findings were suggestive of a contained rupture of an inflamed aorto-bi-iliac prosthesis and the patient underwent immediate surgical treatment.

Table 1 Patient demographics and diagnosis

Patient #	Age	Sex	Location	Histology	Primary diagnosis
1	74	M	Left pulmonary artery	UIS	Pulmonary Embolism
2	45	M	Central pulmonary artery	UIS	Pulmonary Embolism
3	68	M	Descending aorta	UIS	Atheromatous Disease/Chronic Dissection
4	81	M	Abdominal aorta	AS	Contained Aortic Rupture
5	51	F	Right pulmonary artery	UIS	Pulmonary Embolism
6	46	M	Pulmonary vein	LMS	Pneumonia
7	71	M	Distal aortic arch	AS	Congestive Heart Failure/Thrombus
8	49	F	Right pulmonary artery	MFS	Pulmonary Embolism
9	55	F	Right pulmonary artery	UIS	Pulmonary Embolism
10	46	F	Central pulmonary artery	UIS	Pulmonary Hypertension
11	47	F	Central pulmonary artery	UIS	Pulmonary Embolism
12	61	F	Right pulmonary artery	LMS	Pulmonary Embolism
13	54	M	Right pulmonary artery	UIS	Pulmonary Embolism

Imaging characteristic

All available F-18 FDG PET(/CT), MDCT-, MRI- and studies were reviewed with respect to the presence of imaging features suggestive of primary malignancy of the vascular filling defects. In patients with a sarcoma of the pulmonary artery ($n = 8$), we observed the following suspicious imaging features in varying frequency: a filling defect of the entire vessel diameter with vascular distension ($n = 8/8$), a large *unilateral* 'thrombus' ($n = 7/8$), lack of clinical improvement despite adequate anticoagulation without evidence of deep venous thrombosis ($n = 4/8$), an expansion beyond the vessel wall ($n = 2/8$, in the follow-up examination), a heterogeneous enhancement after the intravenous administration of a contrast agent in MRI ($n = 3/4$, MRI was available in 4 patients), metabolic activity as demonstrated by F-18 FDG PET(/CT) ($n = 3/3$, PET was available in 3 patients), a pedunculated appearance ($n = 1/8$), and local or distant metastases ($n = 2/8$).

The semiquantitative analysis of the metabolic activity of the tumors in F-18 FDG PET/CT revealed SUV_{max}-values of 16.1, 8.8 and 14.5, respectively. There was no additional information gathered from the late enhancement sequences. In the patients with sarcomas of the aorta ($n = 3$) we observed comparable imaging features, however, in a different frequency: a pedunculated appearance ($n = 2/3$), an atypical location for a thrombus (n = 2), an expansion beyond the vessel wall ($n = 1/3$), contrast enhancement in MRI ($n = 2/2$, MRI was available in 2 patients) or MDCT (n = 1/1, MDCT was available in 1 patient) and metabolic activity as demonstrated by F-18 FDG PET/CT ($n = 1/1$; $SUV_{max} = 3.6 - 5.5$, PET was available in 1 patient). In the patient with pulmonary vein sarcoma we observed a large filling defect with vascular distension, comparable to the findings as seen in pulmonary artery sarcoma. The related lung parenchyma shows excessive consolidation, consistent with venous infarction.

As deducible from the relative frequency of the above-mentioned findings, we found a *combination* of indicative imaging features in most patients. In the CTA examinations of the pulmonary arteries in three patients, we observed large, unilateral right-sided filling defects in the pulmonary arteries that obturate the whole cross-sectional area of the vessel and lead to a vascular expansion (Figure 1). However, pulmonary embolism was the primary tentative diagnosis in all three cases and the patients received accordant conservative treatment. The follow-up examinations showed a progression of the findings (Figure 1) or at least a lack of improvement, respectively, despite a sufficient anticoagulation therapy and hence strongly suggest a neoplastic nature of the filling defects.

The demonstration of lesion vascularization using first pass perfusion or dynamic contrast-enhanced MRI tech-

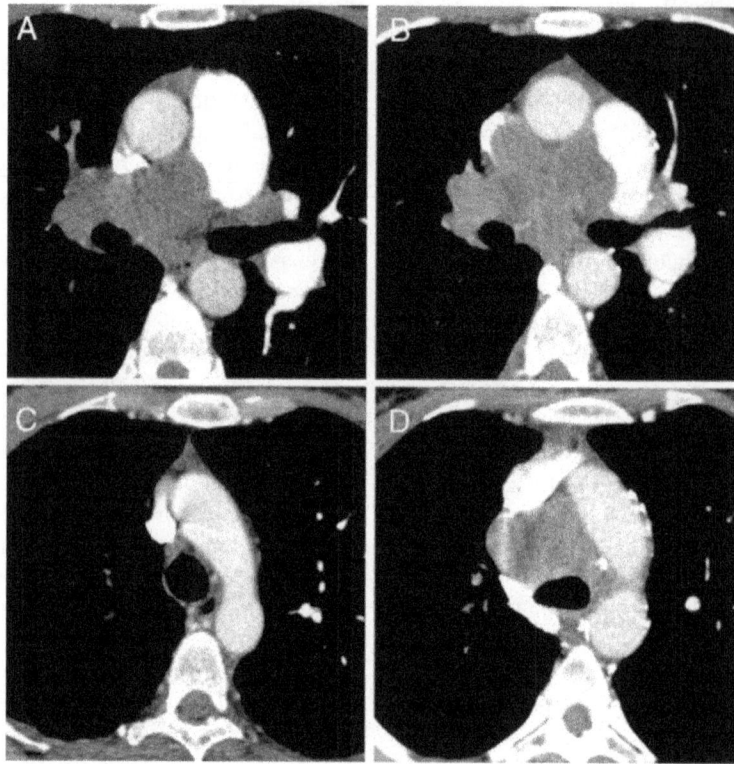

Figure 1 CT pulmonary angiography (CTPA) of a 49-year-old female patient with a myxofibrosarcoma of the right pulmonary artery. Suspicious imaging features were already present in the primary imaging (**A, C**). However, the patient was treated conservatively for suspected pulmonary embolism. A follow-up exam was acquired three month later and demonstrated massive disease progression with tumor expansion beyond the vessel wall and local lymph node metastases (**B, D**)

niques can be challenging. We observed only subtle and inhomogeneous contrast enhancements in our patient cohort. Color-coding of the perfusion images may facilitate the perception of the subtle signal changes (Figure 2).

The evidence of hypermetabolism of the filling defect as shown by F-18 FDG PET/CT, however, could be readily and unequivocally appreciated in all our patients with metabolic imaging (Figures 2, 3) and strengthened the suspicion of malignant disease. Due to the decisive implications of a radical surgical approach, a combination of different imaging studies was requested in many patients of our cohort. The complementary information of morphological, functional and metabolic imaging increases the diagnostic confidence and may facilitate the therapeutic decisions as shown in Figure 3. In equivocal cases, a whole-body staging such as PET/CT may further increase the probability of a malignant disease by revealing distant metastases (Figure 3).

Although few in number, our cases with sarcomas located in the aorta suggest that the typical imaging features are comparable to those seen in tumors occurring in the pulmonary vasculature. Potentially suspicious imaging findings of intraaortal filling defects include an atypical

location for a thrombus, a pedunculated appearance and a subtle enhancement during first-pass perfusion (Figure 4) and hypermetabolism in F-18 FDG PET/CT (Figure 5), consistent with the intraluminal type of aortic sarcoma. Mural-type sarcomas show different imaging characteristics with predominant extraluminal perivascular growth and can be mistaken for inflammatory disease (Figure 6). The findings are summarized in Table 2.

Discussion

As primary malignancies of the great vessels are exceptionally rare, most nuclear medicine specialists and radiologists have no personal experience in diagnosing the disease. This study therefore aimed at identifying typical imaging features of primary sarcomas of the great vessels using MDCT and MRI based on our single-center experience. Furthermore, we report on advanced imaging techniques such as MR perfusion and metabolic F-18 FDG PET/CT imaging that have proven potential as tools for possible diagnosis verification and tumor staging.

To date, about 150 cases of primary aortic sarcomas and approximately 250 cases of primary sarcomas of the pulmonary arteries have been reported in the English-language world literature [1-3]. Many of these reports

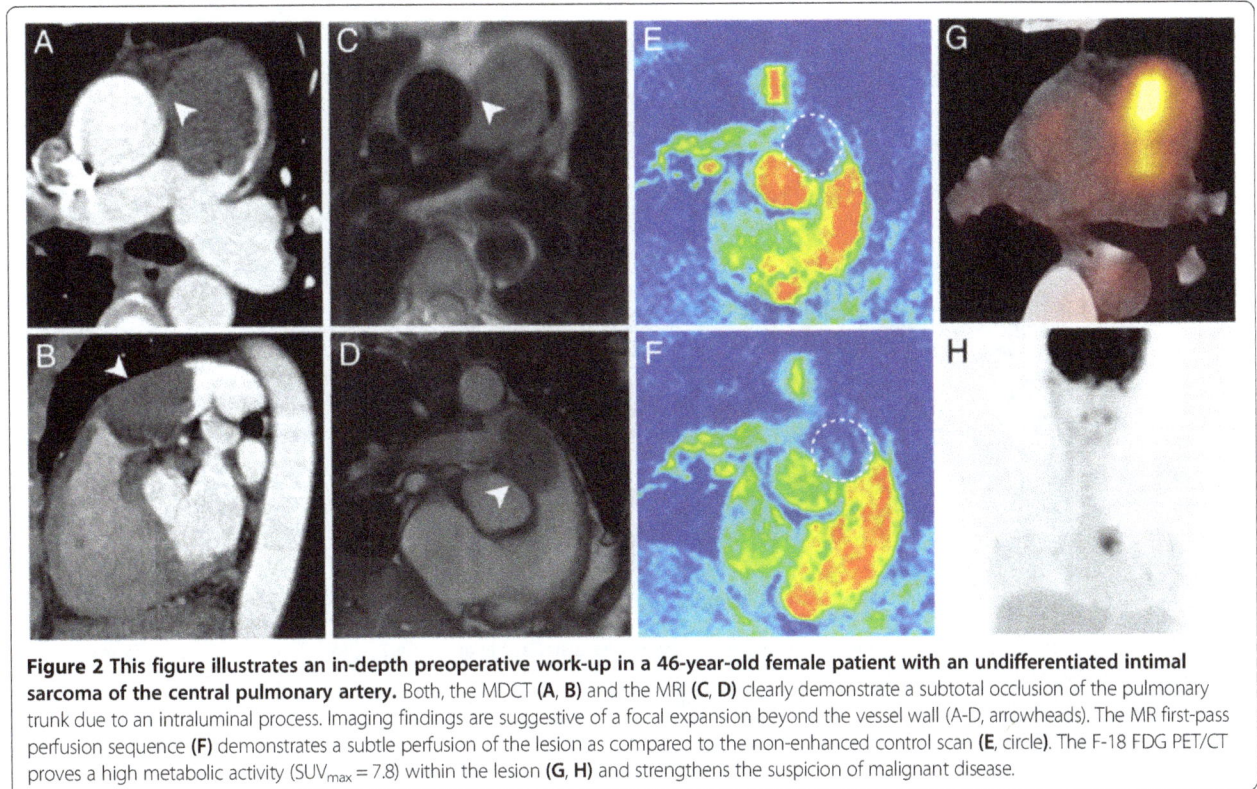

Figure 2 This figure illustrates an in-depth preoperative work-up in a 46-year-old female patient with an undifferentiated intimal sarcoma of the central pulmonary artery. Both, the MDCT (**A**, **B**) and the MRI (**C**, **D**) clearly demonstrate a subtotal occlusion of the pulmonary trunk due to an intraluminal process. Imaging findings are suggestive of a focal expansion beyond the vessel wall (A-D, arrowheads). The MR first-pass perfusion sequence (**F**) demonstrates a subtle perfusion of the lesion as compared to the non-enhanced control scan (**E**, circle). The F-18 FDG PET/CT proves a high metabolic activity (SUV$_{max}$ = 7.8) within the lesion (**G**, **H**) and strengthens the suspicion of malignant disease.

focus on the clinical presentation or pathology. Despite the rareness of these tumors it is important for the radiologist to bear this seldom differential diagnosis in mind, especially when alerted by typical imaging findings that raise the suspicion of a neoplastic origin of an intravascular filling defect as presented in this manuscript.

The overall prognosis of patients with sarcomas of the great vessels is poor. Many patients have a locally advanced state or distant metastases at the time of presentation [1-3]. Hence, a timely diagnosis is essential to identify the patients in a stage of disease where an aggressive surgical therapeutic approach with curative intent is

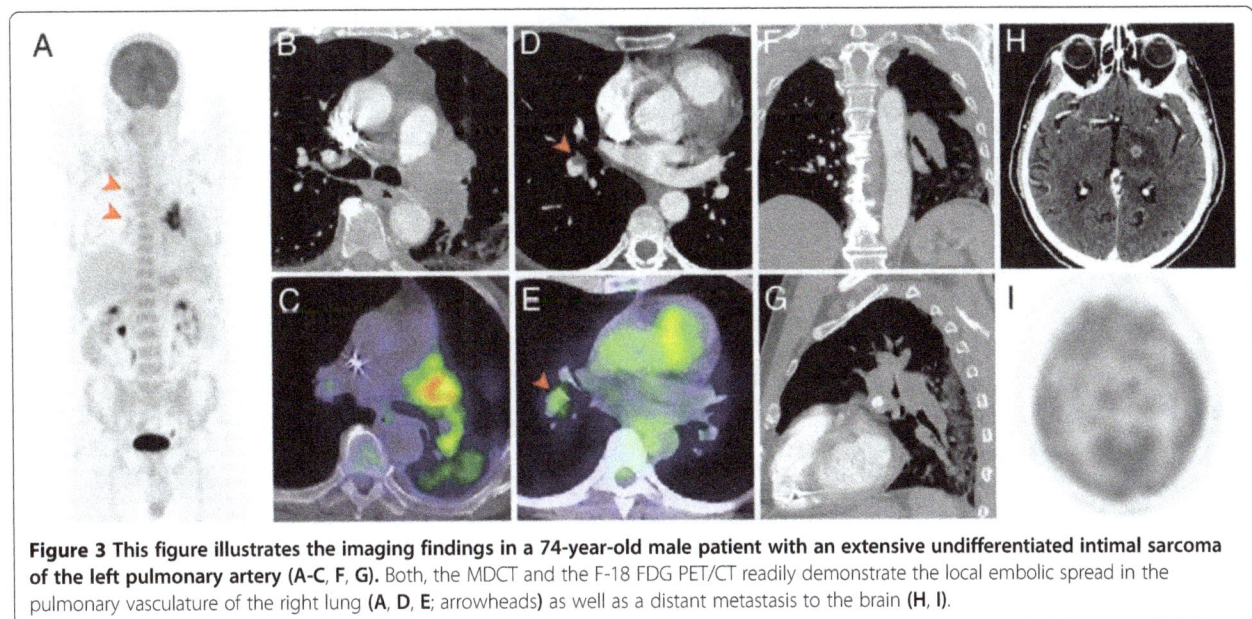

Figure 3 This figure illustrates the imaging findings in a 74-year-old male patient with an extensive undifferentiated intimal sarcoma of the left pulmonary artery (**A-C**, **F**, **G**). Both, the MDCT and the F-18 FDG PET/CT readily demonstrate the local embolic spread in the pulmonary vasculature of the right lung (**A**, **D**, **E**; arrowheads) as well as a distant metastasis to the brain (**H**, **I**).

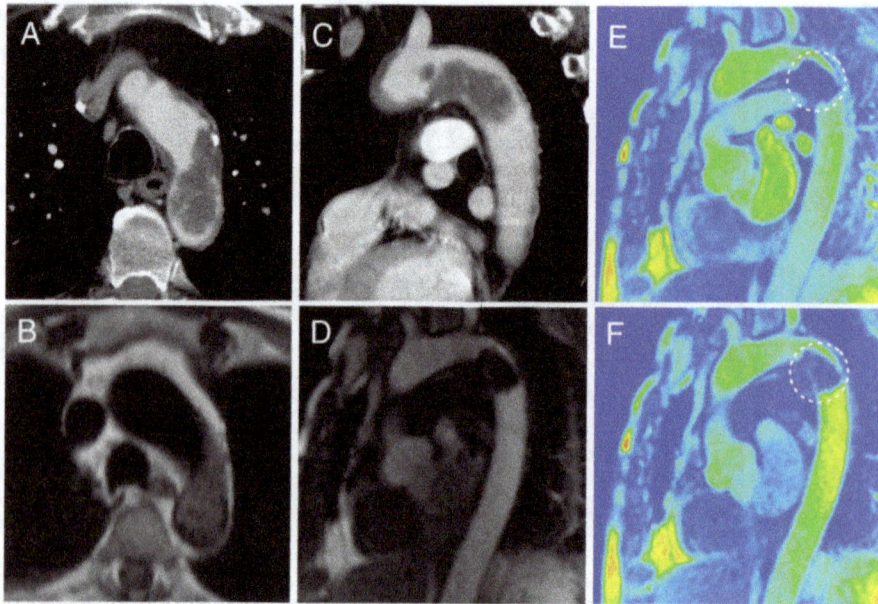

Figure 4 This figure shows an example of an aortic angiosarcoma of the distal aortic arch in a 71-year-old male patient who was treated for congestive heart failure. The MDCT and MRI images **(A-D)** nicely illustrate the typical pedunculated appearance of the lesion in a location that is atypical for atheromatous thrombi. The first pass perfusion sequence **(F)** suggests vascularisation of the lesion as compared to the unenhanced control acquisition **(E**, circle).

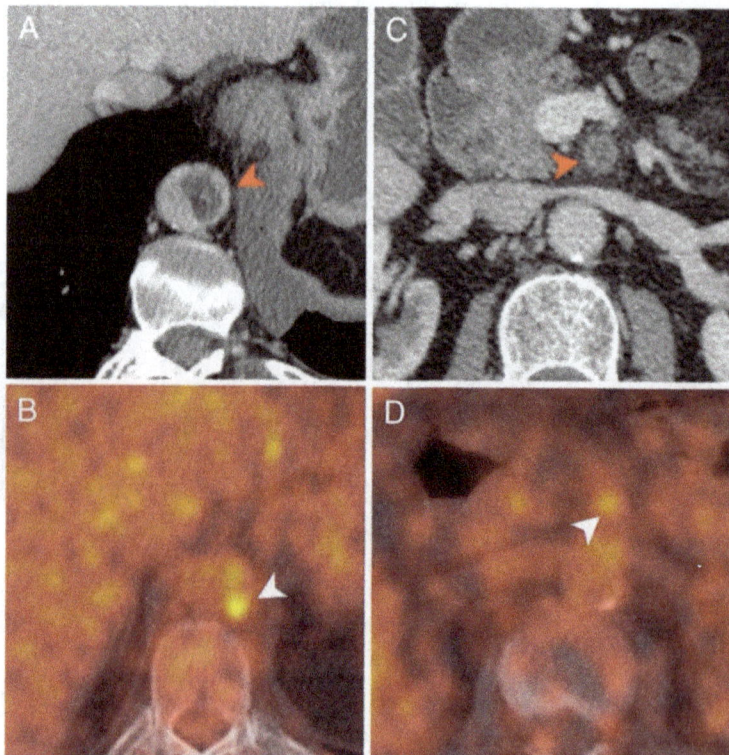

Figure 5 MDCT and PET/CT of a 71-year-old male patient with an undifferentiated intimal sarcoma of the descending aorta and extension into the superior mesenteric artery (A, C). The PET/CT adds valuable information about the metabolic status of vascular filling defect and strengthens the suspicion of malignant disease **(B, D)**.

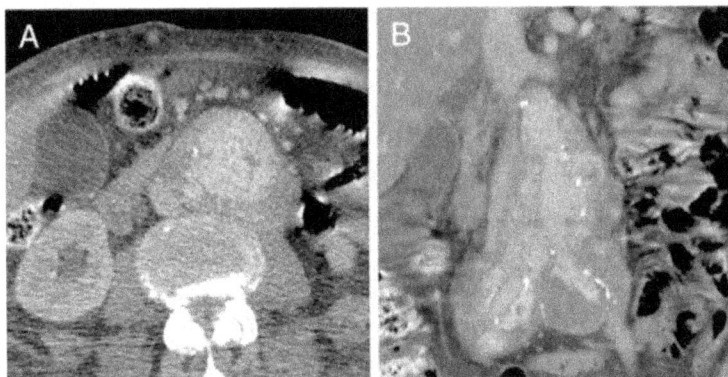

Figure 6 MDCT images in axial (A) and coronal (B) orientation of a 81-year-old patient with an angiosarcoma of the abdominal aorta who had previously undergone open aortic surgery. The extensive extramural tumor formation is clearly visualized and may be confounded with chronic inflammatory disease and contained rupture.

still feasible. We observed a median delay in diagnosis of 11 weeks between the first imaging study and the final diagnosis. The awareness of typical imaging findings presented herein may add to a shortening of this undesirable diagnostic delay. However, the large interval between the first consultation of a physician and the final diagnosis in three of our cases is assumably of higher prognostic relevance, but can hardly be reduced due to the unspecific symptoms that mimic more common diseases such as pulmonary hypertension or congestive heart failure [1,5,7,8].

With regard to primary malignancies of the pulmonary arteries we observed a large filling defect with vascular distension, unilaterality of the filling defect and a lack

Table 2 Imaging features of primary sarcoma of the great vessels

Basic imaging features	
Pulmonary artery sarcoma	Aortic sarcoma
Large *unilateral* obstruction of the main pulmonary arteries	Pedunculated or lobulated appearance
	Unusual location
Vascular distension	
	Expansion beyond the vessel wall
Expansion beyond the vessel wall	
Lack of improvement of a 'pulmonary embolism' despite adequate anticoagulation	
No evidence of a deep-venous thrombosis	
Imaging findings during detailed work-up	
High metabolic activity as demonstrated by F-18 FDG PET or PET/CT	
Lesion vascularization (as demonstrated by contrast-enhanced dynamic or perfusion MRI or CT)	
Distant metastases	

of improvement despite effective anticoagulation as the major imaging findings suggestive of malignant disease. These findings are usually the first 'red flags' that can possibly be encountered in an MDCT scan of the chest usually acquired for unspecific clinical symptoms such as dyspnea or chest pain. Our results are well in concordance with earlier observations in the literature. Yi et al. reported comparable findings in a group of seven patients in a study on the MDCT-appearance of pulmonary artery sarcomas [7]. However, they observed extraluminal expansion in 5 of 7 patients (71%) as compared to 25% (2/8) in our cohort. This difference may be due to an advanced tumor stage in Yi's patient group as the findings occurred in our two patients in the follow-up examinations showing progressive disease. Furthermore, Yi et al. may have had more patients with the mural form of the disease in his patient group as opposed to the exclusively luminal form in our patients. Fasse et al. have also seen comparable findings in five patients [8]. We did not observe a bilateral involvement of the central pulmonary arteries, however, it may occur as shown in a case by Simpson and Mendelson [9].

With respect to sarcomas of the aorta we identified an atypical location of a thrombus and a pedunculated shape as characteristic morphologic imaging features in two patients of our cohort, consistent with the intimal form of aortic sarcoma as described in the literature. Comparable findings have been reported by Bendel et al. [3]. Our single case of a patient with the mural disease pattern who had previously undergone aortic surgery is well in concordance with a few reports in the literature that describe the development of aortic sarcoma in patients after open or endovascular aortic repair. Whether the graft itself or a chronic perigraft infection might contribute to the induction of malignancy in the aortic wall remains subject to discussion, as the number of cases is very limited [10,11]. One patient of our cohort was diagnosed with a sarcoma of the pulmonary vein, which is even less frequently reported in the literature than pulmonary artery sarcoma [12].

When an atypical vascular filling defect is noticed base on the criteria described above, further imaging workup is usually recommended to verify the suspicion of malignant disease. Different imaging modalities such as dynamic MDCT and MRI examinations for the evaluation of lesion vascularization or metabolic imaging using F-18 FDG PET(/CT) are possible examinations whose potential benefits have been sporadically described in the literature. There is only sparse data on the role of F-18 FDG PET (/CT) for the imaging of primary sarcomas of the great vessels, mainly in patients with pulmonary artery involvement. However, the few cases reported in the literature are promising [13-16]. Ito et al. reported on three patients with pulmonary artery sarcomas and demonstrated that the mean SUV_{max} of 7.6 was significantly higher than in patients with pulmonary embolism [13]. Wittram and Scott observed SUV_{max} values in the range from 0.45 to 3.03 for acute pulmonary emboli, which is considerably lower than the SUV_{max} values reported for pulmonary sarcomas [17]. Another small series of three patients was published by Tueller et al. with an SUV_{max} of 5.2 (reported only for one patient) [16]. Treglia et al. recently reported an SUVmax of 13 for a primary pulmonary epitheloid angiosarcoma that presented as an intrapulmonary mass [18]. There is even less experience in patients with aortic sarcoma [19,20] or sarcoma of the pulmonary veins [21]. Our own results on three patients are also encouraging. We observed unequivocal positive findings in all four patients that underwent a F-18 FDG PET or F-18 FDG PET(/CT) examination. Our mean SUV_{max} of 13.1 for patients with pulmonary artery disease was even higher than the values reported in the literature. As PET/CT usually is a whole-body examination it does not only help to decide on the possibly malignant nature of a filling defect, but at the same time serves as a whole-body staging modality. In one of our cases, F-18 FDG PET(/CT) was able to demonstrate embolic metastases in the lungs as well as a peripheral metastasis to the brain (Figure 5).

Although described in most reports of primary sarcomas of the great vessels, there is only few quantitative data on the degree of enhancement or perfusion of these tumors. Kacl et al. reported on dynamic MRI in four patients with sarcomas of the pulmonary arteries and found a 'considerable variability' of the contrast enhancement, which was interpreted as being dependent on the degree of differentiation [22]. Howarth et al. described a single case in which an MRI first-pass perfusion sequence was used to prove the vascularization of the lesion [23]. Fasse et al. reported on MDCT and MRI findings in five patients with sarcomas of the pulmonary

arteries and found only MR imaging suitable for the evaluation of lesion enhancement [8]. However, tumor vascularization cannot be demonstrated in all cases [8]. In our patient population, MR demonstrated a contrast enhancement of the lesions in 3 out of 4 MRI scans of patients with pulmonary disease and in both MRI scans available in the patients with aortic tumors. Notably, the enhancement was subtle in all our patients and required a thorough analysis of the contrast-enhanced sequences. No enhancement was visualized on standard MDCT examinations, except for the patient with the extensive mural aortic sarcoma. However, we did not evaluate the possible value of dedicated MDCT perfusion techniques. Besides the evaluation of possible lesion perfusion, MRI has an additional value in the depiction of the relationship between the tumor and its surrounding structures and may assist the preoperative planning, especially when ECG-gated cine sequences are used.

A number of important limitations of our manuscript need to be addressed. First of all and most obvious, the number of patients in our study is limited and the imaging studies available for our analyses were heterogeneous and do not follow a specific protocol. However, as already outlined above, sarcomas of the great vessels are exceedingly rare and most reports in the literature are therefore limited to descriptions of single cases or small series. To the best of our knowledge, our manuscript represents the largest study group that has been evaluated with respect to the imaging findings. Second, we did not compare our imaging findings to a contrast group such as patients with pulmonary embolic disease or severe aortic atheromatosis. However, the selection of such control groups would be highly artificial. Furthermore, the number of patients in our study is too limited to calculate statistical significances or sensitivities and specificities. In addition, we did not evaluate the potential role of transthoracic or transesophageal echocardiography in our patient cohort. Depending on the location, these modalities may also serve as a viable tool for the depiction of the tumor. However, as the field of view and the capability to characterize soft tissues are limited, echocardiography has its strongest potential in patients with cardiac sarcomas and is inferior to MDCT and MRI in cases of extracardiac disease [3].

Conclusion

In conclusion, if an intraluminal filling defect of a great vessel that is incidentally detected on a routine MDCT or MRI scan shows the characteristic imaging findings outlined in this manuscript, primary sarcoma should be taken into consideration and further diagnostic workup is recommended to avoid any delay in the diagnosis of this rare disease. MR perfusion techniques may add information on the nature of the lesion but the findings may be subtle and equivocal. Based on our limited experience, we see a potential role of F-18 FDG PET/CT in these patients and suggest it to be considered as part of the imaging workup in these patients.

Competing interests
The authors declare that they have no competing interests.

Authors' contributions
CvF, BM and CF designed the study, identified the patients to be included in the study and carried out the analysis. CvF and TR drafted the manuscript. FL carried out the histopathologic studies. FBe, FWa and TR participated in the design and coordination of the study and helped to draft the manuscript. All authors read and approved the final manuscript.

Acknowledgements
The publication of this study is supported by the German Research Foundation project "Open Access Publication".

Author details
[1]Department of Radiology, Hannover Medical School, Hannover 30625, Germany. [2]Department of Cardiothoracic, Transplant and Vascular Surgery, Hannover Medical School, Hannover, Germany. [3]Institute of Pathology, Hannover Medical School, Hannover, Germany. [4]Department of Nuclear Medicine, Hannover Medical School, Hannover, Germany.

References
1. Mayer F, Aebert H, Rudert M, Königsrainer A, Horger M, Kanz L, Bamberg M, Ziemer G, Hartmann JT: **Primary malignant sarcomas of the heart and great vessels in adult patients—a single-center experience.** *Oncologist* 2007, **12:**1134–1142.
2. Burke AP, Virmani R: **Sarcomas of the great vessels. A clinicopathologic study.** *Cancer* 1993, **71:**1761–1773.
3. Bendel EC, Maleszewski JJ, Araoz PA: **Imaging sarcomas of the great vessels and heart.** *Semin Ultrasound CT MR* 2011, **32:**377–404.
4. Restrepo CS, Betancourt SL, Martinez-Jimenez S, Gutierrez FR: **Tumors of the pulmonary artery and veins.** *Semin Ultrasound CT MR* 2012, **33:**580–590.
5. Choong CK, Lawton JS, Moon MR, Damiano RJ Jr: **Failure of medical therapy for pulmonary "thromboembolic" disease: beware the unsuspected primary sarcoma of the pulmonary artery.** *J Thorac Cardiovasc Surg* 2004, **128:**763–765.
6. Fletcher CDM, Unni KK, Mertens F: *World Health Organization classification of tumours: pathology and genetics of tumours of soft tissue and bone.* Lyon: IARC Press; 2002.
7. Yi CA, Lee KS, Choe YH, Han D, Kwon OJ, Kim S: **Computed tomography in pulmonary artery sarcoma: distinguishing features from pulmonary embolic disease.** *J Comput Assist Tomogr* 2004, **28:**34–39.
8. Fasse A, Kauczor HU, Mayer E, Kreitner KF, Heussel CP, Thelen M: **Sarcoma of the pulmonary artery - pre- and postoperative radiologic findings in initial tumor manifestation and recurrence.** *Rofo* 1999, **170:**112–118.
9. Simpson WL Jr, Mendelson DS: **Pulmonary artery and aortic sarcomas: cross-sectional imaging.** *J Thorac Imaging* 2000, **15:**290–294.
10. Alexander JJ, Moawad J, Cai D: **Primary intimal sarcoma of the aorta associated with a dacron graft and resulting in arterial rupture.** *Vasc Endovascular Surg* 2006, **40:**509–515.
11. Weiss WM, Riles TS, Gouge TH, Mizrachi HH: **Angiosarcoma at the site of a Dacron vascular prosthesis: a case report and literature review.** *J Vasc Surg* 1991, **14:**87–91.
12. Oliai BR, Tazelaar HD, Lloyd RV, Doria MI, Trastek VF: **Leiomyosarcoma of the pulmonary veins.** *Am J Surg Pathol* 1999, **23:**1082–1088.
13. Ito K, Kubota K, Morooka M, Shida Y, Hasuo K, Endo H, Matsuda H: **Diagnostic usefulness of F-18 FDG PET/CT in the differentiation of pulmonary artery sarcoma and pulmonary embolism.** *Ann Nucl Med* 2009, **23:**671–676.
14. Chong S, Kim TS, Kim BT, Cho EY, Kim J: **Pulmonary artery sarcoma mimicking pulmonary thromboembolism: integrated FDG PET/CT.** *AJR Am J Roentgenol* 2007, **188:**1691–1693.
15. Ote EL, Oriuchi N, Miyashita G, Paudyal B, Ishikita T, Arisaka Y, Higuchi T, Hirato J, Endo K: **Pulmonary artery intimal sarcoma: the role of** [18]**F-fluorodeoxyglucose positron emission tomography in monitoring response to treatment.** *Jpn J Radiol* 2011, **29:**279–282.
16. Tueller C, Fischer Biner R, Minder S, Gugger M, Stoupis C, Krause TM, Carrel TP, Schmid RA, Vock P, Nicod LP: **FDG-PET in diagnostic work-up of pulmonary artery sarcomas.** *Eur Respir J* 2010, **35:**444–446.
17. Wittram C, Scott JA: **F-18 FDG PET of pulmonary embolism.** *AJR Am J Roentgenol* 2007, **189:**171–176.
18. Treglia G, Cardillo G, Graziano P: **A Rare Case of Primary Pulmonary Epithelioid Angiosarcoma Detected by 18F-FDG PET/CT.** *Clin Nucl Med* 2013. [Epub ahead of print] PubMed PMID: 23657141.
19. Hsiao E, Laury A, Rybicki FJ, Menard MT, Ersoy H: **Images in vascular medicine. Metastatic aortic intimal sarcoma: the use of PET/CT in diagnosing and staging.** *Vasc Med* 2011, **16:**81–82.
20. Sibille L, Ilonca D, Oziol E, Gandilhon P, Micheau A, Vernhet-Kovacsik H, Pascal-Ortiz D: **FDG PET/CT in aortic angiosarcoma.** *Clin Nucl Med* 2010, **35:**134–137.
21. Lin E: **Diagnosis of venous angiosarcoma by FDG PET/CT.** *Clin Nucl Med* 2008, **33:**66–67.
22. Kacl GM, Bruder E, Pfammatter T, Follath F, Salomon D, Debatin JF: **Primary angiosarcoma of the pulmonary arteries: dynamic contrast-enhanced MRI.** *J Comput Assist Tomogr* 1988, **22:**687–691.
23. Howarth NR, Beziat C, Berthezène Y: **Evolution of pulmonary perfusion defects demonstrated with contrast-enhanced dynamic MR perfusion imaging.** *Eur Radiol* 1999, **9:**1574–1576.

19

Assessment of the level of agreement in the interpretation of plain radiographs of lumbar spondylosis among clinical physiotherapists in Ghana

Ajediran I Bello[1*], Eric K Ofori[2], Oluwasegun J Alabi[1] and David N Adjei[3]

Abstract

Background: Objective physical assessment of patients with lumbar spondylosis involves plain film radiographs (PFR) viewing and interpretation by the radiologists. Physiotherapists also routinely assess PFR within the scope of their practice. However, studies appraising the level of agreement of physiotherapists' PFR interpretation with radiologists are not common in Ghana.

Method: Forty-one (41) physiotherapists took part in the cross-sectional survey. An assessment guide was developed from findings of the interpretation of three PFR of patients with lumbar spondylosis by a radiologist. The three PFR were selected from a pool of different radiographs based on clarity, common visible pathological features, coverage body segments and short post production period. Physiotherapists were required to view the same PFR after which they were assessed with the assessment guide according to the number of features identified correctly or incorrectly. The score range on the assessment form was 0–24, interpreted as follow: 0–8 points (low), 9–16 points (moderate) and 17–24 points (high) levels of agreement. Data were analyzed using one sample t-test and fisher's exact test at α = 0.05.

Results: The mean score of interpretation for the physiotherapists was 12.7 ± 2.6 points compared to the radiologist's interpretation of 24 points (assessment guide). The physiotherapists' levels were found to be significantly associated with their academic qualification (p = 0.006) and sex (p = 0.001). However, their levels of agreement were not significantly associated with their age group (p = 0.098), work settings (p = 0.171), experience (p = 0.666), preferred PFR view (p = 0.088) and continuing education (p = 0.069).

Conclusions: The physiotherapists' skills fall short of expectation for interpreting PFR of patients with lumbar spondylosis. The levels of agreement with radiologist's interpretation have no link with year of clinial practice, age, work settings and continuing education. Thus, routine PFR viewing techniques should be made a priority in physiotherapists' continuing professional education.

Keywords: Agreement, Plain radiographs, Interpretation, Clinical physiotherapists

Background

Spondylosis is a degenerative disease which can occur at any level of the spine but commonly detected at the cervical and lumbar regions [1]. It is characterized by a series of degenerative changes at the spinal end-plates, vertebral bodies and intervertebral discs with consequent formation of osteophytes and sclerosis [2]. The clinical deficits of lumbar spondylosis can range from mild to severe pain and from minimal to maximum disability with significant impact on work productivity and the quality of life of the sufferers [3,4].

Plain film radiograph (PFR) is one of the common imaging techniques used to confirm the diagnosis of lumbar spondylosis by the radiologists in most clinical settings in Ghana and it remains the mainstay in most developing African countries given its availability and cost effectiveness.

* Correspondence: iabello@chs.edu.gh
[1]Department of Physiotherapy, School of Allied Health Sciences, College of Health Sciences, University of Ghana, Accra, Ghana
Full list of author information is available at the end of the article

Studies assessing the level of agreement of interpretation of imaging techniques among allied health professionals have been documented in literature. For instance, the outcome of meta-analysis on the degree of agreement between radiographers and radiologists to determine the radiographers' accuracy in radiographic reports revealed accuracy level of the radiographers at 92.6% and 97.7% sensitivity and specificity respectively while nurses working at remote units also showed their respective accuracy levels at 96% for sensitivity and 87% for specificity [5,6]. Although the previous studies have assessed the interpretation of PFR among other allied health professionals, studies on agreement of physiotherapists in the interpretation of PFR are not readily available.

Based on anedoctal observation from the Ghanaian health care setting, at least two orthogonal PFR views (Anterio-posterior and lateral) are commonly examined in the preliminary assessment of patients with lumbar spondylosis by the physicians and orthopaedic specialists. Eventhough the interpretation of PFR remains within the purview of the radiologists, physiotherapists often perform this task either as extended scope of practice or as routine procedure during objective assessment. With the emergence of physiotherapy practice from under the cover of traditional referral system to self-referral methods of health care delivery particularly in wellness and musculoskeletal fields, Ghanaian physiotherapists are required to extend their horizon to be relevant in the ongoing global health reform [7]. Correct interpretation of PFR among physiotherapists becomes necessary in order to identify possible contra-indications to some physiotherapy techniques and/or modification of treatment plans accordingly to change the natural course of the presented conditions [8].

Given the growing reliance on radiographic imaging and the evolvement of first contact practice in some allied health professionals, it is necessary to appraise the skills of the relevant available health care professionals in the interpretation of imaging techniques. This study therefore determined the level of agreement in the interpretation of PFR of lumbar spondylosis between the physiotherapists and radiologists in Ghana.

Methods
Participants
Forty-one (41) clinical physiotherapists participated in this cross-sectional survey. They were recruited through sample of convenience from the Government hospitals and private physiotherapy clinics located at four of the ten Regions in Ghana. Clinical physiotherapists who were registered members of Ghana Physiotherapy Association and those who had practiced for at least one (1) year were included in the study. Retired physiotherapists and those in academics were excluded.

Design of an assessment guide
Three separate PFR (two antero-posterior and one lateral views) were selected from a pool of PFR of patients undergoing physiotherapy for lumbar spondylosis at the selected hospitals and clinics. The selection was based on the clarity of the films, availability of common lumbar spondylosis pathology, coverage of peripheral body segments (bilateral pelvis and hips), and post production period not exceeding three (3) months. The selected films were shown to an experienced independent radiologist who in turn identified the pathological features and listed them as gold standard to serve as an assessment guide (Appendix 1). The listed pathological features were found to be comparable and consistent to that obtained from twenty retrospective radiologists' reports on patients with lumbar spondylosis. A total of 24 features were identified by the radiologist from three PFR with each consisting 8 features. The assessment guide was subjected to test re-tests reliability among seven experienced radiologists whose reports were not included in the retrospective reports to scrutinize the list. A good internal consistency of 0.79 Chrombach's alpha value was obtained through the evaluation process [9]. Correct identification of a pathological feature attracts one (1) point while wrong identification or non-identification attracts 0 point. The score range on the form is 0–24 in which the minimum obtainable score is zero (0) while the maximum obtainable score is 24. The scoring is interpreted as follow: 0–8 points (low level of agreement), 9–16 points (moderate level of agreement) and 17–24 points (high level of agreement).

Procedure
The Ethics and Protocol Review Committee of the School of Allied Health Sciences, University of Ghana approved the proposal for this study. An information sheet containing the title and the intent of the study was made available to the participants and their written consents were obtained. A self-designed data capturing form was used to obtain demographic data such as age, sex and academic qualification and clinical data including number of years of clinical experience, work settings and the number of continuing professional development (CPD) programme attended in the last 5 years (Appendix 2). The three plain film radiographs (PFR) of lumbar spondylosis from which the assessment guide was developed were viewed by the physiotherapists in the presence of the researchers and in no particular order to avoid stereo-typed interpretation. They were required to list the identifiable patho-anatomical features observed in the PFR. A time commitment of 30 minutes was expected of the participants for the completion of the entire procedure. On completion of the interpretation and documentation process, the researchers collected the findings and evaluated each physiotherapist using the assessment guide.

Data analysis

Data were analyzed using the SPSS version 19.0 software. Descriptive statistics of frequency, percentage, mean and standard deviation were used to summarize the data. One sample Kolmogorov-Smirnov test was explored to test the data for normalcy. Comparison of PFR interpretation between the physiotherapists and the radiologist was tested with one sample t test while Fisher's exact test was used to determine the associations between levels of agreement and the physiotherapists' demographic and clinical variables at alpha level of 0.05.

Results

Forty-one (41) physiotherapists participated in this study comprising 17 (41.5%) males and 24 (58.5%) females. The demographic and clinical profiles of the participants are presented in Table 1. Most physiotherapists, 25 (61%) were within the age range 26–30 years and 36 (88%) of them hold bachelor's degree while five (12%) had masters' degree. The study also showed that majority of the physiotherapists 24 (58.5%) worked in teaching hospitals while 3 (7.3%) worked in general hospital. Twenty-five (61%) had been practicing for less than or a total of four (4) years as compared to 16 (39%) who had worked for 5 to 9 years. Twenty-four (58.6%) of the physiotherapists had attended less than or a total of two continuing professional development (CPD) programmes while 6 (14.6%) had attended less than or a total of 6 CPD programmes.

Results of the categorical levels of assessment shows that 4 (9.8%) physiotherapists scored between 0 and 8 points (Low); 35 (85.4%) scored between 9 and 16 points (Moderate); 2 (4.9%) scored between 17 and 24 points (High). The levels of agreement were significantly associated with academic qualification (0.006) and the sex (p = 0.001) of the physiotherapists. However, the levels of agreement were not significantly associated with the age group (p = 0.098), work setting (p = 0.171), year of clinical practice (p = 0.666), preferred PFR views (p = 0.088) and the number of CPD attended (p = 0.069) (Table 2).

Exploration of one sample Kolmogorov-Smirnov test for normalcy of data shows no significant difference in the dataset distribution (p = 0.207) thereby justifying the adoption of one sample t test analysis. The mean score of agreement (12.7 ± 2.6) for the physiotherapists was significantly lower (p = 0.001) than the gold standard point of 24 (Radiologist's score).

Discussion

The main focus of this study was to assess the level of agreement of interpretation of plain radiographs (PFR) between the radiologists and physiotherapists in Ghana. The mean score of interpretation of the physiotherapists compared to that of the radiologists in this study was 12.7 (approximately 50.0% of the total point) which was

Table 1 Demographic and clinical profiles of the physiotherapists

Variable	Number	Percentage
Sex		
Male	17	41.5
Female	24	58.5
Total	41	100
Age group (years)		
21-25	1	2.4
26-30	25	61.0
31-35	11	26.8
36-40	2	4.9
41-45	1	2.4
46-50	1	2.4
Total	41	100.0
Academic qualification		
BSc.	36	87.8
MSc.	5	12.2
Total	41	100
Years of clinical practice		
0-4	25	61.0
5-9	16	39.0
Total	41	100.0
Work setting		
Regional hospital	10	24.4
Teaching hospital	24	58.5
General hospital	3	7.3
Private hospital	4	9.8
Total	41	100.0
CPD programme attendance		
0-2	24	58.6
3-5	11	26.8
≥6	6	14.6
Total	41	100.0
Preference of radiograph view		
Antero-posterior	5	12.2
Lateral	15	36.6
Neither	21	51.2
Total	41	100.0

Key: CPD = Continuing professional development.

statistically lower than the required scores. This finding falls short of expectation giving the high agreement of other health care professionals with the radiologists in the previous studies [5,6]. For instance, Brealey et al. reported high accuracy levels for radiographers at 92.6% and 97.7% sensitivity and specificity respectively [5] while Benger submitted that nurses working in remote units had

Table 2 Fisher's exact analysis for the associations between the physiotherapists' levels of agreement of PFR interpretation and their clinical and demographic characteristics

Variables	Low n (%)	Moderate n (%)	High n (%)	Fisher's exact test p value
Age (years)				
21–25	0 (0.0)	1 (100)	0 (0.0)	0.098
26–30	2 (8.0)	20 (80.0)	3 (12.0)	
31–35	0 (0.0)	11 (100)	0 (0.0)	
36–40	0 (0.0)	2 (100)	0 (0.0)	
41–45	0 (0.0)	0 (0.0)	1 (100)	
46-50	0 (0.0)	1 (100)	0 (0.0)	
Qualification				
B.Sc	2 (5.5)	32 (88.8)	2 (5.5)	0.006*
M.Sc	0 (0.0)	3 (60.0)	2 (40.0)	
Work setting				
Regional hospital	1 (10.0)	8 (80.0)	1 (10.0)	0.171
Teaching hospital	1 (4.1)	21 (87.5)	2 (8.3)	
General hospital	0 (0.0)	2 (66.7)	1 (33.4)	
Private hospital	0 (0.0)	4 (100)	0 (0)	
Years of practice				
0–4	2 (8.0)	22 (88.0)	1 (4.0)	0.666
5-9	0 (0.0)	13 (81.2)	3 (18.7)	
No of CPD attended				
0–2	1 (4.2)	22 (91.7)	1 (4.2)	0.069
3–5	1 (9.0)	9 (81.8)	1 (9.0)	
≥6	0 (0.0)	4 (66.7)	2 (33.4)	
Sex				
Male	0 (0.0)	4 (23.5)	13 (76.4)	0.001*
Female	2 (8.4)	0 (0.0)	22 (91.7)	
Preferred view				
Anterio-posterior view	1 (20.0)	4 (80.0)	0 (0.0)	0.088
Lateral view	0 (0.0)	13 (86.7)	2 (13.4)	
Both	1 (4.7)	18 (85.7)	2 (9.5)	

Key: *Significant at $p < 0.05$.

96% sensitivity and 87% specificity in the interpretation agreement [6]. These variations might not be unconnected with the different settings in which the studies were conducted

In addition, approximately 85.4% of the physiotherapists' scores were within the moderate range (9–16 points) which implies that majority of the participants' performances were within the average in PFR interpretation. Although PFR viewing is a common routine procedure in physiotherapy, it seems little priority has been placed on its techniques in the series of their continuing education programmes. Presumably, they might have acquired their rudimentary skills through personal efforts and interest. These speculations may be justifiable given the crops of young generation of the practicing physiotherapists in Ghana.

In the same vein, the levels of agreement in the interpretation of PFR by the physiotherapists' were significantly associated with their academic qualification and sex. Most of the physiotherapists were first degree holders implying that they were still at the minimum entry level of the profession as stipulated by the World Confederation for Physical Therapy [10]. Post-graduate training programme in the field of physiotherapy is yet to take off in Ghana, thus the few physiotherapists with masters degree had to divert to other fields that may not directly impact on their clinical proficiency. The link between gender and level of agreement may be ascribed to the relative proportion of the sampled male and female physiotherapists in this study. Contrarily, the age, work settings, years of clinical practice and the preferred PFR views have no significant impact on the level of agreements. These findings suggest that the physiotherapists' disposition towards PFR viewing rather than the selected clinical variables are the influencing factors. Further, specialty physiotherapy training and practice in Ghana are yet to be established, hence daily practice cuts across the branches of the profession without specific emphasis on orthopaedics-related cases where x-ray viewing and interpretation are mostly needed.

A shift in the focus of health care delivery from the hospital to the community, are placing increased demands on physiotherapists to embrace primary-care systems. Available evidence suggests that physiotherapists' involvements in the primary health care setting are beneficial to patients suffering from musculoskeletal problems such as arthritis and low back pain [11]. Indeed, the convergence of rising health care costs and physician shortages have made health care transformation a priority in many developing countries resulting in the emergence of new models of care that often involve the extension of the scope of practice for most allied health professionals. Physiotherapists in extended scope roles must emerge as key providers in such new models, especially in settings providing services to patients with musculoskeletal disorders [12].

Limitation of the study

The findings from this study are limited by the use of very few plain film radiographs of patients suffering from lumbar spondylosis with which the participants were assessed. Sampling over sufficient numbers of patients' x-rays would have ensured external validity of the results. These observations should be the focus of the future study.

Conclusions

We conclude that the sampled Ghanaian physiotherapists had disproportionate level of agreement in the interpretation of PFR of patients with lumbar spondylosis compared to that of the Radiologist. The sex and academic qualification of the sampled physiotherapists had significant bearing on their level of agreement. The outcomes of this study thus underscore the urgent need to include basic training in the interpretation of plain radiographs into the continuing professional development programme of physiotherapists in Ghana.

Appendix 1

Assessment guide

The underlisted three plain film radiographs (PFR) A, B, and C contain the common degenerative features found in patients diagnosed with lumbar spondylosis in two views (anterio-posterior and lateral):

  PFR A: Lumbar spine only (anterio-posterior view)
  PFR B: Lumbar spine + Pelvis (anterio-posterior view)
  PFR C: Lumbar spine only (Lateral view)

The following (8) features were the pathological features found in each of the PFR.
1. Marginal osteophytes on lumbar vertebrae
2. Decreased vertebral body height
3. Decreased lumbar intervertebral disc space
4. End plate sclerosis of articular surfaces in the lumbar region
5. Scoliotic lumbar vertebrae
6. Exaggerated lumbar lordosis
7. Straightening of the lumbar spine (reduced normal lumbar lordosis)
8. Vacuum phenomenon

Mark each correctly identified pathological feature as 1 point and wrong identification or non-identification as 0 point. The total score is 24 ranging from 0–24 in which the minimum obtainable score is zero (0) while the maximum obtainable score is 24. The scoring is interpreted as follow: 0–8 scores (low level of agreement), 9–16 scores (moderate level of agreement) and 17–24 scores (high level of agreement).

Appendix 2

Data capturing form

Instruction: Kindly supply the following information as applicable to you

Section A: Demographics
1. AGE: 21–25 □ 26–30 □ 31–35 □ 36–40 □ 41–45 □ 46–50 □ 51–55 □ 55 □
2. SEX: Male □ Female □
3. ACADEMIC QUALIFICATIONS (kindly tick more than one if applicable)
   Diploma □ B. Sc. □ M. Sc. □ Ph. D □
   Others (specify)..
1. Are you a registered member of the Ghana Association of Physiotherapists?
   Yes □ No □

Section B: Clinical variables
1. In which of the following work settings do you practise?
   Teaching Hospital □ General Hospital □ Regional Hospital □ Private □
1. How many years of Clinical experience (excluding internship) do you have? ....
2. How many Orthopaedics related Continuous Professional Development (C.P.D.) programme (workshop, seminar, conference e.t.c.) have you attended in the last 5 years? ....
3. Which view of the plain Radiograph would you request for when assessing a patient suspected to have Lumbar spondylosis?
   Antero-Posterior □ Lateral □

Competing interests
The authors declare that they have no competing interests.

Authors' contributions
AB responsible for the design of the manuscript for intellectual presentation. He also contributed to the collection, management, analysis and interpretation of data. EO, assisted in the collection, management, analysis and interpretation of data. OA, participated in the collection of data and final editing of the manuscript. DA participated in data interpretation and analysis. All authors read and approved the final manuscript.

Acknowledgement
We sincerely acknowledge the immense contributions of the Radiologists from the selected hospitals for their readiness to assist in the design of the assessment form. Special tribute also goes to Dr Harriet Obeng for her time in interpreting the three plain film radiographs used in developing the assessment guide.

Author details
[1]Department of Physiotherapy, School of Allied Health Sciences, College of Health Sciences, University of Ghana, Accra, Ghana. [2]Department of Radiography, School of Allied Health Sciences, College of Health Sciences, University of Ghana, Accra, Ghana. [3]Department of Medical Laboratory Sciences, School of Allied Health Sciences, College of Health Sciences, University of Ghana, Accra, Ghan.

References
1. Gibson JNA, Waddell G: **Surgery for degenerative lumbar spondylosis.** *Spine* 2005, **20**:2312–2320.
2. Emery SE, Ringus VM: **Osteoarthritis of the Spine.** In *Osteoathritis: Diagnosis and Medical/Surgical Management.* 4th edition. Edited by Moskowitz RW, Altman RD, Hochberg MC, Buckwalter JA, Goldberg VM. Philadelphia: Lippincott Williams and Wilkins; 2007:427–452.
3. Haldeman S, Chapman SD, Peterson DM: **Diagnostic Imaging of Lumbar Dics Herniations.** In *Guidelines for Chiropractic Quality Assurance and Practice Parameters.* Edited by Haldeman S, Chapman SD, Peterson DM. Gaithersburg MD: Aspen; 1995.
4. Middleton K, Fish DE: **Lumbar spondylosis: clinical presentation and treatment approaches.** *Curr. Rev Musculoskelet Med* 2009, **2**:94–104.
5. Brealey S, Scally A, Halm S, Thoma N, Godfrey C: **Accuracy of Radiographers' plain radiograph reporting in clinical practice: a meta-analysis.** *J Clin Radiol* 2005, **60**:232–241.
6. Benger JR: **Can nurses working in remote units accurately request and interpret radiographs?** *Emerg Med J* 2002, **19**(1):68–70.
7. Litchfield R, MacDougall C: **Professional issues for physiotherapists in familty-centered and community-based settings.** *Aust J Physiother* 2002, **48**:105–112.
8. Jarvik JG, Hollingworth W, Martin B, Emerson SS, Gray DT, Overman S, Robinson D, Staiger T, Wessbecher F, Sullivan SD, Kreuter W, Deyo RA: **Rapid magnetic resonance imaging versus radiographs for patients with Low back pain: a randomized controlled trial.** *J Am Med Assoc* 2003, **4 289**(21).2810.
9. Tavacol M, Dennick R: **Making sense of Cronbach's alpha.** *Int J Med Educ* 2011, **2**:53–55. doi:10.511/ijme.4dfb.8dfd.
10. World Confederation for Physical Therapy (2012): *Entry Education Programmes in Physical Therapy.* WCPT Reports; 2012. Available online at http://www.wcpt.org.
11. Cott CA, Mandoda S, Landry MD: **Models of integrating physical therapists into family health teams in Ontario, Canada: challenges and opportunities.** *Physiother Can* 2011, **63**(3):265–275. doi:10.3138/ptc.2010-01.
12. Desmeules F, Roy JS, Woodhouse LJ: **Advanced practice physiotherapy in patients with musculoskeletal disorders: a systematic review.** *BMC Musculoskelet Disord* 2012, **13**:107.

20

Atypical localization of intraosseous angioleiomyoma in the rib of a pediatric patient

Goran Djuričić[1]* (iD), Zorica Milošević[2], Tijana Radović[1], Nataša Milčanović[1], Predrag Djukić[1], Marko Radulovic[2] and Jelena Sopta[3]

Abstract

Background: This is the first reported case of a primary intraosseous angioleiomyoma and the second case of a primary leiomyoma of the rib, irrespective of age. Angioleiomyomas mostly occur in patients of advanced age, in any part of the body, particularly the lower extremities and present as painful, slow-growing nodules in the dermis, subcutaneous fat or deep fascia. Other localizations, especially bone, are considered extremely rare, as well as their occurrence in paediatric patients.

Case presentation: A 10-year-old girl was admitted to the orthopaedic surgery department for further assessment of a pain localized in the posterior part of the right hemithorax. After magnetic resonance imaging (MRI) and surgical biopsy, intraosseus angioleiomyoma of the fourth rib was diagnosed by histopathology examination. Atypical costal localization of this type of a benign tumour presents diagnostic difficulty, especially in children. The differential diagnoses included cartilaginous tumours, Ewing sarcoma, fibrous dysplasia, Langerhans cell histiocytosis, intraosseous haemangioma and metastatic tumours. We report a detailed diagnostic procedure including MRI, selective angiography and histopathologic examination.

Conclusion: Diagnosis of intraosseous angioleiomyoma is difficult due to the extreme rarity of this tumour and absence of pathognomonic radiological signs. Although very rarely identified in bones and young age group, radiographers and reporting doctors should be aware of this possible angioleiomyoma presentation and supported by the provided detailed diagnostic information.

Keywords: Intraosseous angioleiomyoma, Rib, Bone tumour, Paediatric

Background

Angioleiomyoma is a rare benign tumour, occurring in the soft tissues (dermis and subcutaneous fat) of the lower extremities in middle-aged women between fourth to sixth decade of life [1] It can arise from the tunica media of a blood vessel in any part of the body and is found in the dermis, subcutaneous fat or deep fascia [1]. The most frequent localization is in the extremities, especially the lower leg (50–70%) [2]. The majority of these lesions appear as solitary, small (< 20 mm), freely moving, subcutaneous, slow-growing nodules, with painful tenderness in approximately 60% of the patients [2, 3]. They occur extremely rarely in bones, where they incite painful swelling [4]. The reported cases of bone localization include the gnathic region, especially the mandible in middle-aged patients [5]. The rarity of intraosseous angioleiomyomas, especially in the pediatric population, renders them very hard to diagnose, occasionally even by histopathological examination.

In our paediatric patient case, primary intraosseus angioleiomyoma was localized in a rib and to our knowledge, this is the first reported case thus far with rib localization and the second case of a primary leiomyoma in the rib. We describe the differential diagnosis of angioleiomyoma at this atypical localization considering the common costal tumour pathologies in children, such

---

* Correspondence: gorandjuricic@gmail.com
[1]Department of Radiology, University Children's Hospital, Belgrade, School of Medicine, University of Belgrade, Tiršova 10, 11000 Belgrade, Republic of Serbia
Full list of author information is available at the end of the article

as cartilaginous tumours, Ewing sarcoma, fibrous dysplasia, Langerhans cell histiocytosis, intraosseous haemangioma and metastatic tumours.

Case presentation

A 10-year-old girl was admitted to the orthopaedic surgery department for further assessment of a pain localized in the posterior part of the right hemithorax. According to the physical examination, there was no evidence of a palpable chest wall mass, but the patient reported worsening of symptoms during palpation. Skin and subcutaneous tissue showed no swelling or discoloration. Laboratory values, including serum levels of tumour markers, were all within the normal reference ranges. The initial chest X-ray performed in another institution has been lost. We opted for MRI instead of the CT as the next diagnostic procedure in order to avoid additional exposure of the young patient to ionizing radiation.

Magnetic resonance imaging (MRI) of the thorax revealed a spherical, lobulated tumour, located in the posterior arch of the right fourth rib and the adjacent chest wall, 10 mm from its costovertebral junction. The lesion measured $30 \times 50 \times 20$ mm in all three diameters and showed heterogeneous signal intensity. It was mostly hyperintense relative to the muscle on non-contrast T1-weighted (T1W) fast spin echo (FSE) images (Fig. 1a), with prominent postcontrast enhancement on T1-weighted (T1W) fast spin echo (FSE) images (Fig. 1b) and hyperintense on T2W-weighted fat-suppressed (T2W FS) images (Fig. 1c, d). Compression of the adjacent lung parenchyma and thickening of the adjacent pleura was observed as the tumour showed endogenous growth but without signs of lung parenchyma invasion. Vascularization was observed as two vessel branches, 2.5 mm in diameter, arising from the intercostal blood vessels, while the clarity of another feeding branch from the thoracic aorta was limited and only suspected (Fig. 1d). In Fig. 1 (a - d), branching feeding vessels are noted in the center of the lesion. This observation was suggestive of an apparently vascular tumour mass with three feeding arteries but can also be interpreted as distended vascular structure. Those structures are optimally presented in contrast-enhanced T1W in the coronal plane, however, contrast-enhanced T1W was in this case performed only in the axial plane.

The patient underwent a surgical biopsy. After an opening of the cortical layer, abnormal bleeding from the rib was seen. Macroscopically, the tumour lesion corresponded to an aneurysmal bone cyst. A specimen was collected, and the material sent for histopathological analysis (Fig. 2). Pathohistological analysis of the tumuor has revealed its numerous blood vessels with a thick wall of smooth muscle layers and partially irregular lumina.

Atypical or mitotic smooth muscle cells were not detected. Foci of adipose metaplasia were present in between the blood vessels. The smooth muscle antigen (SMA) immunoreactivity was observed for proliferating perivascular smooth muscle cells and the muscular wall of thick blood vessels, whereas endothelial cells were CD34 positive. These observations were sufficient to establish the diagnosis of intraosseous angioleiomyoma – venous type.

Following the histopathologic diagnosis, selective arteriography was performed in order to plan adequate surgical treatment. The right femoral artery was the route and contrast agent was injected into three catheter tip positions: the ascending aorta, brachiocephalic trunk and descending aorta, in order to visualize all the potential feeding vessels. Non-homogeneous tumour enhancement was obtained only after contrast agent application in the ascending aorta. The three feeding arteries were also visualized – two of them were proximal and very thin, less than 1 mm in diameter, while the distal artery was 2.2 mm in diameter (Fig. 1e). Embolization and surgery were finalized through resection and confirmation on histopathology.

Discussion and conclusions

This case highlights the extremely unusual angioleiomyoma rib localization and patient age group, with pain without swelling [6]. The absence of a visible or palpable chest mass was yet another unusual trait, possibly due to the endothoracic propagation of the tumour lesion. Intraosseous angioleiomyomas usually arise in the jaw, maxillary tooth socket and the temporal bone [5]. The appendicular skeleton including angioleiomyomas of the tibia, ulna and femoral neck is rarely implicated [7–9]. Therefore, the observed rib localization was striking. Leiomyoma with costal localization was the only reported case of a histologically similar tumour [6].

Chest computed tomography (CT) and MRI are the diagnostic modalities of choice. Whereas CT provides high diagnostic sensitivity for bone and lung parenchyma, MRI is more optimal for assessment of soft tissue propagation. Because of its non-invasiveness, chest MRI has lately become the first step in the diagnostics sequencing of the chest wall tumour assessment for pediatric population. Angioleiomyoma MRI presents as a well-demarcated and strongly enhancing mass with an isointense to slightly hyperintense signal compared to muscle on T1W images and hyperintense signals on T2W images [10]. MRI features of the angioleiomyoma localized in soft tissues of the extremities were described in a series of 8 cases by *Yoo* et al. [11]. According to this study, all the masses were isointense or slightly hyperintense on T1W, whereas they showed slightly higher signal intensity on T2WI relative to

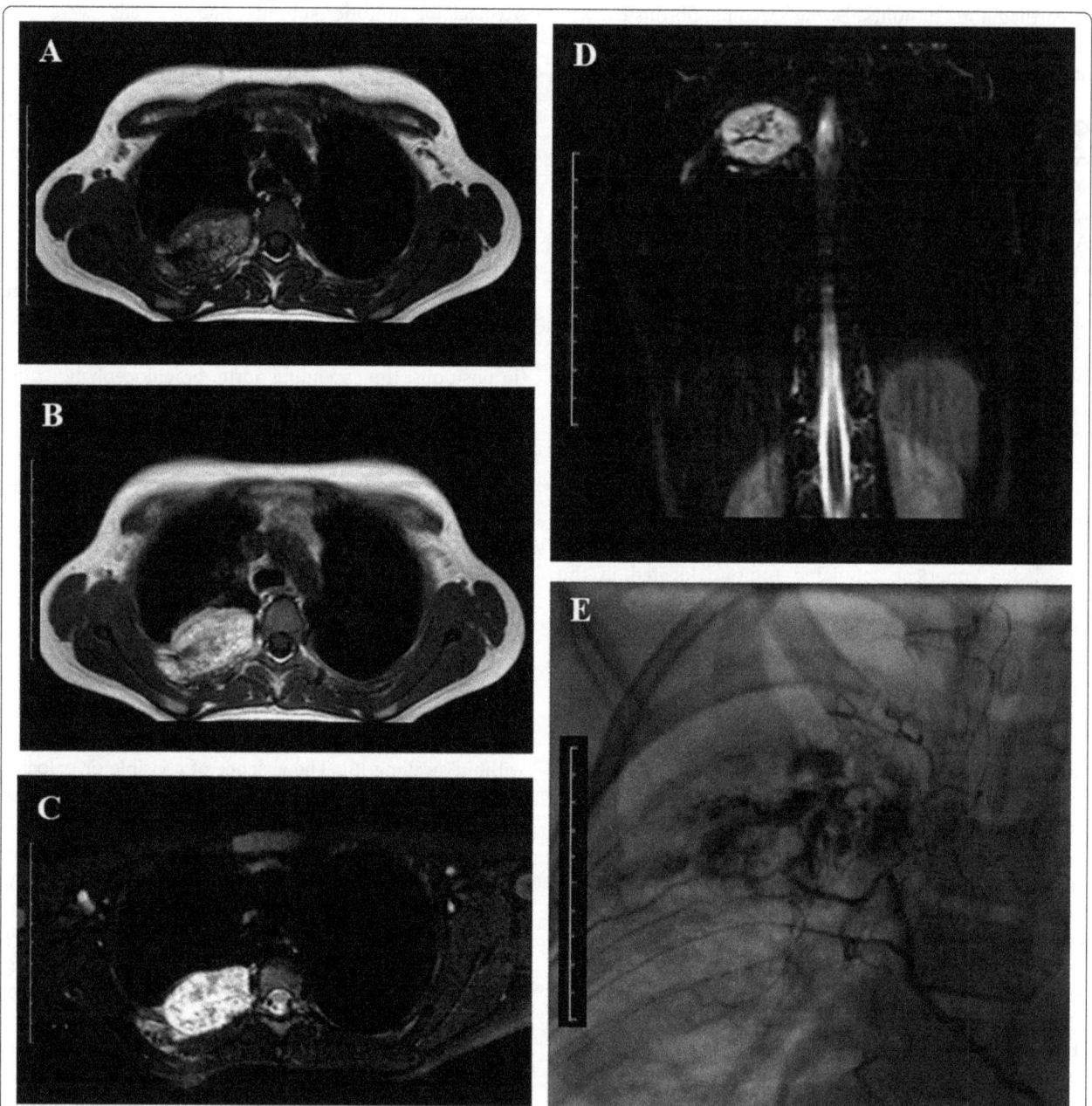

Fig. 1 MRI of the thorax reveals a spherical tumour lesion. Rib tumour lesion is presented with lobulated contours, measuring $30 \times 50 \times 20$ mm, located at the medial sector of the posterior arch of the fourth right rib and the adjacent chest wall, at the level of the costovertebral junction. A loss of normal bone structure is notable in the described sector. **a**, Heterogeneous lesion is slightly hyperintense, dominantly isointense to muscle on FSE T1W images; **b**, Intravenous administration of paramagnetic contrast agent resulted in tumour enhancement on T1W images; **c**, On fat-suppressed T2W image a heterogeneous hyperintensity to muscle is obvious; **d**, On fat-suppressed T2W image, two tubular structures, 2.5 mm in size, were seen arising from intercostal blood vessels adjacent to the tumour mass; **e**, Selective angiography revealed a non-homogeneous vascular tumour mass supplied by the three feeding arteries, two of which were proximal and very thin, less than 1 mm in diameter. The diameter of the largest, distal artery was 2.2 mm. *Scale bar*: 10 cm

skeletal muscle. Moreover, almost all lesions showed homogeneous and good enhancement on postcontrast T1W. Tubular structures adjacent to the masses were found in almost all patients, suggestive of vascular structures, similarly to the case described in the current study [11]. Taken together, all MRI characteristics of the masses were identical to a case described in the current report.

The only case of leiomyoma in the rib was published by *Ganyusufoglu* et al. [6]. They showed MRI characteristics of the mass detected in the 7th left rib with low signal intensity similar to muscle on T1W, whereas the

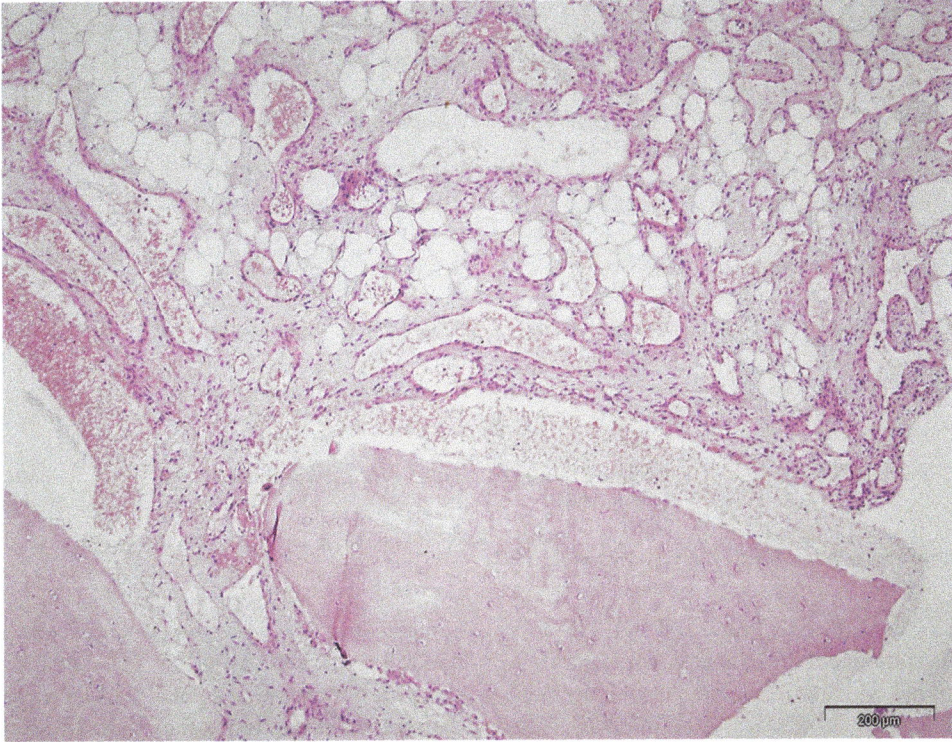

Fig. 2 Histological appearance of intraosseous angioleiomyoma, with numerous blood vessels, thick smooth muscle layer and partially irregular lumina. Smooth muscle cells showed no cellular atypia or mitoses. Foci of adipose metaplasia are visible between the blood vessels. *Scale bar:* 200 μm

lesion in the current case report showed mostly high signal intensity. In both cases, signal intensity on T2W was prominently high compared to adjacent muscle. Also, both lesions showed homogenous contrast enhancement. However, tubular formations highly suspected of vascular structures were seen only in our case.

Atypical costal localization of angioleiomyoma created a diagnostic challenge, considering that the rib is the common site of several tumours in children, such as cartilaginous tumour, Ewing sarcoma, fibrous dysplasia, Langerhans cell histiocytosis, intraosseous haemangioma and metastatic tumours [12].

Table 1 presents the radiological properties of the described case in comparison to the six plausible diagnoses. Fibrous dysplasia (FD) has been taken into diagnostic consideration as the most frequent benign tumour of the ribs, representing 30% of all benign tumours of the thoracic wall. Up to 20% of the monostotic FD affects ribs, whereby it most frequently affects 2nd rib [13]. That was not the case with our patient whose 4th rib was affected. Good demarcation, heterogeneity and high MRI signal intensity on T2W of the tumour in our patient counted in favor of FD. However, considering that the other typical FD characteristics such as hypo- to isointense lesion on T1W and a sclerotic rim as a hypointense area that surrounds the lesion could not be

observed in our patient, FD was excluded as a differential diagnosis [13, 14].

Enchondroma was also taken into consideration as a differential diagnosis, having in mind that it is the second most frequent tumour of the ribs [13] and that its MRI characteristics for the most part match the MRI characteristics of the lesion in our patient. Enchondroma is a lesion that consists of a hyaline cartilage lobulus with calcifications within it. It is seen on MRI as a well-defined expansive mass with lobulated contours that is T1W-hypointense and T2W-hyperintense with possible hypointense foci that match calcifications. Due to peripherally localized fibrovascular tissue and presence of avascular hyaline lobes in enchondroma, tumour appearance is contrast-enhanced in a typical "ring and arc" pattern. Since this characteristic of enchondroma was in opposition to a pronounced contrast-enhanced MRI signal intensity of the lesion in our patient, enchondroma was also excluded from differential diagnosis considerations [15–17].

In addition to the most frequent benign rib tumours in children, the most frequent malignant tumours with the same localization in children were also taken into consideration – Ewing sarcoma and metastatic tumours. Ewing sarcoma is the second most frequent malignant bone tumour in children, with a peak incidence in the

Table 1 Radiological properties of the presented case compared to five considered differential diagnoses[a]

	Demarcation	Sclerotic rim	T1W	T2W	T2WFS	Calcification	Postcontrast
Our patient case	Well defined	No	Isointense to slightly hyperintense signal	Hyperintense	Hyperintense	No	Homogenous; Prominently enhanced
Fibrous dysplasia	**Well demarcated**	Yes	Hypointense to isointense	**Hyperintense**	intermediate to high	Yes	Variable contrast enhancement (from mild to marked in degree)
Enchondroma	**Well defined**	**No**	Hypointense	**Hyperintense**	Predominantly high signal	Yes	"Rim and arc" pattern
Ewing sarcoma	Poorly defined	**No**	Hypointense to isointense	Variable signal intensities	Variable signal intensities	**No**	Heterogeneous; Prominently enhanced
Langerhans cell histiocytosis	**Well defined**	**No**	Hypointense to isointense	**Hyperintense**	**Hyperintense**	**No**	Diffusely enhanced
Intraosseous hemangioma	**Well defined**	**No**	Low to intermediate signal intensity (with regions of high signal)	**Hyperintense**	**Hyperintense (with regions of low signal)**	**No**	Heterogeneous Increased enhanced
Angioleiomyoma	Well defined	No	**Isointense to slightly hyperintense signal**	Hyperintense	Hyperintense	No	**Homogenous; Prominently enhanced**

[a]Radiological properties matching the presented patient case are marked in bold

second decade of life [18, 19]. In general, the extraosseous soft tissue component of Ewing sarcoma tends to be larger compared with its intramedullary component, especially when the flat bones are involved [20]. Heterogenous appearance and hypo- to isointensity on T1W are typical characteristics of Ewing sarcoma that partially matched our case with mostly high signal intensity on T1W. However, unclear demarcation of Ewing sarcoma, "hair on end" appearance of periosteal or reactive bone formation and elevated levels of tumour markers were characteristics that did not match our case. Heterogeneity of a tumour in all sequences could be the result of haemorrhage and tissue necrosis. On fluid sensitive sequences Ewing sarcoma typically shows variable signal intensity, with possible hypointense appearance related to muscles as a consequence of high tumour cellularity, with pronounced contrast-enhanced MRI signal intensity. In our case we observed a notable contrast-enhancement, but with a dominant homogenous contrast-enhanced appearance of the tumour lesion [21, 22].

Langerhans cell histiocytosis matched our case by several MRI characteristics: a demarcated lesion with hyperintense appearance on fluid-sensitive sequences and diffuse contrast enhancement. However, the predominantly hyperintense lesion on T1W in our patient diverged from the typical hypo- to isointense Langerhans cell histiocytosis appearance on T1W [23].

Because of the highly suspected vascular tumour, intraosseous hemangioma was also included in the differential diagnosis. Hemangiomas with bone localization are rare and include less than 1% of all bone tumours [24]. Our case shares similar MRI characteristics with the case published by *Tew* et al. [25]. They reported the case of expansile mass in the right 5th rib proved to be a

hemangioma. The lesion was well-defined with a heterogeneous intermediate signal on T1W, a heterogeneous high signal on fat-suppressed T2W and increased contrast enhancement. In contrast to our case, within the lesion there were small areas with signal characteristics of fat [25].

Diagnosis of intraosseous leiomyoma is difficult not only due to the extreme rarity of a tumour but also the absence of pathognomonic radiological signs. The exact diagnosis is thus only achieved by histopathological examination and immunostaining [26]. Differential histopathological diagnosis of angioleiomyoma and other vascular lesions is based on its very consistent case-to-case appearance. Angioleiomyomas are classified into three histological categories: solid (the most common type in soft tissues), venous and cavernous. All three patterns are often observed within the same tumour. These tumours typically exhibit well-defined smooth muscle tissue nodules interspersed with thick-walled blood vessels. The walls of these vessels are composed of the inner and outer layers, while their lumens are partially open. Usually, the smooth muscles of the vessel inner layers are organized in the circumferential pattern. However, the outer layers of the smooth muscles are swirled away from the vessel and integrated with muscle cells at the periphery. It is difficult to determine blood vessels as veins or arteries in these tumours. Although intraosseous localisation is very rare, angioleiomyoma of the bone exhibits similar typical histological features as soft-tissue angioleiomyomas. The use of immunohistochemical staining was helpful for differential diagnosis because the tumour cells were strongly positive for muscle markers, SMA and desmin, thus confirming this tumour's smooth muscle origin. CD34 was positive in endothelial cells, but negative in the tumour neoplastic cells.

In conclusion, this case emphasizes that atypical intraosseous angioleiomyoma, especially in the ribs of paediatric patients, could mislead the referring physician to more common pathologies in this region. Besides its extreme rarity, diagnosis of intraosseous angioleiomyoma is further complicated by the absence of any pathognomonic radiological signs. Its diagnosis is thus reliably achieved by histopathological examination combined with immunostaining. We expect that the detailed description of this unusual presentation of angioleiomyoma would provide a valuable resource to facilitate diagnosis of such untypical presentations in the future.

Abbreviations
CE: Contrast enhanced; CT: Computerized tomography; FD: Fibrous dysplasia; FSE: Fast spin echo; LCH: Langerhans cell histiocytosis; MRI: Magnetic resonance imaging; SMA: Smooth muscle antigen; T1W: T1 weighted; T2W: T2 weighted

Acknowledgements
The authors would like to thank colleagues from the Department of Paediatric Orthopaedic Surgery of the University Children's Hospital in Belgrade for their support and collaboration.

Funding
This work was supported by the Ministry of Education, Science and Technological Development of the Republic of Serbia, grant ON175068. This funding source had no role in in the design of the study, collection, analysis and interpretation of data, or in writing the manuscript.

Authors' contributions
All authors significantly contributed to the conception and design of the study. GD, NM, JS and TR were in charge of data acquisition, analysis and interpretation. PD was responsible for manuscript drafting. ZM and JS made a major contribution to study conception and design. MR provided a substantial critical revision of intellectual content. All authors contributed to the manuscript preparation, read and approved the final text and agree to be accountable for all aspects of work ensuring integrity and accuracy.

Consent for publication
Publication consent has been obtained from the parents of the patient in a written form.

Competing interests
The authors declare that they have no competing interests.

Author details
[1]Department of Radiology, University Children's Hospital, Belgrade, School of Medicine, University of Belgrade, Tiršova 10, 11000 Belgrade, Republic of Serbia. [2]Institute of Oncology and Radiology of Serbia, School of Medicine, University of Belgrade, Pasterova 14, 11000 Belgrade, Republic of Serbia. [3]Institute of Pathology, School of Medicine, University of Belgrade, Dr Subotica 1, 11000 Belgrade, Republic of Serbia.

References
1. Woo KS, Kim SH, Kim HS, Cho PD. Clinical experience with treatment of angioleiomyoma. Arch Plast Surg. 2014;41(4):374–8 Epub 2014/07/31.
2. Cigna E, Maruccia M, Malzone G, Malpassini F, Soda G, Drudi FM. A large vascular leiomyoma of the leg. J Ultrasound. 2012;15(2):121–3 Epub 2013/02/12.
3. Calle S, Louis D, Westmark R, Westmark K. Angioleiomyoma of the falx. J Radiol Case Rep. 2016;10(4):8–15 Epub 2016/05/21.
4. Salunke AA, Vala PC, Singh H, Parwani R, Gandhi S, Shah D. Intraosseous leiomyoma of the calcaneum: an unusual bone tumor of foot and review of literature. J Clin Orthop Trauma. 2016;7(Suppl 1):61–4 Epub 2016/12/27.
5. Loyola AM, Araujo NS, Zanetta-Barbosa D, Mendes VC, Jordao-Silva C, Bittar TO. Intraosseous leiomyoma of the mandible. Oral Surg Oral Med Oral Pathol Oral Radiol Endod. 1999;87(1):78–82 Epub 1999/02/02.
6. Ganyusufoglu AK, Ayalp K, Ozturk C, Sakallioglu U, Ozer O. Intraosseous leiomyoma in a rib. A case report. Acta Orthop Belg. 2009;75(4):561–5 Epub 2009/09/25.
7. Aisner SC, Blacksin M, Patterson F, Hameed MR. A painful tibial mass in a 37-year-old man. Clin Orthop Relat Res. 2008;466(3):756–9 Epub 2008/01/19.
8. Tomoda K, Iyama K. A case of intraosseous angioleiomyoma. Acta Orthop Scand. 1992;63(5):568–70 Epub 1992/10/01.
9. Lau SK. Intraosseous angioleiomyoma the tibia: a case report. Pathol Res Pract. 2014;210(5):321–4 Epub 2014/03/19.
10. Jeung MY, Gangi A, Gasser B, Vasilescu C, Massard G, Wihlm JM, et al. Imaging of chest wall disorders. Radiographics. 1999;19(3):617–37 Epub 1999/05/21.
11. Yoo HJ, Choi JA, Chung JH, Oh JH, Lee GK, Choi JY, et al. Angioleiomyoma in soft tissue of extremities: MRI findings. AJR Am J Roentgenol. 2009;192(6):W291–4 Epub 2009/05/22.
12. Marden FA, Calilao GC, Guzman G, Roy SS. Glossal angiomyoma: imaging findings and endovascular treatment. Head Neck. 2004;26(12):1084–8 Epub 2004/11/06.
13. Walsh M, Jacobson JA, Kim SM, Lucas DR, Morag Y, Fessell DP. Sonography of fat necrosis involving the extremity and torso with magnetic resonance imaging and histologic correlation. J Ultrasound Med. 2008;27(12):1751–7 Epub 2008/11/22.
14. Berquist TH, Ehman RL, King BF, Hodgman CG, Ilstrup DM. Value of MR imaging in differentiating benign from malignant soft-tissue masses: study of 95 lesions. AJR Am J Roentgenol. 1990;155(6):1251–5 Epub 1990/12/01.
15. Heiken JP, Lee JK, Smathers RL, Totty WG, Murphy WA. CT of benign soft-tissue masses of the extremities. AJR Am J Roentgenol. 1984;142(3):575–80 Epub 1984/03/01.
16. White RI Jr, Pollak J, Persing J, Henderson KJ, Thomson JG, Burdge CM. Long-term outcome of embolotherapy and surgery for high-flow extremity arteriovenous malformations. J Vasc Interv Radiol. 2000;11(10):1285–95 Epub 2000/12/01.
17. van Rijswijk CS, Geirnaerdt MJ, Hogendoorn PC, Taminiau AH, van Coevorden F, Zwinderman AH, et al. Soft-tissue tumors: value of static and dynamic gadopentetate dimeglumine-enhanced MR imaging in prediction of malignancy. Radiology. 2004;233(2):493–502 Epub 2004/10/02.
18. Alaggio R, Coffin CM, Vargas SO. Soft tissue tumors of uncertain origin. Pediatr Dev Pathol. 2012;15(1 Suppl):267–305 Epub 2012/05/11.
19. Fogli KD, Quiogue T, Moser RP Jr. Ewing's sarcoma. Radiol Clin N Am. 1993;31(2):325–37 Epub 1993/03/01.
20. Kransdorf MJ, Smith SE. Lesions of unknown histogenesis: Langerhans cell histiocytosis and Ewing sarcoma. Semin Musculoskelet Radiol. 2000;4(1):113–25 Epub 2000/11/04.
21. Brisse H, Ollivier L, Edeline V, Pacquement H, Michon J, Glorion C, et al. Imaging of malignant tumours of the long bones in children: monitoring response to neoadjuvant chemotherapy and preoperative assessment. Pediatr Radiol. 2004;34(8):595–605 Epub 2004/04/23.
22. George JC, Buckwalter KA, Cohen MD, Edwards MK, Smith RR. Langerhans cell histiocytosis of bone: MR imaging. Pediatr Radiol. 1994;24(1):29–32 Epub 1994/01/01.
23. Abdelaal AH, Yamamoto N, Hayashi K, Takeuchii A, Tsuchiyai H. Intraosseous leiomyoma of the tibia. A case report. J Orthop Case Rep. 2016;6(2):81–5 Epub 2016/10/06.
24. Clements RH, Turnage RB, Tyndal EC. Hemangioma of the rib: a rare diagnosis. Am Surg. 1998;64(11):1027–9 Epub 1998/11/03.
25. Tew K, Constantine S, Lew WY. Intraosseous hemangioma of the rib mimicking an aggressive chest wall tumor. Diagn Interv Radiol. 2011;17(2):118–21 Epub 2010/08/03.

21

Adding attenuation corrected images in myocardial perfusion imaging reduces the need for a rest study

Elin Trägårdh[*], Sven Valind and Lars Edenbrandt

Abstract

Background: The American Society of Nuclear Cardiology and the Society of Nuclear Medicine conclude that incorporation of attenuation corrected (AC) images in myocardial perfusion scintigraphy (MPS) will improve diagnostic accuracy. The aim was to investigate the value of adding AC stress-only images for the decision whether a rest study is necessary or not.

Methods: 1,261 patients admitted to ^{99m}Tc MPS were studied. The stress studies were interpreted by two physicians who judged each study as "no rest study necessary" or "rest study necessary", by evaluating NC stress-only and NC + AC stress-only images. When there was disagreement between the two physicians, a third physician evaluated the studies. Thus, agreement between 2 out of 3 physicians was evaluated.

Results: The physicians assessed 214 more NC + AC images than NC images as "no rest study necessary" (17% of the study population). The number of no-rest-study-required was significantly higher for NC + AC studies compared to NC studies (859 vs 645 cases (p < 0.0001). In the final report according to clinical routine, ischemia or infarction was reported in 23 patients, assessed as "no rest study necessary" (22 NC + AC cases; 8 NC cases), (no statistically significant difference). In 11 of these, the final report stated "suspected/possible ischemia or infarction in a small area".

Conclusions: Adding AC stress-only images to NC stress-only images reduce the number of unnecessary rest studies substantially.

Keywords: Tc99m MPS, Ischemic cardiac disease, Attenuation correction, Stress-only studies

Background

Stress myocardial perfusion scintigraphy (MPS) is widely regarded as a clinically useful non-invasive imaging modality for diagnosing patients with suspected coronary artery disease. The diagnostic accuracy is high, and risk stratification has been well validated [1-3]. However, Compton scatter and depth-dependent reduction of spatial resolution degrade MPS image quality and decrease test accuracy. In addition, localized soft-tissue attenuation by the breasts, lateral chest wall, and abdomen may create artefacts that mimic true perfusion abnormalities and decrease test specificity [4,5].

Several studies have reported an increase in the diagnostic accuracy (through higher specificity) for the detection of coronary artery disease when MPS is attenuation corrected (AC) [6-12]. The American Society of Nuclear Cardiology and the Society of Nuclear Medicine conclude in their joint position statement from 2004 [6] that incorporation of AC in addition to ECG gating with MPS images will improve image quality, interpretive certainty, and diagnostic accuracy. These combined results are anticipated to have a substantial impact on improving the effectiveness of care and lowering health care costs.

One of the problems with attenuation is that it reduces laboratory efficiency by requiring comparison of stress and rest image sets to distinguish perfusion abnormalities from attenuation artefacts. If a stress study is considered completely normal, there is no need for a rest study, thus increasing laboratory efficiency and reducing the radiation dose to the patient. Heller et al. [13] investigated the clinical value of attenuation correction in

* Correspondence: elin.tragardh@med.lu.se
Clinical Physiology and Nuclear Medicine Unit, Skåne University Hospital, Lund University, Entrance 44, 205 05 Malmö, Sweden

stress-only MPS and found that attenuation corrected images significantly increased the ability to interpret studies as definitely normal or abnormal and reduced the need for rest imaging.

The aim of the present study was to investigate the value of adding AC stress-only images for the decision whether a rest study is necessary or not.

Methods

Study population

All patients admitted to Tc-99m MPS at the Department of Clinical Physiology and Nuclear Medicine, Skåne University Hospital, Malmö, Sweden in 2007 were included. In total, 1283 patients were considered. Of these, 22 patients were excluded due to missing MPS data files. The study complies with the Declaration of Helsinki and was approved by the local research ethics committee at Lund University.

Stress-only assessment (Evaluations between NC only and NC + AC)

All stress studies were interpreted by two experienced physicians who judged each study as "no rest study necessary" or "rest study necessary". When there was disagreement between the physicians, a third physician evaluated the studies. Thus, agreement between 2 out of 3 physicians was evaluated. The physicians evaluated two sets of images for each patient: NC images only, and both NC and AC images. The studies were blinded so that the evaluation for NC images only was not known when evaluating both NC and AC images. Stress and gated images were available for this interpretation, but not clinical information or electrocardiogram findings. The EXINI heart™ software package (EXINI Diagnostics AB, Lund, Sweden) was used to aid the interpretation.

Clinical final report

The final reports according to clinical routine were compared to the results from the stress-only assessment described above. All cases with infarction or ischemia present or probably present were categorized as requiring a rest study, whereas all other cases were categorized not requiring a rest study. Rest (NC and AC), stress (NC and AC), gated images, clinical information, and electrocardiogram findings were available for this interpretation, which was performed according to clinical routine by the physician in charge of the study, not knowing that the patient was included in a study. In clinical routine in our department, the physician in charge evaluates the stress images, and decides whether a rest study is necessary or not. In the study population used in this study, 44% of the studies were stress-only studies. The EXINI heart™ software package was used for the visual interpretation.

Radionuclide imaging

The MPS studies were performed using a 2-day gated stress/non-gated rest Tc-99m-tetrofosmin protocol, starting with injection of 600 MBq Tc-99m-tetrofosmin at stress. Patients were stressed using either maximal exercise on an ergometer or pharmacological test with adenosine. The exercise was continued for at least 1 min after the injection of the tracer and the adenosine infusion at least 2 min after the injection of the tracer. Normal findings at stress were not followed by a rest study. Not definitely normal stress studies were followed by a rest study with injection of 600 MBq Tc-99m-tetrofosmin. The need for a rest study was determined by the physician in charge of the study according to clinical routine.

Stress and rest acquisition began about 60 min after the end of the injection of Tc-99m-tetrofosmin. Images were obtained according to established clinical protocols, using SPECT over 180° elliptical, autocontour rotations from the 45° right anterior oblique position, with a dual-head gamma camera, e.cam (Siemens AG Medical Solutions, Erlangen, Germany). Patients were imaged in the supine position. Low energy high-resolution collimator and a zoom factor of 1.0 were used. We obtained 64 (32 views per camera) projections in a 128×128 matrix, with an acquisition time of 25 s per projection. Stress images were gated to the electrocardiogram using 8 frames per cardiac cycle. No automatic motion-correction program was applied; instead the acquisition was repeated if motion was detected. If motion was apparent on the repeated examination as well, a motion-correction program was used. Tomographic reconstruction and calculation of short and long axis slice images were performed using e.soft (Siemens AG Medical Solutions, Erlangen, Germany). NC images were reconstructed with filtered back-projection. A 2D Butterworth pre-reconstruction filter was used with critical frequency of 0.45, order 5. AC images were reconstructed with an iterative algorithm, 6 iterations [14] where a ramp filter was applied on the error projection prior to backprojection. A Butterworth filter with a cut-off frequency of 0.40, order 5, was applied for regularization. Attenuation maps were generated from simultaneous transmission measurement using a Gd-153 multiple-line source (Siemens AG Medical Solutions, Erlangen, Germany) [15].

Statistical analysis

The McNemar test was used to analyze the differences in classification of patients between the NC only group and the NC + AC images group. The level of statistical significance was set at 0.05. Analyses were carried out using Analyse-it® for Microsoft Excel (Analyse-it Software Ltd, Leeds, UK).

Results

The number of no-rest-study-required cases was significantly higher using the NC + AC studies compared to the NC studies (859 vs 645 cases (p < 0.0001). In 634 cases (50%) the evaluations for both NC and NC + AC stress images were no-rest-study-required and in 391 cases (31%) that a rest study was required. In 11 cases (1%), the physicians did not want a rest study when evaluating NC images, but wanted a rest study when evaluating NC + AC images. In 225 cases (18%), the physicians thought it was necessary to perform a rest study when evaluating NC images, but not when evaluating NC + AC images.

961 studies (76%) were considered normal (i.e. no ischemia or infarction present) based on the final report according to clinical routine. In 8 of the 645 (1.2%) NC stress images classified as no-rest-study-required, ischemia/infarction was present on the final report. The corresponding results for the NC + AC images were 22 of 859 (2.6%) and this difference was not statistically significant. Cases classified as rest-study-required were more often interpreted as ischemia/infarction in the final report for the NC + AC images (69%) than the NC images (47%) (p < 0.0001). The numbers are shown in Table 1A and B.

Patients with abnormal MPS (final report) that were missed on stress-only images

In total, 23 patients had ischemia and/or infarction on the final reports, but were regarded as "no-rest-study-required" on either NC or NC + AC stress image evaluation; thus would falsely have been sent home without a rest study. Of these, 1 patient was missed when evaluating NC images, 15 when evaluating NC + AC images and 7 patients were missed for both evaluations. In 11 of the 23 cases, the final report stated "suspected/possible ischemia or infarction in a small area of the left ventricle"; in 9 cases "ischemia or infarction in a small area of the left ventricle"; and in 3 cases "ischemia

Table 1 The distribution of the evaluations from NC images (A) and NC + AC images (B)

		Final report		
		Normal	Abnormal	
A				
NC only	No rest	637	8	**645**
	Rest	324	292	**616**
		961	**300**	**1261**
B				
AC + NC	No rest	837	22	**859**
	Rest	124	278	**402**
		961	**300**	**1261**

in a moderately large area of the left ventricle". Two of the patients with moderately large ischemia underwent coronary angiography within 6 months after the MPS, and both received percutaneous coronary intervention (PCI). The third patient underwent coronary angiography with PCI of the right coronary artery 4 years after the MPS. Three of the 9 patients with "ischemia/infarction in a small area" underwent coronary angiography; two without any need of PCI and one with PCI of the left ascending coronary artery and the left circumflex artery. Only 1 patient with "suspected ischemia" underwent coronary angiography, with subsequent PCI of a diagonal branch. This patient got a dissection in the left main coronary artery during the angiography.

Discussion

In the present study we investigated the accuracy for determining the need for a rest study when using NC images or NC + AC images. We found that adding AC images were superior to using only NC images. When using NC + AC compared to NC images, 214 more patients (17% of the study population) could avoid a rest study. The advantages of being able to reduce the number of rest studies are substantially reduced radiation exposure, lower costs by eliminating unnecessary imaging time and radiopharmaceutical doses, and improved laboratory efficiency by freeing up camera time to study additional patients.

In this material, when using NC images, 1.2% of the patients would have been sent home without a rest study, when a rest study was needed according to the final report. The number for AC images was 2.6% (no statistically significant difference). The reasons for this could be either that the final report was not always correct or that the physicians who evaluated the stress studies did not have access to the clinical information (as stated in the study limitations section) or that can be difficult to see small perfusion abnormalities on stress-only images in some cases. The number of missed certain ischemia/infarction due to a normal interpretation on stress-only images was very low in this study (less than 1%), but the goal is not to miss any patients with ischemia or infarction. In a study by Johansson et al. [16], trying to decide whether nuclear medicine technologists are able to determine the necessity for a rest study, 2.6% of the patients would have been sent home without a rest study, when a rest study was needed according to gold standard (ischemia or infarction on combined stress-rest interpretation). Thus, their results were similar to the ones found in the present study.

The stress-only approach has been investigated in several studies. Worsley et al. [17] demonstrated that rest images were not required if normal imaging findings had been obtained after exercise or pharmacologic stress. This was later confirmed by Schroeder-Tanka et al. [18] in a larger study. Heller et al. [13] found that AC applied to studies with stress-only ^{99m}Tc MPS significantly increased the ability to interpret studies as definitely normal or abnormal and reduced the need for rest imaging. In their study, ten experienced nuclear cardiologists independently interpreted 90 stress-only MPS in a sequential fashion: MPS alone, MPS plus ECG-gated data, and AC MPS with ECG-gated data. Images were interpreted for diagnostic certainty (normal, probably normal, equivocal, probably abnormal, abnormal, and perceived need for rest imaging). Adding AC data increased the number of studies characterized as definitely normal or abnormal to 84% (37% for MPS data alone) and reduced the perceived need for rest imaging from 77% for MPS data only to 43% for the addition of AC data. Heller et al., however, included far fewer patients than the present study, and only included patients with either known coronary artery disease or patients with a 5% or lower likelihood of coronary artery disease. The ten independent readers also interpreted the studies in a sequential manner. The fact that only patients with known coronary artery disease or patients with a very low likelihood of coronary artery disease in combination with the sequential interpretation could be the reason for the larger difference in the number of rest studies needed when adding AC images compared to NC images only found in their study compared to the present study.

Current guidelines also recommend the stress study to be performed first, since the rest study can be omitted if the stress study is interpreted as normal [19]. Thus a rest study should only be performed in patients with equivocal or clearly abnormal studies. Chang et al. [20] investigated whether a normal stress-only MPS confers the same prognosis as a normal MPS on the bases of evaluation of stress and rest images. They found that patients who had a normal MPS on the basis of stress imaging alone have a similar mortality rate as those who have a normal MPS on the basis of evaluation of both stress and rest images.

Study limitations

In the present study the final reports according to clinical routine was used to compare the results from the stress-only assessment by the three study physicians. This might not be the optimal since physicians with different levels of experience interpreted the studies, and because there is always inter-observer variability when interpreting studies.

The physicians who evaluated the NC and AC stress studies did not have any clinical information about the patients. It is possible that fewer patients would have been falsely regarded as "no-rest-study-required" if the

clinical information was available, as it is in the true clinical setting.

A third limitation is that in clinical routine at our department, physicians already evaluate the need for a rest study after the stress study (based on NC and AC stress images, gated images and clinical information). In 44% of the cases, no rest study is performed, and "no ischemia or infarction" is stated on the final report. If any mistakes were done in the clinical assessment, the final report used in the present study could be wrong.

Conclusion

Adding AC stress-only images to NC stress-only images reduce the number of unnecessary rest studies substantially. The risk that a patient sent home without a rest study would have been diagnosed with definite infarction or ischemia using the combined stress-rest interpretation was low. 214 more patients (17% of the study population) did not require a rest study when adding AC images. We conclude that adding AC images will improve laboratory efficiency.

Competing interests
LE is employed by and stockholder of EXINI Diagnostics.

Authors' contributions
ET participated in the design of the study, acquired and evaluated the data, performed the statistical analysis and drafted the manuscript. SV evaluated the data and helped to draft the manuscript. LE participated in the design of the study, evaluated the data and helped to draft the manuscript. All authors read and approved the final manuscript.

Acknowledgement
This study was supported by the Medical Faculty at Lund University.

References
1. Hachamovitch R, Berman DS, Kiat H, Cohen I, Cabico JA, Friedman J, Diamond GA: Exercise myocardial perfusion SPECT in patients without known coronary artery disease. *Circulation* 1996, 93:905–914.
2. Hachamovitch R, Berman DS, Shaw LJ, Kiat H, Cohen I, Cabico JA, Friedman J, Diamond GA: Incremental prognostic value of myocardial perfusion single photon emission computed tomography for the prediction of cardiac death. *Circulation* 1998, 97:535–543.
3. Iskander S, Iskandrian AE: Risk assessment using single photon emission computed tomography technetium-99 m-sestamibi imaging. *J Am Coll Cardiol* 1998, 32:57–62.
4. DePuey EG, Garcia EV: Optimal specificity of thallium-201 SPECT through recognition of imaging artefacts. *J Nucl Med* 1989, 30:441–449.
5. Corbett JR, Ficaro EP: Clinical review of attenuation-corrected cardiac SPECT. *J Nucl Cardiol* 1999, 6:54–68.
6. Heller GV, Links J, Bateman TM, Ziffer JA, Ficaro E, Cohen MC, Hendel RC: American Society of Nuclear Cardiology and Society of Nuclear Medicine joint position statement: attenuation correction of myocardial perfusion SPECT scintigraphy. *J Nucl Cardiol* 2004, 11:229–230.
7. Gallowitsch HJ, Sykora J, Mikosch P, Kresnik E, Unterweger O, Molnar M, Grimm G, Lind P: Attenuation-corrected thallium-201 single-photon emission tomography using a gadolinium-153 moving line source: clinical value and the impact of attenuation correction on the extent and severity of perfusion abnormalities. *Eur J Nucl Med* 1998, 25:220–228.
8. Hendel RC, Merman DS, Cullom SJ, Follansbee W, Heller GV, Kiat H, Groch MW, Mahmarian JJ: Multicenter clinical trial to evaluate the efficacy of correction

for photon attenuation and scatter in SPECT myocardial perfusion imaging. *Circulation* 1999, **99**:2742–2749.

9.   Links JM, Becker LC, Rigo P, Taillefer R, Hanelin L, Anstett F, Burckhardt D, Mixon L: **Combined corrections for attenuation, depth-dependent blur, and motion in cardiac SPECT: a multicenter trial.** *J Nucl Cardiol* 2000, **7**:414–425.

10. Links JM, DePueyo EG, Taillefer R, Becker LC: **Attenuation correction and gating synergistically improve the diagnostic accuracy of myocardial perfusion SPECT.** *J Nucl Cardiol* 2002, **9**:183–187.

11. Thompson RC, Heller GV, Johnson LL, Case JA, Cullom SJ, Garcia EV, Jones PG, Moutray KL, Bateman TM: **Value of attenuation correction on ECG-gated SPECT myocardial perfusion imaging related to body mass index.** *J Nucl Cardiol* 2005, **12**:195–202.

12. Masood Y, Liu YH, Depuey G, Taillefer R, Araujo LI, Allen S, Delbeke D, Anstett F, Peretz A, Zito MJ, Tsatkin V, Wackers FJ: **Clinical validation of SPECT attenuation correction using x-ray computed tomography-derived attenuation maps: multi-center clinical trial with angiographic correlation.** *J Nucl Cardiol* 2005, **12**:676–686.

13. Heller GV, Bateman TM, Johnson LL, Cullom SJ, Case JA, Galt JR, Garcia EV, Haddock K, Moutray KL, Poston C, Botvinick EH, Fish MB, Follansbee WP, Hayes S, Iskandrian AE, Mahmarian JJ, Vandecker W: **Clinical value of attenuation correction in stress-only Tc-99m sestamibi SPECT imaging.** *J Nucl Cardiol* 2004, **11**:273–281.

14. Wallis JW, Miller TR: **Rapidly converging iterative reconstruction algorithms in single-photon emission computed tomography.** *J Nucl Med* 1993, **34**:1793–1800.

15. Hawman EG, Ray M, Xu R, Vija AH: **An attenuation correction system for a dedicated small FOV, dual head, fixed-90° cardiac gamma camera using arrays of Gd-153 line sources.** *IEEE Nucl Science Symposium Conference Record* 2006, **3**:1806–1810.

16. Johansson L, Lomsky M, Gjertsson P, Sallerup-Reid M, Johansson J, Ahlin NG, Edenbrandt L: **Can nuclear medicine technologists assess whether a myocardial perfusion rest study is required?** *J Nucl Med Technol* 2008, **36**:181–185.

17. Worsley DF, Fung AY, Coupland DB, Rexworthy CG, Sexsmith GP, Lentle BC: **Comparison of stress-only vs. stress/rest with technetium-99 m methoxyisobutylisonitrile myocardial perfusion imaging.** *Eur J Nucl Med* 1992, **19**:441–444.

18. Schroeder-Tanka JM, Tiel-van Buul MM, van der Wall EE, Roolker W, Lie KI, van Royen EA: **Should imaging at stress always be followed by imaging at rest in Tc-99m MIBI SPECT? A proposal for a selective referral and imaging strategy.** *Int J Card Imaging* 1997, **13**:323–329.

19. Hesse B, Tägil K, Cuocolo A, Anagnostopoulos C, Bardies M, Bax J, Bengel F, Busemann Sokole E, Davies G, Dondi M, Edenbrandt L, Franken P, Kjaer A, Knuuti J, Lassmann M, Ljungberg M, Marcassa C, Marie PY, McKiddie F, O'Connor M, Prvulovich E, Underwwod R, van Eck-Smit B: **EANM/ESC procedural guidelines for myocardial perfusion imaging in nuclear cardiology.** *Eur J Nucl Med Mol Imaging* 2005, **32**:855–897.

20. Chang SM, Nabi F, Xu J, Raza U, Mahmarian JJ: **Normal stress-only versus standard stress/rest myocardial perfusion imaging: similar patient mortality with reduced radiation exposure.** *J Am Coll Cardiol* 2010, **55**:221–230.

22

An automated method for analysis of microcirculation videos for accurate assessment of tissue perfusion

Sumeyra U Demir[1], Roya Hakimzadeh[1], Rosalyn Hobson Hargraves[1,2,4], Kevin R Ward[1,4,5,6], Eric V Myer[1] and Kayvan Najarian[1,3,4,5*]

Abstract

Background: Imaging of the human microcirculation in real-time has the potential to detect injuries and illnesses that disturb the microcirculation at earlier stages and may improve the efficacy of resuscitation. Despite advanced imaging techniques to monitor the microcirculation, there are currently no tools for the near real-time analysis of the videos produced by these imaging systems. An automated system tool that can extract microvasculature information and monitor changes in tissue perfusion quantitatively might be invaluable as a diagnostic and therapeutic endpoint for resuscitation.

Methods: The experimental algorithm automatically extracts microvascular network and quantitatively measures changes in the microcirculation. There are two main parts in the algorithm: video processing and vessel segmentation. Microcirculatory videos are first stabilized in a video processing step to remove motion artifacts. In the vessel segmentation process, the microvascular network is extracted using multiple level thresholding and pixel verification techniques. Threshold levels are selected using histogram information of a set of training video recordings. Pixel-by-pixel differences are calculated throughout the frames to identify active blood vessels and capillaries with flow.

Results: Sublingual microcirculatory videos are recorded from anesthetized swine at baseline and during hemorrhage using a hand-held Side-stream Dark Field (SDF) imaging device to track changes in the microvasculature during hemorrhage. Automatically segmented vessels in the recordings are analyzed visually and the functional capillary density (FCD) values calculated by the algorithm are compared for both health baseline and hemorrhagic conditions. These results were compared to independently made FCD measurements using a well-known semi-automated method. Results of the fully automated algorithm demonstrated a significant decrease of FCD values. Similar, but more variable FCD values were calculated using a commercially available software program requiring manual editing.

Conclusions: An entirely automated system for analyzing microcirculation videos to reduce human interaction and computation time is developed. The algorithm successfully stabilizes video recordings, segments blood vessels, identifies vessels without flow and calculates FCD in a fully automated process. The automated process provides an equal or better separation between healthy and hemorrhagic FCD values compared to currently available semi-automatic techniques. The proposed method shows promise for the quantitative measurement of changes occurring in microcirculation during injury.

* Correspondence: knajarian@vcu.edu
[1]Signal Processing Technologies LLC, Richmond, VA, USA
[3]Department of Emergency Medicine, Virginia Commonwealth University, Richmond, VA, USA
Full list of author information is available at the end of the article

Background

Understanding the distribution and circulation of blood in capillaries has been considered a key aspect for assessment of tissue perfusion [1]. Visualization and quantification of changes in microcirculation has been proposed as a potential tool in diagnosis and treatment of illnesses and diseases such as sepsis [2], sickle cell disease [3,4], chronic ulcers, diabetes mellitus and hypertension [5,6]. In each of these diseases, several characteristics of the microcirculation such as the structure of capillaries and quality of blood flow in the capillaries change over time [7-11]. A recent study suggests there is value in monitoring the microcirculation for titrating vasodilators in perioperative use [12]. Monitoring microcirculation during resuscitation could also be envisioned as a tool to prevent over and under resuscitation of victims of hemorrhage and other critical illness and injuries such as sepsis. Therefore, quantitative and accurate analysis of the microcirculation is likely to be essential if microcirculatory imaging is to be adopted as useful tool in clinical monitoring [13].

Orthogonal polarization spectral (OPS) imaging [1,2,5] and side-stream dark field (SDF) imaging [13,14] have been extensively employed in the field of clinical microcirculatory research. OPS and SDF imaging are both non-invasive imaging modalities and have been used to track changes in the microcirculation on mucosal surfaces. Most studies have used the sublingual surfaces of the oral cavity. These imaging techniques use green polarized light with wavelength of 550 nm which is absorbed by hemoglobin and makes red blood cells visible [15,16].

To analyze microcirculatory images and videos, several software tools have been developed. However currently available software is unable to perform real or near real time analysis of the videos and require manual intervention to ensure accurate results. Researchers in the field have stated the need for improvements of current software to expedite clinical bedside use [17]. The computer-assisted image analysis system CapImage (Zeintl, Heidelberg, Germany) was originally developed for traditional intravital microscopy [18], but is capable of analysis of SDF and OPS images [19]. It uses a Line Shift Diagram Method for measurement of velocity and real-time movement correlation. This software tool is capable of measuring different properties of the microcirculation such as blood cell velocity and capillary density. However, it is only capable of detecting straight blood vessels which limits its efficacy since the microvascular geometry is complex. Expert users of CapImage claim that analysis of microcirculation with CapImage is time consuming and may only be performed off-line [20].

CapiScope, a system for the measurement of capillary morphology and capillary blood cell velocity, requires stable images, but lacks a stabilization function [21].

JavaCap and Capilap Toolbox are two other available software tools which use triangulation methods to calculate intercapillary distance [22,23].

Automated Vascular Analysis (AVA)—also known as MAS (Microvascular Analysis Software, Microvision Medical BV)—is the most current commercial software tool developed by Dobbe et al [24] for analysis of microcirculation videos. The method is the most accurate among the existing systems and performs a semi-automated process based on image stabilization, center-line detection and space time diagram. Despite all the capabilities provided by AVA, it does not provide full automation which leaves the burden of selecting the areas of interest, configuration, initialization, filtering of many false positives, dealing with many false negatives, and addressing of connectivity to the user. In addition, according to the developers of AVA, the software provides neither automatic vessel detection nor vessel diameter and blood flow calculation [24]. The system, while an improvement, requires manual editing which can take over 20 minutes for a typical video sequence.

The aim of this study is to automate the analysis of microcirculatory video recordings and the derivation of Functional Capillary Density (FCD). FCD is defined as the ratio of the area of functionally active capillaries to the entire area of the image. FCD has been considered an important measurement of the microcirculation to indicate the quality of tissue perfusion [25]. Image processing algorithms are designed for this study to automatically detect capillaries and small blood vessels in order to derive diagnostically useful information that may assist clinicians and medical researchers in the future.

Methods

The methodology behind the proposed algorithm to quantify the assessment of the microcirculation is summarized in Figure 1. The process—which is not shown in the schematic diagram—starts with the stabilization of the video frames. The weighted mean of consecutive frames from the stabilized video is calculated for each five-frame block. Pre-processing, multi-thresholding and vessel segmentation are the following steps and are highlighted in the diagram. A more detailed diagram is provided in Figure 2 to describe pre-processing, multi-thresholding and segmentation algorithm. After performing morphological operations such as filling and opening, the binary images resulting from segmentation are unioned together. If a pixel is segmented as vessel in more than one frame, it is assigned the label of "vessel". Post processing includes additional morphological operations (e.g., bridge, spur, fill) and region growing to eliminate any possible discontinuities. Vessels with blood flow—perfused vessels—are identified in the last step and FCD is calculated accordingly.

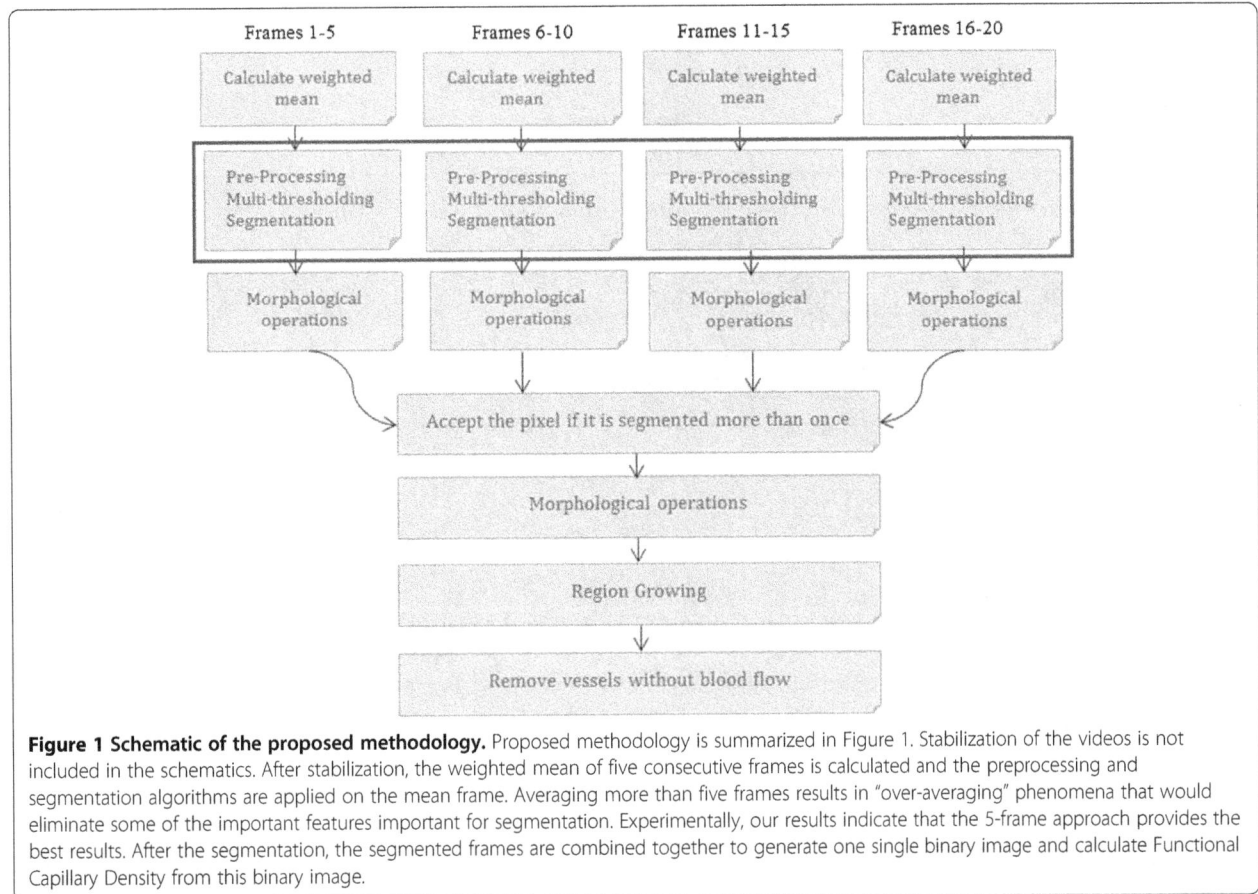

Figure 1 Schematic of the proposed methodology. Proposed methodology is summarized in Figure 1. Stabilization of the videos is not included in the schematics. After stabilization, the weighted mean of five consecutive frames is calculated and the preprocessing and segmentation algorithms are applied on the mean frame. Averaging more than five frames results in "over-averaging" phenomena that would eliminate some of the important features important for segmentation. Experimentally, our results indicate that the 5-frame approach provides the best results. After the segmentation, the segmented frames are combined together to generate one single binary image and calculate Functional Capillary Density from this binary image.

Stabilization

The microcirculatory videos are captured by a commercially available hand-held SDF device (Microscan, Microvision Medical, BV). Because it is hand-held and is highly susceptible to motion artifacts due to movement of subject and/or device, we developed a stabilization algorithm to eliminate these motion artifacts. A block matching algorithm is developed that calculates cross-correlation coefficients to measure the similarity of the blocks. Block matching algorithms use a predefined size of windows-blocks or even entire images to estimate motion vectors. One of the disadvantages of block matching methods is defined as 'remarkableness' of the window content [26]. If a window does not contain distinctive details, there is a high probability of mismatch. To avoid errors caused by 'remarkableness' issues, i.e. using points for matching that have no significant image-processing values (e.g. regular pixels inside the background) the processed blocks are checked to ensure they include blood vessels using Laplacian of Gaussian filtering. The stabilization process is described in detail in a previously published study [27]. Gradients of the frames are calculated using the first order derivative of the Gaussian function. Gradient of the Gaussian enhances images and improves visibility of blood vessels. Distinctive features of

the images, which are typically the branching points of blood vessels, are selected and assigned as control points to overcome remarkableness issues. Control points are selected which are known to belong to capillaries to calculate the transformation between two consecutive frames. For this purpose, a 3-by-3 Laplacian filter which calculates second order derivatives is applied to the output of the Gaussian Gradient.

The maximum values from seven areas of the frame are selected as control points. Then, around the control points, 25×25 pixel windows are selected as sub-regions. The cross-correlation is calculated between these sub-regions in the current frame and a 40×40 pixel window around these sub-regions in the following frame. The size of the windows discussed above was optimized based on a previous visual empirical assessment of the algorithm over a set of microcirculation videos. The frames are registered according to the results of correlation calculations. Since the control points are defined for the first frame and they are tracked through adjacent frames, Laplacian filtering is not repeated throughout the algorithm. If any of the defined control points leaves the current frame due to excessive motion, new control points are defined using the same method.

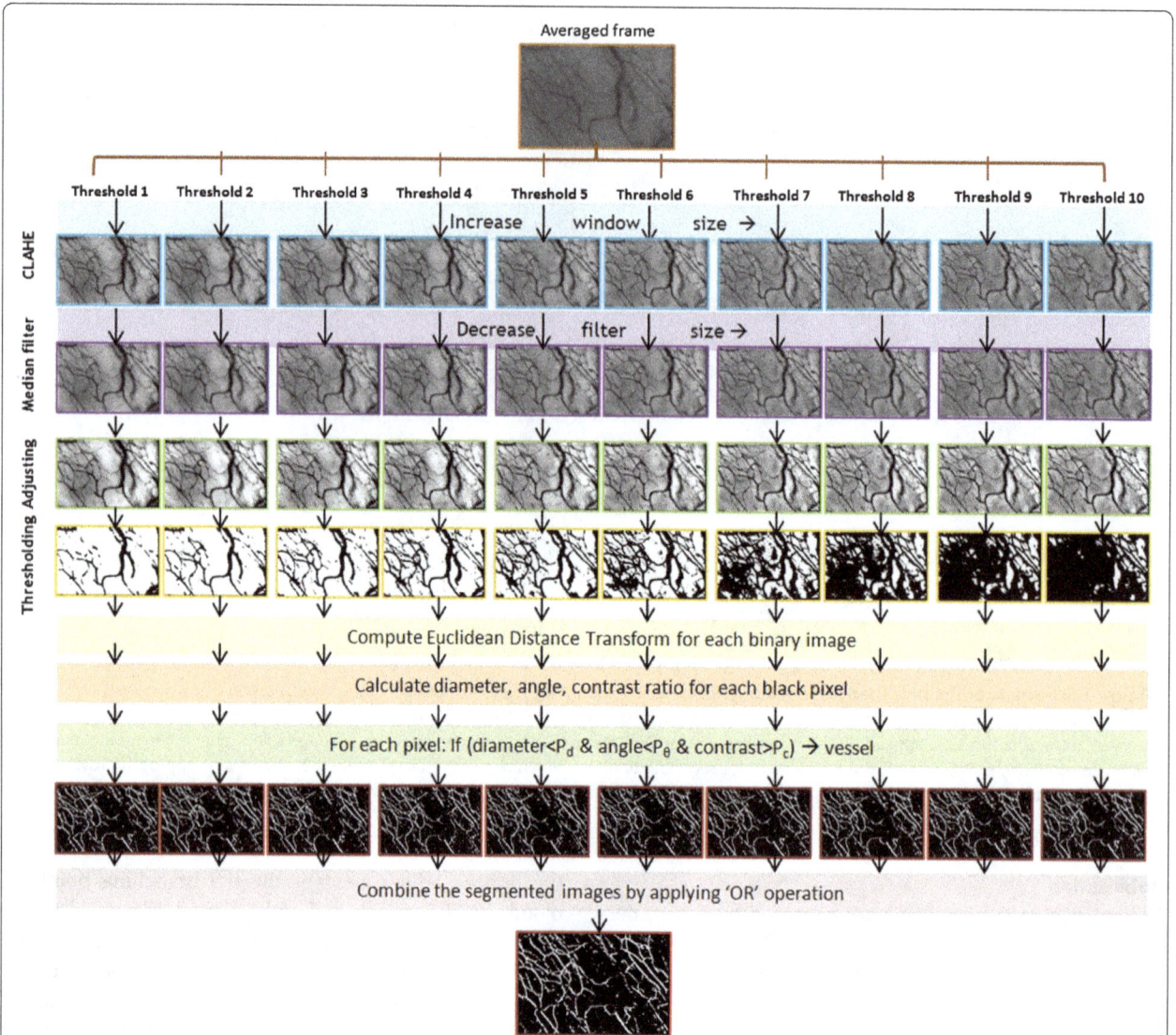

Figure 2 Detailed diagram of pre-processing and vessel segmentation. Figure 2 provides a detailed diagram of preprocessing and segmentation steps for different threshold levels. It starts with the averaged frame. For 10 different threshold levels, the parameters of CLAHE (Contrast Limited Adaptive Histogram Equalization) and median filter vary throughout the process. For the first threshold level, the window size of CLAHE is kept small. Median filter is applied right after histogram equalization with a small filter size such as 3 × 3. Median filtering is followed by image adjustment. The preprocessed image is converted to binary image using the first threshold level. Euclidean Distance Transform (EDT) is calculated for the binary image. Diameter and angle parameters are extracted from EDT and with the addition of contrast ratio; three parameters are used to determine if a pixel belongs to a vessel.

Preprocessing, multi-thresholding, and segmentation

After the stabilization of the video recordings, the weighted mean of five consecutive frames is calculated to improve connectivity of the blood vessels. The frame in the middle has the highest weight in this process. Averaging the frames is followed by preprocessing algorithms. The vessel extraction algorithm is based on multiple level thresholding. Preprocessing is repeated at each threshold with different parameters.

Video contrast and clarity vary widely from source to source and necessitate preprocessing in order to generate images that will yield accurate results. To enhance the local contrast, Contrast Limited Adaptive Histogram Equalization (CLAHE) is performed on microcirculation images. CLAHE partitions the image into small regions, called 'tiles', and applies histogram equalization to each tile in order to even out the overall gray level distribution of the image [28]. Histogram equalization is followed by median filtering. To remove noise, median filtering is a widely preferred method in the literature [29]. In this application, the purpose of applying median filtering is smoothing.

The window sizes of adaptive histogram equalization and median filtering are subject to change at each threshold level. At low threshold levels, in order to include only wide and clear vessels, histogram equalization is applied in smaller windows. The median filter size is kept large at these low threshold levels. As the threshold level increases, the result of the process is a darker binary image with almost all vessels and background included. Window size of adaptive histogram equalization is increased and median filter size is reduced to enhance the thinner vessels. Without these steps results will suffer as vessels may not be fully segmented and flow correctly detected. This preprocessing is followed by thresholding.

Vessel segmentation is based on verifying each pixel at multiple threshold levels as vessel. The method is modified from a pixel verification method proposed by Jiang et al. using retinal images [30]. The pre-processed images are converted to binary images using multiple threshold levels resulting in multiple binary images. Euclidean Distance Transform (EDT) is created for each binary image. EDT calculates the distance of nearest background pixel for each object pixel. The coordinates of the nearest background pixel is the second output of the transform. For each pixel of each binary image, three different features are calculated using the outputs of the EDT and the gray-level intensity values of the pixels. Two of these parameters are the diameter P_d and the angle P_θ of the vessel, which are considered as geometrical features. The gray level intensity values of pre-processed images are used to calculate the third feature, P_C, which is the contrast ratio identifying the ratio of intensity across background and blood vessel pixels. These three features serve to determine if a pixel in the image is indeed a vessel pixel. Pd limits the size of the vessel to ensure it is a capillary. P_θ ensures curvilinear structure to the pixel, and excludes any anomalous pixels because of physiological improbabilities. Pc, ensures contrast between background and vessel pixels.

Figure 3 provides a visual depiction of these parameters. 5*5 neighborhood of a candidate pixel is included in the calculations. The current pixel is referred to as 'p', which is a vessel candidate. Its 24 neighbors are defined as $N_1 - N_{24}$. The nearest background pixel to 'p' is 'b_p' and the nearest background pixels to each of the 24 neighbors are '$b_{n1} - b_{n24}$'. The b_{n1-24} having the greatest distance from 'b_p' is considered the opposite background pixel, b_{max}. The maximum Euclidean distance from 'b_p' to '$b_{n1}-b_{n24}$' is decided to be the diameter of the candidate pixel:

$$d = \max_{bj \in b_{n1} - b_{n24}} \left\| b_p, \bar{b}_j \right\| \qquad (1)$$

where $\left\| b_p, \bar{b}_j \right\|$ is the distance between b_p and b_j. The parameter θ is the angle between the background pixels 'b_p' and '$b_{n1}-b_{n24}$' according to Figure 3. The angle is calculated using the cosine rule. If d is less than P_d then

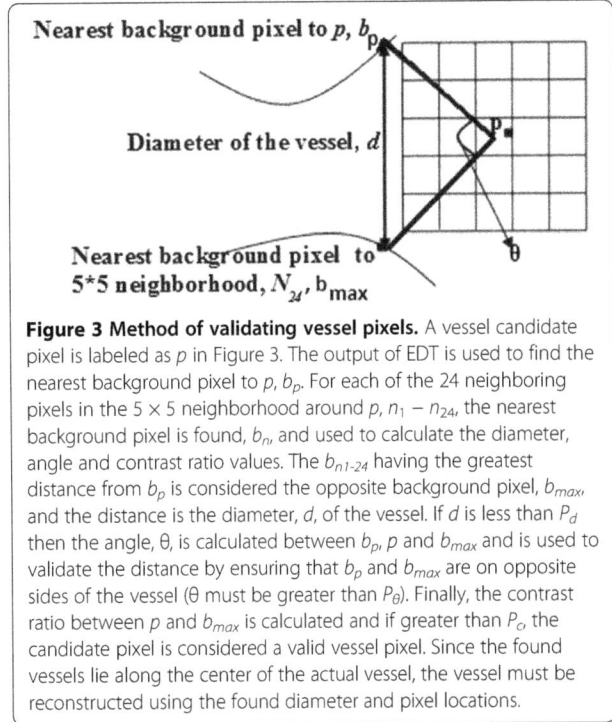

Figure 3 Method of validating vessel pixels. A vessel candidate pixel is labeled as p in Figure 3. The output of EDT is used to find the nearest background pixel to p, b_p. For each of the 24 neighboring pixels in the 5×5 neighborhood around p, $n_1 - n_{24}$, the nearest background pixel is found, b_n, and used to calculate the diameter, angle and contrast ratio values. The b_{n1-24} having the greatest distance from b_p is considered the opposite background pixel, b_{max}, and the distance is the diameter, d, of the vessel. If d is less than P_d then the angle, θ, is calculated between b_p, p and b_{max} and is used to validate the distance by ensuring that b_p and b_{max} are on opposite sides of the vessel (θ must be greater than P_θ). Finally, the contrast ratio between p and b_{max} is calculated and if greater than P_c, the candidate pixel is considered a valid vessel pixel. Since the found vessels lie along the center of the actual vessel, the vessel must be reconstructed using the found diameter and pixel locations.

the angle, θ, is calculated between b_p, p and b_{max}. The maximum angle derived from the 24 neighbor pixels is used as 'θ':

$$\theta = \max_{bj \in b_{n1} - b_{n24}} \cos^{-1} \left(\frac{\left\| p, \bar{b}_p \right\|^2 + \left\| p, \bar{b}_j \right\|^2 - d^2}{2 \left\| p, \bar{b}_p \right\| \left\| p, \bar{b}_j \right\|} \right) \qquad (2)$$

Finally the third feature is the ratio of gray level values of nearest background pixels and the vessel candidate 'p':

$$C = \max_{bj \in b_{n1} - b_{n24}} \frac{GL(b_j)}{GL(p)} \qquad (3)$$

where $GL(p)$ is the gray-level intensity value of current pixel 'p'. To calculate contrast ratio, images with enhanced contrast are used. Therefore, GL in Equation 3 stands for the gray level of the output of the CLAHE.

To verify the vessel candidate pixel, 'd' needs to be less than pre-defined P_d to avoid large vessels, 'θ' needs to be larger than P_θ to assure curvilinear structure and the calculated contrast ratio needs to be higher than P_C to remove background noise. If the pixel in the binary image is black and it meets the criteria defined by three parameters P_d, P_θ and P_C, it is verified to be a vessel pixel. After repeating the same procedure for all threshold levels, the segmented images of each threshold level are combined resulting in one segmented binary image for each frame.

The parameters, P_d, P_θ and P_C were selected from multiple experiments using a set of training videos. P_d controls the maximum diameter of the blood vessels to accept. It is determined based on the diameter of blood vessels and capillaries to be included in the microcirculation. P_θ is another geometric parameter to ensure curvilinear structure of the vessels and is empirically derived.

Region growing

Since the segmentation algorithm is based on pixel verification, it is possible to have isolated pixels in the result. To prevent that, binary morphological operators are used before region growing. The morphological operators include filling the isolated interior pixels and opening.

The region growing algorithm is developed to overcome disconnectivity of blood vessels. First, the final segmented image is divided into $35*35$ windows to determine the orientation of segmented vessel within the window. The vessel is allowed to grow in the computed direction if the gray level is within the range of average gray level of vessel pixels in the window $\pm 0.5*standard$ $deviation$.

FCD calculation

Segmentation processes described up until this stage detect all blood vessels at each frame of the video recording. To provide quantitative information on blood flow, the vessels through which blood is flowing must be identified. To that end, the difference of consecutive segmented frames is calculated pixel by pixel. If the summation of difference for twenty segmented frames is higher than a threshold value, the pixel is assigned as an active blood vessel.

FCD is currently one of the main parameters used to evaluate the microcirculation. FCD can be calculated using two different approaches: one is completely manual by gridding the frame and counting the number of vessels crossing the grid lines; the second approach calculates the ratio of perfused vessels to the total surface using a software tool [31]. FCD is calculated automatically in this study by dividing the area of active vessels to the total area of interest. It is much easier to form the skeleton of the network of active capillaries and calculate the length of this skeleton to form the density measure. However, since the width/thickness of capillaries along this network would be inconsistent (on the actual sublingual surface, the captured video, and in the processed image), the density measure calculated on this length would be the least reliable measure, as it does not incorporate the changes in the thickness of the capillary and therefore the true extent of circulation inside the capillary. The area-based density measure, on the other

hand, since it incorporates the thickness of the capillaries into the calculation, is not susceptible to this issue. We have also included the length-based FCD calculation in this paper for comparison with the output from AVA.

Results and discussion
Results

The proposed experimental algorithm and the software product Microcirculation Analyzer (MCA) were applied to videos acquired from a library of microcirculatory videos of a previous animal study. The protocol was approved by the Virginia Commonwealth University Institutional Animal Care and Use Committee in accordance with the National Institutes of Health Guide for the Care and Use of Laboratory Animals (National Institutes of Health Publication 86-23, revised 1996). In this animal study, sublingual microcirculatory videos were taken from nine healthy juvenile swine at baseline as well as after 40% of the animal's blood was removed. All animals were under a state of general anesthesia. Twenty frames from each video were used for the assessment of the video recordings. The parameters at multi-thresholding stage are defined empirically. Specifically, a series of videos were used as the training set in which we change the values of these parameters over a reasonable range and choose the values that give the parameters providing the best segmentation results. In this study, "the best segmentation result" was visually evaluated. According to this process the image features are obtained; P_d =13, P_θ =130 and P_C = 1.17. The angle is calculated in degrees. In order to capture desired vessels and avoid segmenting larger structures like venules, P_d =13 corresponds to a vessel diameter of about 20 μm at the resolution captured by the test camera. An original frame from sublingual microcirculatory video of a healthy subject is displayed in Figure 4. Active capillaries segmented using MCA are highlighted in Figure 5.

FCD parameters are calculated from SDF videos for nine subjects in both baseline (PPV = 1) and hemorrhage (PPV < 1) conditions. As expected, a significant decrease in FCD is noticed during hemorrhage recordings with respect to baseline videos. For MCA, a paired-samples t-test was conducted to compare FCD values of healthy baseline and hemorrhage video recordings. There was a significant difference in the scores for healthy baseline (μ = 12.68, σ = 1.479, area-based; μ = 3.26 × 10^{-5}, σ = 5.93 × 10^{-6}, length-based) and hemorrhage (μ = 7.35, σ = 2.139, area-based; μ = 1.99 × 10^{-5}, σ = 5.53 × 10^{-6}, length-based) conditions; with t_8 = 6.50 and p-$value$ = .000189. These results suggest that the proposed algorithm, MCA, can successfully derive quantitative information from microcirculation videos. Specifically, the results suggest that microcirculatory alterations caused by hemorrhage can be identified by analyzing sublingual microcirculatory video recordings.

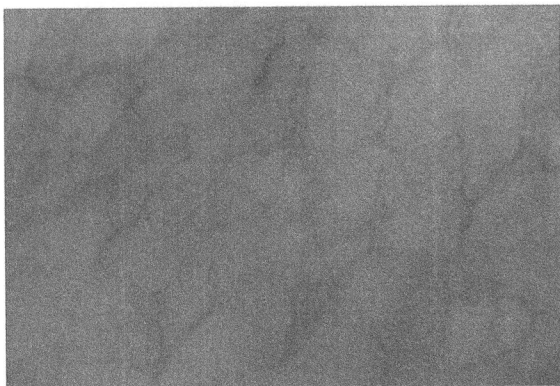

Figure 4 An example frame from a healthy subject. An example frame from a sublingual microcirculatory video captured from a healthy baseline subject is presented.

FCD percentages for nine subjects for healthy baseline and hemorrhage conditions are shown in Table 1.

The same videos were analyzed using the currently available semi-automated tool, AVA, with manual editing. Analysis was performed using the method described in the manufacture's tutorial of the product. All videos were analyzed in an identical format. The microcirculation videos are first automatically analyzed using the software tools and then manual interaction with the software for manipulation of the segmentation results must be performed to remove the large vessels, false positives, and vessels without flow. Figure 6 provides and example of the microcirculation after hemorrhage and can be compared to the healthy (baseline) microcirculation in Figure 4.

Videos were analyzed by two experts previously trained with AVA and the results for each video averaged in the analysis of FCD. These individuals were blinded to FCD values derived from the fully automated method. The analysis resulted in a Kappa coefficient of 0.9 (very good

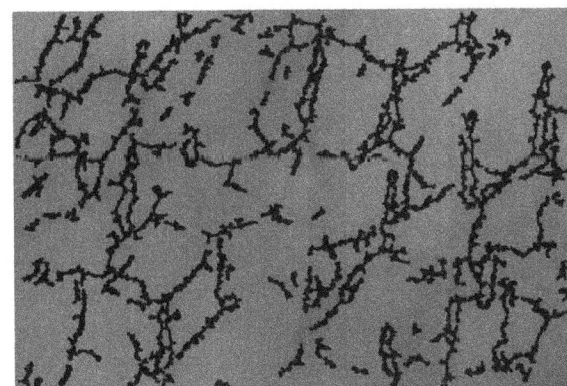

Figure 5 Segmented active capillaries of the frame in Figure 4. The result of the proposed algorithm highlights all active capillaries from the original frame in Figure 4.

agreement). The Kappa coefficient is a statistical measure of inter-rater agreement. The FCD results of this analysis are provided in Table 2. A significant difference is also noticed in these scores for healthy baseline conditions ($\mu = 12.26$, $\sigma = 1.759$, area-based; $\mu = 1.65 \times 10^{-5}$, $\sigma = 5.485 \times 10^{-6}$, length-based) versus hemorrhage conditions ($\mu = 8.56$, $\sigma = 1.432$, area-based; $\mu = 1.20 \times 10^{-5}$, $\sigma = 4.124 \times 10^{-6}$, length-based); with $t_8 = 4.19$ and *p-value* = 0.003.

It should be pointed out that even though AVA allows manual interaction, the version we had access to does not allow the user to draw the capillaries to be included. If the user sees that a capillary has not been identified, the user must define an area that the vessel resides in and then have the program outline the vessel. However, in some instances, the program will still not outline the vessel for inclusion in the FCD calculations. The user cannot manually force the outlining of vessels.

To clearly understand the results generated by the proposed experimental algorithm (MCA) and heavily edited AVA, a chart is generated showing the FCD values for healthy baseline and hemorrhage conditions. Figure 7 shows the results from the heavily edited AVA software. The FCD values from subjects in the healthy baseline condition (PPV = 1) are labeled as baseline. Results of MCA are displayed in Figure 8. The decrease in FCD values for hemorrhage (PPV < 1) is clearly visible for each subject for the FCD values calculated by the experimental MCA automated algorithm. Figures 9 and 10 provide an example of the overlay between MCA and the edited semi-automated AVA method. However, comparing the compilation of data shown in Figures 7 and 8 and Tables 1 and 2, we conclude that MCA provides a better separation of FCD values between healthy baseline and hemorrhage. Furthermore, a Bland-Altman comparison of heavily edited AVA vs. fully-automated MCA (Figure 11) shows that MCA is capable of producing results in line with those achieved from edited AVA.

Discussion

This study presents an entirely automated method, MCA, to derive quantitative information from microcirculatory videos in near real-time. Currently available techniques for analysis of the microcirculation, in their present state, do not appear to be practical in the clinical setting due to the need for significant manual interaction with the software in order to process the image and determine FCD. The significant difference in calculated FCD values across healthy baseline and hemorrhage shows that MCA has the potential for analyzing microcirculation videos in the clinical settings. Although the sample size of this study is relatively small, the algorithm demonstrates promise in its ability to rapidly provide quantitative information. Future studies will test the MCA algorithm on larger datasets—including human microcirculation videos—and improved accordingly.

Table 1 Calculated FCD values using the automated MCA algorithm, including both area and length based results

	Baseline (PPV = 1)		Hemorrhagic (PPV < 1)		Difference	
	FCD (Area) %	FCD (Length) mm/mm^2	FCD (Area) %	FCD (Length) mm/mm^2	FCD (Area) %	FCD (Length) mm/mm^2
Subject 1	12.16	2.35×10^{-5}	9.72	1.42×10^{-5}	2.44	9.28×10^{-6}
Subject 2	14.99	3.35×10^{-5}	7.32	1.48×10^{-5}	7.67	1.87×10^{-5}
Subject 3	13.97	3.10×10^{-5}	11.38	3.26×10^{-5}	2.59	-1.54×10^{-6}
Subject 4	11.95	2.56×10^{-5}	5.92	1.97×10^{-5}	6.03	5.91×10^{-6}
Subject 5	10.21	3.10×10^{-5}	7.58	2.02×10^{-5}	2.63	1.08×10^{-5}
Subject 6	13.81	3.75×10^{-5}	4.41	2.12×10^{-5}	9.40	1.63×10^{-5}
Subject 7	11.90	4.01×10^{-5}	7.38	1.65×10^{-5}	4.52	2.36×10^{-5}
Subject 8	13.49	4.04×10^{-5}	7.05	1.77×10^{-5}	6.44	2.28×10^{-5}
Subject 9	11.65	3.11×10^{-5}	5.37	2.26×10^{-5}	6.28	8.52×10^{-6}
Mean	12.68	3.26×10^{-5}	7.35	1.99×10^{-5}	5.33	1.27×10^{-5}

To overcome the variance among different video recordings, machine learning techniques, in particular neural networks and support vector machines that show superior performance in detection of elongated vessel-like objects in both biomedical image processing applications [32,33] as well as other image processing applications [34], will be applied and algorithm parameters adjusted accordingly. The use of machine learning techniques provide for a means to compensate for variations due to differences in factors such as lighting, pressure, video quality and specific machine/camera used for imaging. Notwithstanding the small sample size, the results show promise for an automated system that derives diagnostically important information from microcirculation videos.

MCA and semi-automated AVA both show a significant decrease in FCD values for the hemorrhagic subjects. Even though FCD values calculated using semi-automated AVA are statistically different for the healthy and hemorrhagic cases ($\mu=3.78$, $\sigma=2.267$, t8=5.0, p-value = $1.1 \times 10{-}3$), the difference is not consistent (Figure 7). As noted in Figure 9, the overlay of analyzed results

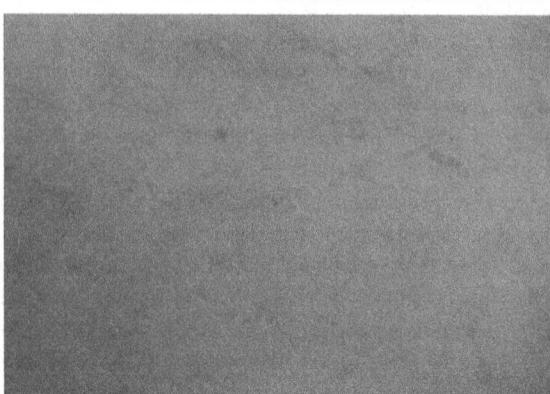

Figure 6 Example of hemorrhage subject video source. An original frame from sublingual microcirculatory video of a hemorrhage subject.

demonstrates very close performance between the automated MCA algorithm and that of the heavily edited AVA method. FCD values during hemorrhage generated by MCA were consistently lower than FCD values from the healthy baseline state (Figure 8). Visual inspection of the videos confirmed the ability of MCA to identify more vessels without flow and thus not include them in the determination of FCD. A potential limitation to this finding is new version of AVA that reportedly allows users to add missed vessels by manual drawing. We did not have access to this version. While use of this newer version may have reduced the differences between semi-automated AVA and the fully automated MCA, this improved version of AVA still requires editing and interaction of the user with the software.

While the approach taken with MCA cannot be considered actual real-time, the 20 second wait for results versus the 20-40 minutes of manual interaction required with semi-automated AVA makes the use of MCA near real-time and may thus be appropriate in the future for bedside point-of-care decision making. Additionally, the use of MCA would negate the considerable training that must be provided to the AVA user in order for them to be able to properly identify the active vessels in the results. This is in contrast to the proposed automated system, which incorporates that knowledge in the algorithm.

In the future, the automated method could be easily integrated into existing SDF or OPSI hardware systems which would allow real-time bedside determinations of FCD and potentially other microcirculatory parameters such as flow quantification. It is likely that in order to use SDF or OPSI derived FCD measures to affect care, an automated and reproducible software approach to analysis will be required for regulatory approval of such an approach.

Recent automated capillary detection methods such as Bezemer et al. [35] demonstrated impressive speed in its analysis. The authors of this method, however, indicate that

Table 2 Calculated FCD values using semi-automated software, AVA

	Baseline (PPV = 1)		Hemorrhagic (PPV < 1)		Difference	
	FCD (Area) %	FCD (Length) mm/mm²	FCD (Area) %	FCD (Length) mm/mm²	FCD (Area) %	FCD (Length) mm/mm²
Subject 1	13.77	1.63×10^{-5}	9.72	9.52×10^{-6}	4.05	6.73×10^{-6}
Subject 2	14.50	2.15×10^{-5}	7.32	1.47×10^{-5}	7.18	6.80×10^{-6}
Subject 3	10.81	1.72×10^{-5}	11.39	1.62×10^{-5}	-0.58	9.75×10^{-7}
Subject 4	11.95	2.41×10^{-5}	6.68	1.91×10^{-5}	5.27	5.00×10^{-6}
Subject 5	9.44	2.18×10^{-5}	9.21	9.65×10^{-6}	0.23	1.22×10^{-5}
Subject 6	13.38	1.00×10^{-5}	7.47	8.29×10^{-6}	5.91	1.72×10^{-6}
Subject 7	10.15	1.75×10^{-5}	8.36	1.43×10^{-5}	1.79	3.15×10^{-6}
Subject 8	13.23	1.23×10^{-5}	8.06	8.22×10^{-6}	5.17	4.08×10^{-6}
Subject 9	13.07	8.18×10^{-6}	8.82	8.04×10^{-6}	4.25	1.35×10^{-7}
Mean	12.26	1.65×10^{-5}	8.56	1.20×10^{-5}	3.70	4.53×10^{-6}

performance is limited by high cell densities and velocities, which severely impede the applicability of this method in real SDF images. We believe this is due to the fact that many factors and thresholds in this method were set to fixed numbers and that they require adjustment from one video to another (just as in AVA). Again, these issues form the basis for the MCA approach as a means of reaching true automation. While we used a binary assessment of flow (flow or no-flow) in identifying functional capillaries, improvements in assessing flow beyond this simple method may be helpful.

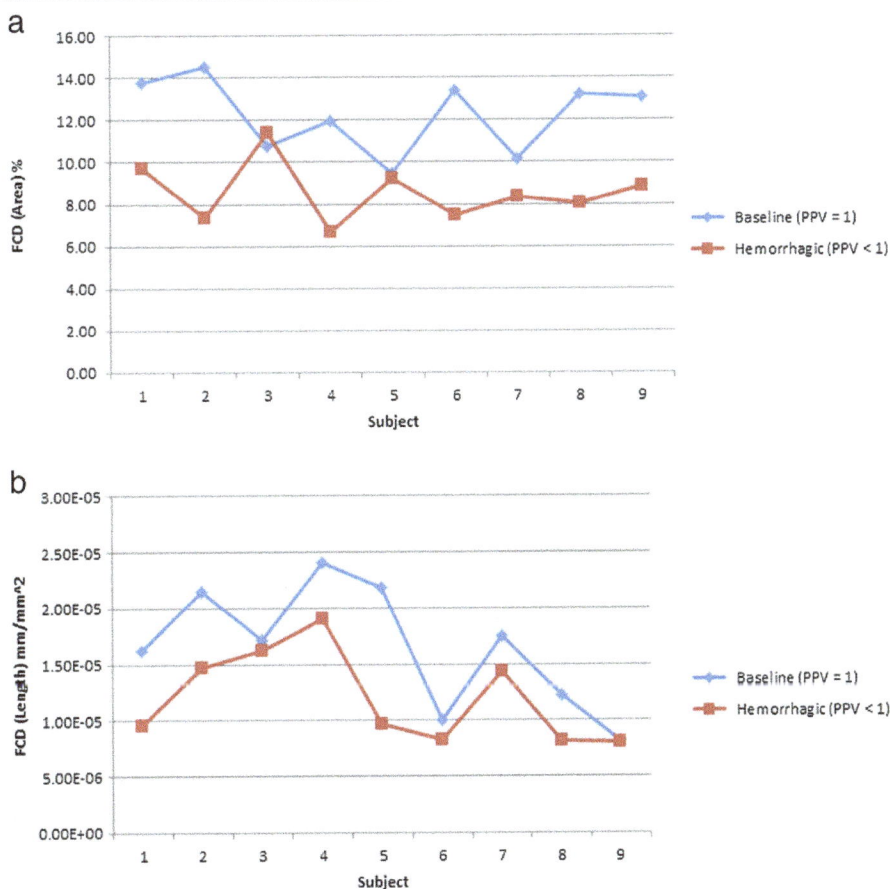

Figure 7 FCD results calculated from heavily edited AVA. The FCD values calculated from heavily edited AVA for both healthy baseline and hemorrhage conditions are displayed. The healthy condition FCD values are labeled as baseline. The change in FCD values during hemorrhage is not consistent. **a**: FCD results (area based) from heavily edited AVA show inconsistent separation between the healthy (baseline, PPV = 1) and hemorrhagic (PPV < 1) cases. **b**: FCD results (length based) from heavily edited AVA.

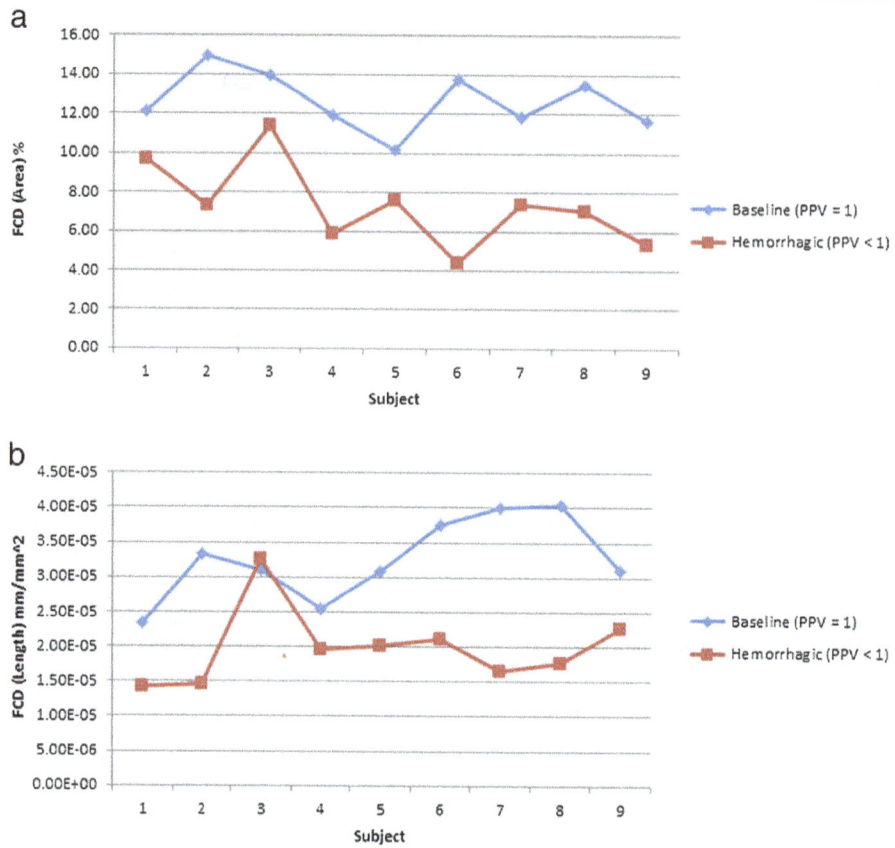

Figure 8 FCD results calculated using the proposed algorithm (MCA). The FCD values calculated using the proposed algorithm for both healthy baseline and hemorrhage conditions are displayed. The healthy condition FCD values are labeled as baseline. The decrease in FCD values for each subject during hemorrhagic is obvious in the provided figure. **a**: FCD results (area based) from the proposed automated system show better and consistent separation between healthy (baseline, PPV = 1) and hemorrhagic (PPV < 1) cases. **b**: FCD results (length based) from the proposed automated system show good separation, but demonstrate the problem with length based FCD calculation where vessel width is not taken into consideration as it is with area based FCD.

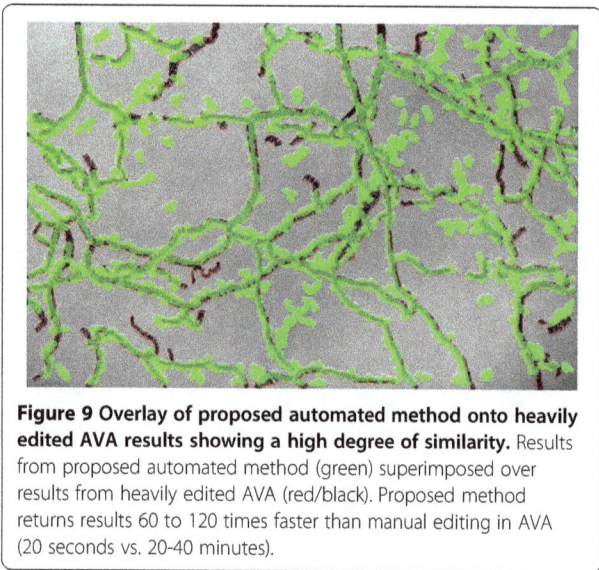

Figure 9 Overlay of proposed automated method onto heavily edited AVA results showing a high degree of similarity. Results from proposed automated method (green) superimposed over results from heavily edited AVA (red/black). Proposed method returns results 60 to 120 times faster than manual editing in AVA (20 seconds vs. 20-40 minutes).

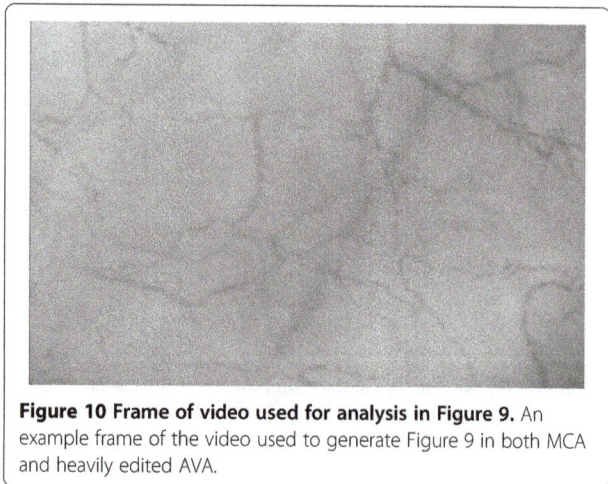

Figure 10 Frame of video used for analysis in Figure 9. An example frame of the video used to generate Figure 9 in both MCA and heavily edited AVA.

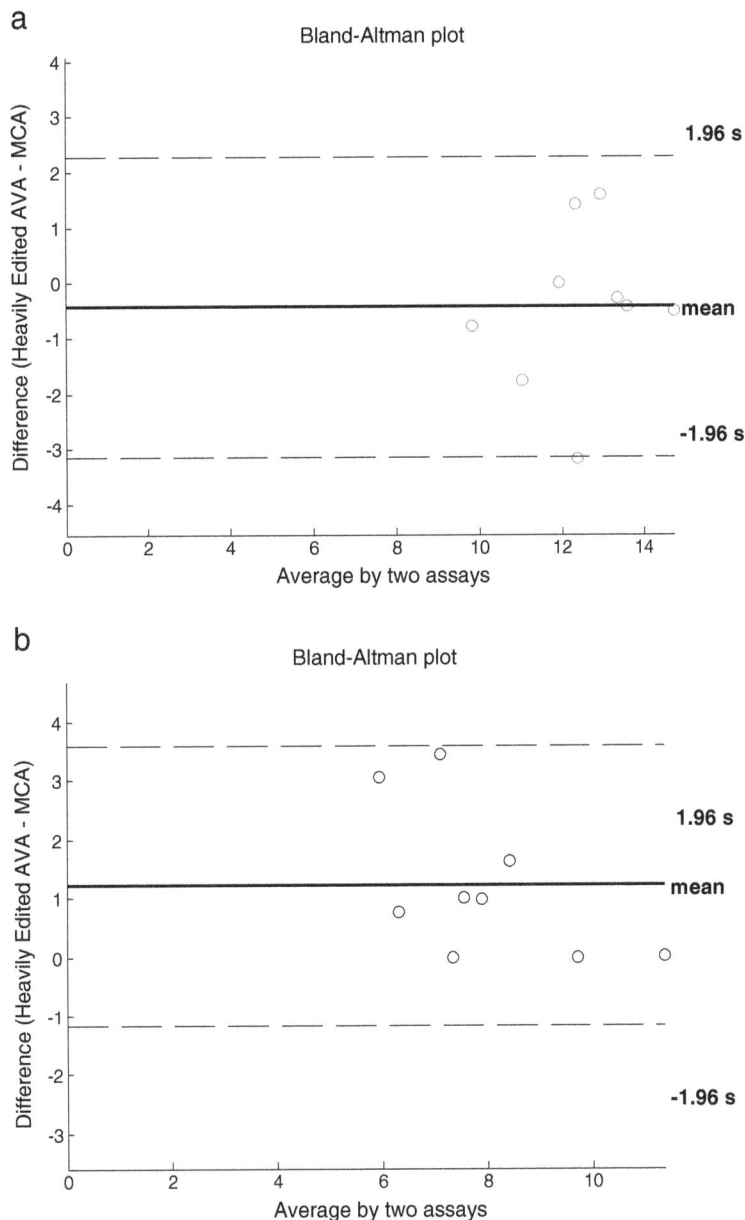

Figure 11 Bland-Altman plots showing validity of fully-automated MCA as a measurement tool vs. current "gold standard" of heavily edited AVA (baseline (a) and hemorrhagic (b). a: Bland-Altman plot showing correlation between heavily edited AVA and fully-automated MCA for baseline (PPV = 1) subjects. **b**: Bland-Altman plot showing correlation between heavily edited AVA and fully-automated MCA for hemorrhagic (PPV < 1) subjects.

This might result in improved accuracy and compensation for some of the mechanical shortcomings of image acquisition using the camera technology, which, is capable of producing pressure related flow artifacts.

Conclusions

A suggested algorithm to analyze microcirculation video recordings based on advanced machine learning is proposed which is capable of identifying active capillaries and calculating FCD parameters automatically. The approach is capable of detecting significant changes in FCD produced by hemorrhage and are comparable to a heavily manually edited commercially available software product. Future work will focus on adjusting the algorithm parameters on larger datasets and improving accuracy as well as developing improved methods of quantifying blood flow. It is hoped that these expanded methods and analyses will lead to the ability to derive diagnostically important decisions from the microcirculatory video recordings as well as to guide therapeutic interventions.

Competing interests

Dr. Demir has intellectual property including pending patents on the technology discussed in this manuscript through Virginia Commonwealth University. She also has served as an employee of Signal Processing Technologies, LLC.

Dr. Hakimzadeh has intellectual property including pending patents on the technology discussed in this manuscript. She also is a co-owner/share-holder of Signal Processing Technologies, LLC which received an NSF SBIR grant for this research. She also serves as Chief Executive Officer at the company.

Dr. Hargraves has intellectual property including pending patents on the technology discussed in this manuscript. She also is a co-owner/share-holder of Signal Processing Technologies, LLC and serves as Chief Technology Officer at the company.

Dr. Ward has intellectual property including pending patents on the technology discussed in this manuscript through Virginia Commonwealth University. He also has serves as an uncompensated consulted to Signal Processing Technologies (SPT), LLC. Dr. Ward used to serve as Chief Medical Officer for SPT with ownership interest but currently he neither has any ownership in SPT nor serves as an officer for this company.

Mr. Myer has intellectual property including pending patents on the technology discussed in this manuscript through Virginia Commonwealth University. He has also served as an employee of Signal Processing Technologies, LLC.

Dr. Najarian has intellectual property including pending patents on the technology discussed in this manuscript through Virginia Commonwealth University. His wife is a co-owner/share-holder of Signal Processing Technologies, LLC, which received an NSF SBIR grant for this research. Dr. Najarian has also served as a technology advisor for Signal Processing Technology LLC.

Authors' contributions

Dr. SUD participated in the design of the image reprocessing algorithms, implemented the algorithms and processed the videos using the proposed algorithm. Dr.RH supervised the coordination of the entire study and the design and testing of the software. Dr. RHH co-supervised the design, implementation, testing and validation of the vessel detection algorithms and identification of pixels in vessels based on angle, intensity and width. Dr. KRW formed the guidelines for data collection, provided the data, outlined the clinical objectives of the study, and assessed the results from physiological and clinical standpoint and oversaw the general development and refinement of the image processing algorithm. Mr. EVM designed the improvements to the per-processing steps, participated in conducting the comparison between the proposed method and other methods, and carries out the statistical analysis. Dr. KN supervised the design of the entire image processing algorithm, in particular stabilization and region growing. All authors' read and approved the final manuscript.

Acknowledgments

This material is based upon work supported by the National Science Foundation under Grant No. 1046521. All authors equally contributed to this work. The dataset used in this research was provided by Virginia Commonwealth University, Department of Emergency Medicine. In addition, the authors would like to thank Dr. Hakam Tiba and Gerard Draucker from the Virginia Commonwealth University Reanimation Engineering Science Center (VCURES) for their participation in sample preparation, data collection and verification of the results.

Author details

[1]Signal Processing Technologies LLC, Richmond, VA, USA. [2]Department of Electrical Engineering, Virginia Commonwealth University, Richmond, VA, USA. [3]Department of Emergency Medicine, Virginia Commonwealth University, Richmond, VA, USA. [4]Virginia Commonwealth University Reanimation Engineering Science (VCURES), Richmond, VA, USA. [5]Department of Computer Science, Virginia Commonwealth University, Richmond, VA, USA. [6]Department of Emergency Medicine, Michigan Center for Integrative Research in Critical Care, University of Michigan, Ann Arbor, MI, USA.

References

1. Cěrný V, Turek Z, Pařízková R: Orthogonal polarization spectral imaging: a review. *Physiol Res* 2007, **56:**141–147.
2. Bateman R, Sharpe M, Ellis C: Bench-to-bedside review: microvascular dysfunction in sepsis: hemodynamics, oxygen transport and nitric oxide. *Crit Care Med* 2003, **7:**359–373.
3. Hebbel R, Osarogiagbon R, Kaul D: The endothelial biology of sickle cell disease; inflammation and chronic vasculopathy. *Microcirculation* 2004, **11:**129–151.
4. Stuart M, Nagel R: Sickle cell disease. *Lancet* 2004, **364:**1343–1360.
5. Levy B, Ambrosio G, Pries A, Struijker-Boudier H: Microcirculation in hypertension: a new target for treatment? *Circulation* 2001, **104:**735–740.
6. Verdant C, Backer DD: Monitoring of the microcirculation may help us at the bedside. *Curr OpinCrit Care* 2005, **11**(3):240–244.
7. Nath K, Katusic Z, Gladwin M: The perfusion paradox and instability in sickle cell disease. *Microcirculation* 2004, **11:**179–193.
8. Kaul D, Farby M: In vivo studies of sickle red blood cells. *Microcirculation* 2004, **11:**153–156.
9. Touyz R: Intracellular mechanisms involved in vascular remodeling of resistance arteries in hypertension: role of angiotensin II. *Exp Physiol* 2005, **90:**449–455.
10. Serne E, Gans R, ter Maaten J, Tangelder G, Donker A, Stehouwer C: Impaired skin capillary recruitment in essential hypertension is caused by both functional and structural capillary rarefaction. *Hypertension* 2001, **38:**238–242.
11. Creager M, Luscher T, Cosentino F, Bechkman J: Diabetes and vascular disease: pathophysiology, clinical consequences, and medical therapy: part I. *Circulation* 2003, **108:**1527–1532.
12. Atasever B, Boer C, van der Kuil M: Quantitative imaging of microcirculatory response during nitroglycerin-induced hypotension. *J Cardiothorac Vasc Anesth* 2011, **25**(1):140–144.
13. Balestra G, Bezemer R, Boerma E, Yong Z, Sjauw K, Engstrom A, Koopmans M, Ince C: Improvement of sidestream dark field imaging with an image acquisition stabilizer. *BMC Med Imaging* 2010, **10:**15.
14. Ince C: Sidestream dark field imaging: an improved technique to observe sublingual microcirculation. *Crit Care* 2005, **9:**72.
15. Groner W, Winkelman JW, Harris AG, Ince C, Bouma GJ, Messmer K, Nadeau RG: Orthogonal polarization spectral imaging: a new method for study of the microcirculation. *Natmed* 1999, **5:**1209–1212.
16. Goedhart PT, Khalilzada M, Bezemer R, Merza J, Ince C: Sidestream dark field (SDF) imaging: a novel stroboscopic LED ring-based imaging modality for clinical assessment of the microcirculation. *Opt Express* 2007, **15:**15101–15114.
17. Awan ZA, Wester T, Kvernebo K: Human microvascular imaging: a review of skin and tongue videomicroscopy techniques and analysing variables. *Clin Physiol Funct Imaging* 2010, **30:**79–88.
18. Klyscz T, Junger M, Jung F, Zeintl H: Cap image: a new kind of computer-assisted video image analysis system for dynamic capillary microscopy. *Biomed Tech (Berl)* 1997, **42:**168–175.
19. Genzel-Boroviczeny O, Strotgen J, Harris AG, Messmer K, Christ F: Orthogonal polarization spectral imaging (OPS): a novel method to measure the microcirculation in term and preterm infants transcutaneously. *Pediatr Res* 2002, **51:**386–391.
20. Bauer A, Kofler S, Thiel M, Elfert S, Christ F: Monitoring of the sublingual microcirculation in cardiac surgery using orthogonal polarization spectral imaging. *The American Society of Anesthesiologists* 2007, **107**(6):939–945.
21. Schaudig S, Dadasch B, Kellam K, Christ F: Validation of an analysis software for OPS-imaging used in humans. In *Proceedings of the 7th World Congress for Microcirculation*. Sydney: Australian and New Zealand Microcirculation Society; 2001:2–59.
22. Zhong J, Asker C, Salerud E: Imaging, image processing and pattern analysis of skin capillary ensembles. *Skin Res Technol* 2000, **6:**45–57.
23. Sainthillier J, Gharbi T, Muret P, Humbert P: Skin capillary network recognition and analysis by means of neural algorithms. *Skin Res Technol* 2005, **11:**9–16.
24. Dobbe J, Streekstra G, Atasever B, van Zijderveld R, Ince C: The measurement of functional microcirculatory density and velocity distributions using automated image analysis. *Med BiolEngComput* 2008, **46**(7):659–670.
25. Nolte D, Zeintl H, Steinbauer M, Pickelmann S, Messmer K: Functional capillary density: an indicator of tissue perfusion? *Int J MicrocircClinExp* 1995, **15:**244–249.

26. Zitov_a B, Flusser J: Image registration methods: a survey. *Image and Vision Computing* 2003, **21**(11):977–1000.

27. Demir S, Mirshahi N, Tiba M, Draucker G, Ward K, Hobson R, Najarian K: Image processing and machine learning for diagnostic analysis of microcirculation. In *ICME International Conference on Complex Medical Engineering (CME 2009): 9-11 April 2009; Tempe*: IEEE; 2009:1–5.

28. Zuiderveld K: Contrast limited adaptive histogram equalization. In *Graphics Gems IV*. Edited by Heckbert PS. San Francisco: Morgan Kaufmann; 1994:474–485.

29. Najarian K, Splinter R: *Biomedical Signal and Image Processing*. Boca Raton: The CRC Press; 2005.

30. Jiang X, Mojon D: Adaptive local thresholding by verification-based multithreshold probing with application to vessel detection in retinal images. *IEEE Trans Pattern Anal Mach Intell* 2003, **25**:131–137.

31. Backer DD, Hollenberg S, Boerma C, Goedhart P, Büchele G, Ospina-Tascon G, Dobbe I, Ince C: How to evaluate the microcirculation: report of a round table conference. *Crit Care* 2007, **11**(5):R101.

32. Chen W, Smith R, Ji SY, Ward K, Najarian K: Automated ventricular systems segmentation in brain CT images by combining low-level segmentation and high level template matching. *BMC Med Inform Decis Mak* 2009, **9**(Suppl 1):S4.

33. Ji SY, Smith R, Huynh T, Najarian K: A comparative analysis of multi-level computer-assisted decision making systems for traumatic brain injuries. *BMC Med Inform Decis Mak* 2009, **9**:2.

34. Muralikrishnan B, Najarian K, Raja J: Surface wavelength based clustering using neural networks for manufacturing process mapping. *Int J Mach Tool Manuf* 2003, **43**(4):369–477.

35. Bezemer R, Dobbe J, Bartels S, Boerma C, Elbers P, Heger M, Ince C: Rapid automatic assessment of microvascular density in sidestream dark field images. *Med Biol Eng Comput* 2011, **49**:1269–1278.

23

Determining optimal medical image compression: psychometric and image distortion analysis

Alexander C Flint*

Abstract

Background: Storage issues and bandwidth over networks have led to a need to optimally compress medical imaging files while leaving clinical image quality uncompromised.

Methods: To determine the range of clinically acceptable medical image compression across multiple modalities (CT, MR, and XR), we performed psychometric analysis of image distortion thresholds using physician readers and also performed subtraction analysis of medical image distortion by varying degrees of compression.

Results: When physician readers were asked to determine the threshold of compression beyond which images were clinically compromised, the mean image distortion threshold was a JPEG Q value of 23.1 ± 7.0. In Receiver-Operator Characteristics (ROC) plot analysis, compressed images could not be reliably distinguished from original images at any compression level between $Q = 50$ and $Q = 95$. Below this range, some readers were able to discriminate the compressed and original images, but high sensitivity and specificity for this discrimination was only encountered at the lowest JPEG Q value tested ($Q = 5$). Analysis of directly measured magnitude of image distortion from subtracted image pairs showed that the relationship between JPEG Q value and degree of image distortion underwent an upward inflection in the region of the two thresholds determined psychometrically (approximately $Q = 25$ to $Q = 50$), with 75 % of the image distortion occurring between $Q = 50$ and $Q = 1$.

Conclusion: It is possible to apply lossy JPEG compression to medical images without compromise of clinical image quality. Modest degrees of compression, with a JPEG Q value of 50 or higher (corresponding approximately to a compression ratio of 15:1 or less), can be applied to medical images while leaving the images indistinguishable from the original.

Keywords: Medical image compression, JPEG, Lossy, Psychometrics, Image analysis

Background

Medical images are increasingly displayed on a range of devices connected by distributed networks, which place bandwidth constraints on image transmission. As medical imaging has transitioned to digital formats such as DICOM and archives grow in size, [1] optimal settings for image compression are needed to facilitate long-term mass storage requirements.

One definition of optimal medical image compression is a degree of compression that decreases file size substantially but produces a degree of image distortion that is not clinically significant. A more conservative definition of optimal image compression would require a degree of image distortion that cannot be perceived by the viewer at all. Other methods that have been used to distinguish degrees of medical image compression include pixel analysis and blinded measurements of diagnostic accuracy [2].

We assessed the crossover point for distortion of grayscale medical images (CT, MR, and XR modalities) by JPEG compression according to two different definitions: (1) the point at which distortion is clinically significant to the viewer and (2) the point at which any distortion can be reliably discriminated by the viewer. We additionally performed analysis of subtracted images to correlate the accumulation of increasing error pixel burden at lower JPEG Q values with the thresholds determined psychometrically.

Correspondence: alexander.flint@interconnectmedical.com
Interconnect Medical, LLC, Menlo Park, CA 94025, USA

Methods

Test Images

40 fully anonymized test images without any identifying features in DICOM format were subjected to JPEG compression as described in detail below using ImageJ64 software (version 1.45, http://rsbweb.nih.gov/ij/index.html). Single representative images with or without pathological features were chosen across a range of modalities and body regions, including CT, MR, and XR imaging modalities (Figure 1, Additional file 1). Clinically standard window/level settings for each modality/body region were chosen for presentation. All images were grayscale, at 8-bit depth (0 to 255 gray values), at source pixel dimensions (minimum pixel dimensions 512 x 512, maximum pixel dimensions 2328 x 2320).

Image Viewing by Clinicians

Because this study aimed to determine thresholds for image distortion by JPEG compression during viewing of images in a range of clinical contexts (e.g. on a personal or clinical office computer, using a web browser, or using a portable electronic device), test images were displayed to subjects using Macintosh and Windows PCs and using both image analysis software and HTML5-compatible web browsers. Because background lux levels can impact radiological image interpretation [3,4], background lux levels were measured using a Mastech MS8229 lux meter and maintained throughout viewing in the range of 25–100 lux.

For the presentation of continuous 100 to 1 JPEG Quality image stacks, images were presented using ImageJ64

software on a Macintosh computer with LCD screen dimensions of 1280 x 800 pixels, with images rendered at full size up to the screen resolution. Image stacks consisted of 100 images created by successively compressing an original single DICOM image into the full range of JPEG compression from JPEG Quality 100 to 1. Viewers were instructed to view the entire range of image compression from JPEG Quality 100 to 1 by scrolling through the image stack continuously using left/right arrows on the computer keyboard or scroll gestures on the computer touchpad. Viewers did not have feedback as to the degree of compression while performing this task; determinations were made solely on the basis of image appearance.

For the presentation of pairwise image comparisons, images were displayed using LCD monitors with screen resolutions of 1280 x 800 to 1280 x 1024 pixels with image presentation by way of an HTML5-compatible web browser (Google Chrome version 15) with images displayed at full size up to the screen resolution. For each pairwise comparison, viewers used the left/right arrows on the computer keyboard to rapidly switch back and forth between the two images being compared.

Clinicians in the study were practicing physicians with board certification in their primary medical specialty (Radiology, Neurology, Neurosurgery, Pulmonary/Critical Care Medicine, and Internal Medicine). A total of 8 clinicians participated in the continuous compression experiment, and a total of 10 clinicians participated in the pairwise image comparison experiment. Clinician subjects were blinded to all aspects of study design and any indicators of image compression other than intrinsic image characteristics.

Psychometric Measurements

Viewers assessed distortion thresholds in two different experiments: (1) determination of clinically important distortion by assessment of continuous JPEG compression from JPEG Q Value 100 to 1, and (2) determination of the level of compression that can be reliably perceived by the viewer, by assessment of a range of differently compressed image pairs.

For the continuous assessment of JPEG compression, viewers scrolled through stacks of 100 images constructed as described above with a range of JPEG compression from JPEG Q Value 100 to 1. Viewers were asked to determine the approximate point at which the image was felt to be distorted to any clinically meaningful extent, and the Q Value corresponding to this point was recorded. Viewers were allowed as much time as needed to make this determination. Each viewer assessed 40 image stacks.

For the pairwise comparison of images, viewers were shown 7 pairs of images for 8 images randomly chosen from the overall set of 40 images. For each image pair,

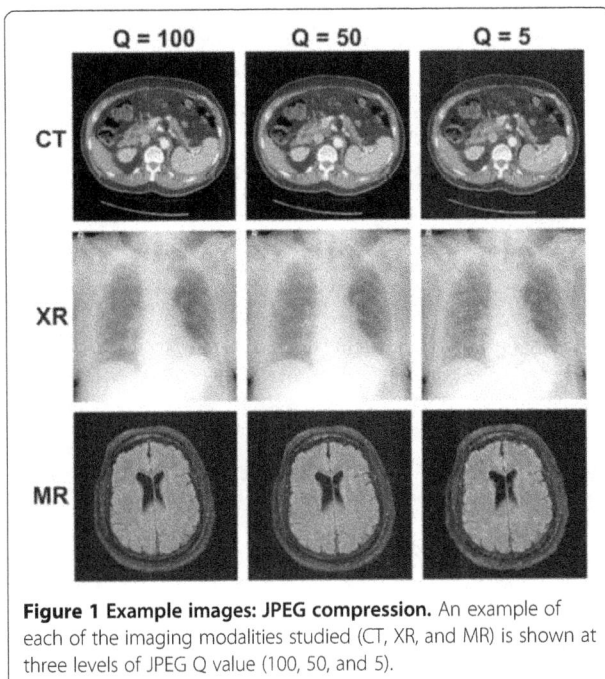

Figure 1 Example images: JPEG compression. An example of each of the imaging modalities studied (CT, XR, and MR) is shown at three levels of JPEG Q value (100, 50, and 5).

one image was JPEG Quality = 100 and the other image was JPEG Quality = (5, 20, 35, 50, 65, 80, or 95). Each viewer was shown 7 image pairs presented in randomly chosen order and asked to determine which image of each pair (also presented in randomly chosen order) was the lower quality image. Viewers were instructed to choose an image even if they could not tell the images apart (to guess if required), and also to indicate whether they felt that their choice was a guess or not.

Random choices for image selection and order of image presentation were made with the use of a true random number generator (www.random.org).

For ROC plot analysis, sensitivity and specificity were calculated based on correct or incorrect identification of "image 0" or "image 1" from each image pair. Because the presentation of image pairs was chosen by random number generator, the labeling of "image 0" or "image 1" for ROC analysis was randomly chosen and the subject's response of "image 0" or "image 1" was determined by whether the subject correctly identified the compressed image or not.

Image Pixel Difference Measurements

To determine the degree of absolute pixel differences between compressed images and a source JPEG Q Value 100 image, we performed subtraction of whole images across the range of JPEG compression from Q Value 99 to 1 using ImageJ64 software. Each successively compressed image was subtracted from the source image, yielding a stack of difference images from (Q Value 100–99) to (Q Value 100–1). Measurements were taken of the total density of difference pixels across each image in the stack, and this operation was then performed on all 40 images viewed by the subject as described above. The mean ± standard deviation total image pixel differences across the 40 images were displayed after normalization to the maximal difference in each image stack.

The conduct of this study was fully compliant with the World Medical Association (WMA) Declaration of Helsinki. Fully anonymized images without any identifying features were shown to physicians who volunteered their own time to participate. No identifying data about the individual physicians was used, stored, or transmitted as part of the study. Based on these specific study characteristics, the study was exempt from IRB review. Exempt status was confirmed by the Kaiser Foundation Research Institute IRB.

Results

Psychometric Experiment 1: Clinically important distortion

When physician readers were asked to determine the degree of compression beyond which images were clinically compromised, the mean image distortion threshold was a JPEG Q value of 23.1 ± 7.0 (Figure 2). The distribution of the data about this mean Q value was approximately Gaussian (Figure 2A, mean = 23 ± 8.1). The task in this experiment was a subjective one (determination of the point at which the reader felt the image was unacceptably distorted), so not surprisingly, there was variation in crossover point values from reader to reader (Figure 2B, $P < 0.001$, Kruskal-Wallis test). Despite this, the highest crossover point for any image or reader was a JPEG Q value of 44.

Psychometric Experiment 2: ROC plot analysis of discrimination between compressed and original image pairs

In ROC plot analysis, compressed images could not be reliably distinguished from original images at any compression level between Q = 50 and Q = 95 (Figure 3A). For Q values 50, 65, 80, and 95, the 95 % confidence intervals (CI) of the sensitivity and specificity estimates each crossed the line of unity where (sensitivity = [1 - specificity]), indicating no reliable discrimination between image pairs (Figure 3A). At a

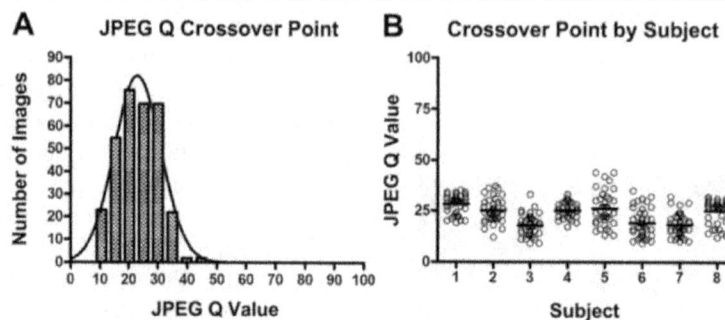

Figure 2 Analysis of "acceptable image" crossover point. A. Histogram of n = 320 crossover points from 8 readers, displayed in bins 5 JPEG Q points wide (hatched bars, mean = 23.1 ± 7.0), with a Gaussian curve fit to the data (solid line, mean = 23 ± 8.1). B. Crossover points according to subject. Subjects (1–8) are displayed on the x axis; each data point shows the crossover point for each of the 40 image stacks shown to each subject. Solid horizontal lines show the mean crossover point for each subject.

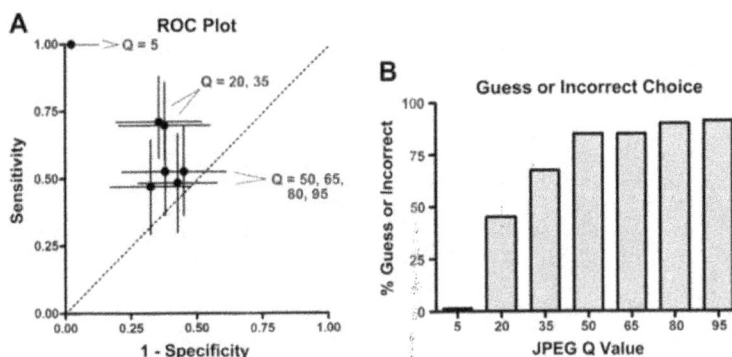

Figure 3 Pairwise image comparisons: ROC plot and "guess or incorrect" analysis. A. ROC plot showing sensitivity and (1 - specificity) at each of the levels of compression tested in pairwise (compressed vs. original) image comparisons (Q values of 5, 20, 35, 50, 65, 80, and 95 compared to 100). Point estimates for each Q value (see labels) are solid circles; 95% CI for sensitivity are shown as vertical bars and 95% CI for specificity are shown as horizontal bars. The dotted oblique line represents the "line of unity" where sensitivity = (1 - specificity): points on a ROC plot along this line represent a cut point at which no reliable discrimination has been found. B. Plot of guess or incorrect choice as a function of Q value for the compressed image. The percentage of responses representing an incorrect choice or a known guess are shown at each of the Q values for the compressed image in each randomly presented image pair.

Q level of 20 or 35, discrimination between the compressed and original images improved beyond chance (sensitivity and specificity increased and the 95% CI no longer crossed the line of unity, Figure 3A). However, high sensitivity and specificity for image discrimination was only encountered at the lowest JPEG Q value tested (Q = 5, Figure 3A).

As viewers were additionally asked in this experiment to record whether they felt that their choice was a guess, we also analyzed the relationship between JPEG Q value and the rate at which readers guessed or made the incorrect choice (Figure 3B). Consistent with the ROC plot analysis, the rate of guessing or incorrect choice rose steeply across the Q = 5 to Q = 50 range, then plateaued (Figure 3B).

Direct analysis of distortion pixels by image subtraction

To determine whether basic features of the JPEG compression algorithm might potentially explain the thresholds encountered in the psychometric experiments above, we performed software analysis of the magnitude of image distortion in subtracted image pairs across the full range of JPEG compression from Q = 99 to Q = 1. A visual demonstration of the effect of image subtraction to reveal error pixels is shown in Figure 4. Direct measurements of subtracted images showed that, as expected, the degree of total pixel error increased across the full range from Q = 99 to Q = 1 (Figure 5). However, this increase in the degree of pixel error had a low slope at Q values above 50, and only at higher levels of compression did the slope show an upward inflection (Figure 5). About 25% of the error pixel accumulation occurred between Q = 50 and Q = 99, while the remaining 75% of error pixel accumulation occurred between Q = 1 and Q = 50.

Discussion

Our data show that lossy JPEG compression can be applied to medical images without clinical image compromise. More subtle lossy JPEG compression (Q values of 50 or higher, roughly a compression ratio of 15:1 or less) can be applied without giving expert viewers the ability to reliably distinguish between the compressed image and the original.

The medical literature on JPEG image compression has typically presented data on compression ratios (e.g. 8:1 or 30:1). However, the software control of compression in the JPEG standard allows for direct manipulation only of Q values, not compression ratio; the compression ratio varies from image to image at a given Q value, depending on the complexity of the source image [5-7]. Since the relationship between Q value and compression ratio for a given image cannot be known *a priori*, it is more reasonable to present data on Q values, assuming software adherence to the standards of the Independent JPEG Group (www.ijg.org).

Previous work in this field has focused on relatively subtle degrees of medical image compression. For example, based on a review of the literature on compression of medical images, one group recommended a range of JPEG compression from 5:1 to 8:1. Another review of prior studies recommended this same range of compression.[8] Similarly, consensus-based approaches have yielded estimates of acceptable compression from 5:1 to 15:1 [9]. Another group tested higher degrees of compression following their own literature review[10], but they were unable to perform ROC analysis because the chosen range of compression ratios was too conservative [11]. Of note, in the same study, JPEG compression appeared to perform better than JPEG 2000 compression at the higher levels of compression tested

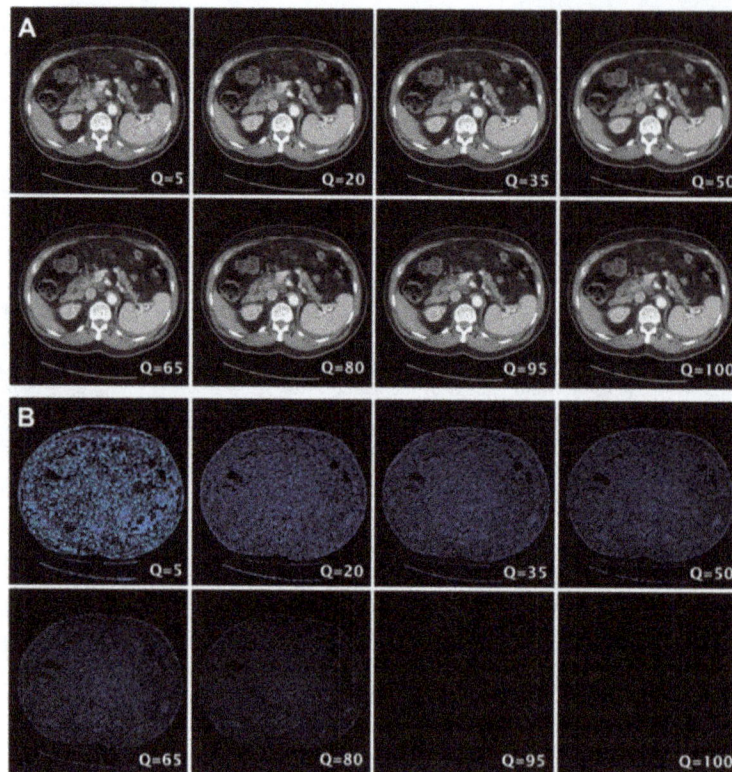

Figure 4 Visual demonstration of the process of image subtraction to reveal error pixels created by JPEG compression. A. A range of 8 example JPEG images from an abdominal CT scan, with compression Q values ranging from 5 to 100. B. A range of 8 images created by subtracting each of the images in (A) from the Q = 100 image. If the same window level as the original images in (A) is used, the error pixels are difficult to appreciate, so the images have been pseudocolored with a black to blue lookup table (LUT) and the contrast has been increased to better show the error pixels.

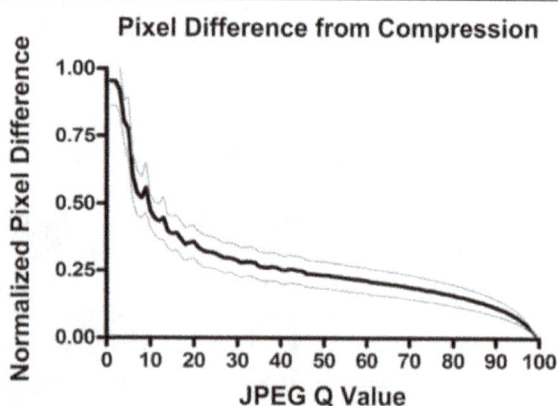

Figure 5 Normalized average pixel error across the range of JPEG Q values. Total difference pixel gray values were determined for the range of JPEG Q values from 1 to 99 by subtracting away the original JPEG Q = 100 image and measuring the total value of all difference pixels for each subtracted image. Measurements were averaged after normalization to the maximum difference value for a given difference image stack. The mean normalized pixel difference is shown as a solid black curve flanked by the +/− standard deviation of the mean in solid gray curves.

[11]. This observation led us to choose JPEG compression (in contrast to JPEG 2000 compression) for our experiments.

Some work has suggested that higher degrees of compression may be acceptable. For example, one study examined the impact of JPEG 2000 compression on interpretation of mammographic digital images and found that images with compression ratios up to 60:1 were not distinguishable from source images [12].

Our study has limitations. We chose to focus on CT, MR, and XR modalities, all of which are grayscale, and therefore one cannot necessarily extrapolate our results to other imaging modalities, particularly color images. We also chose an approach to determine thresholds of clinically acceptable compression and the ability of readers to discriminate a compressed and original image; therefore, we did not specifically examine the ability of readers to distinguish pathology from normal anatomy, which represents a fundamentally different task.

From the data presented here and data from prior studies,[8,9,11-15] it is reasonable to conclude that a modest degree of JPEG compression is acceptable for many applications, particularly those involving network transmission of images.

Conclusion

It is possible to apply lossy JPEG compression to medical images (including CT, MR, and XR modalities) without significant compromise of clinical image quality. Regardless of whether one uses a threshold of clinically acceptable quality or a threshold of inability to distinguish the compressed image from the original, use of a JPEG Q value of 50 to 100 (an approximate compression ratio of 15:1 or lower) can be viewed as generally safe. Within the range of JPEG Q values from 50 to 100, trade-offs between quality and file size should be assessed based on the specific application or clinical need.

Competing interests

The author is Co-Founder and Chief Medical Officer of Interconnect Medical, LLC, a company that designs web-based software for sharing medical imaging.

References

1. Schreiber D: **Swelling archives warrant closer look at compression.** *Radiol Manage* 2003, **25**:36–39.
2. Erickson BJ: **Irreversible compression of medical images.** *J Digit Imaging* 2002, **15**:5–14.
3. Brennan PC, McEntee M, Evanoff M, Phillips P, O'Connor WT, Manning DJ: **Ambient Lighting: Effect of Illumination on Soft-Copy Viewing of Radiographs of the Wrist.** *American Journal of Roentgenology* 2007, **188:** W177–W180.
4. Chawla AS, Samei E: **Ambient illumination revisited: a new adaptation-based approach for optimizing medical imaging reading environments.** *Med Phys* 2007, **34**:81–90.
5. Fidler A, Likar B, Skaleric U: **Lossy JPEG compression: easy to compress, hard to compare.** *Dentomaxillofac Radiol* 2006, **35**:67–73.
6. Fidler A, Skaleric U, Likar B: **The impact of image information on compressibility and degradation in medical image compression.** *Med Phys* 2006, **33**:2832–2838.
7. Fidler A, Skaleric U, Likar B: **The effect of image content on detail preservation and file size reduction in lossy compression.** *Dentomaxillofac Radiol* 2007, **36**:387–392.
8. Braunschweig R, Kaden I, Schwarzer J, Sprengel C, Klose K: **Image data compression in diagnostic imaging: international literature review and workflow recommendation.** *Rofo* 2009, **181**:629–636.
9. Loose R, Braunschweig R, Kotter E, Mildenberger P, Simmler R, Wucherer M: **Compression of digital images in radiology - results of a consensus conference.** *Rofo* 2009, **181**:32–37.
10. Koff DA, Shulman H: **An overview of digital compression of medical images: can we use lossy image compression in radiology?** *Can Assoc Radiol J* 2006, **57**:211–217.
11. Koff D, Bak P, Brownrigg P, Hosseinzadeh D, Khademi A, Kiss A, Lepanto L, Michalak T, Shulman H, Volkening A: **Pan-Canadian evaluation of irreversible compression ratios ("lossy" compression) for development of national guidelines.** *J Digit Imaging* 2009, **22**:569–578.
12. Kang BJ, Kim HS, Park CS, Choi JJ, Lee JH, Choi BG: **Acceptable compression ratio of full-field digital mammography using JPEG 2000.** *Clin Radiol* 2011, **66**:609–613.
13. Kim KJ, Kim B, Lee KH, Kim TJ, Mantiuk R, Kang H-S, Kim YH: **Regional difference in compression artifacts in low-dose chest CT images: effects of mathematical and perceptual factors.** *AJR Am J Roentgenol* 2008, **191:** W30–37.
14. Kim KJ, Lee KH, Kim B, Richter T, Yun ID, Lee SU, Bae KT, Shim H: **JPEG2000 2D and 3D reversible compressions of thin-section chest CT images: improving compressibility by increasing data redundancy outside the body region.** *Radiology* 2011, **259**:271–277.
15. Kim TJ, Lee KH, Kim B, Kim KJ, Chun EJ, Bajpai V, Kim YH, Hahn S, Lee KW: **Regional variance of visually lossless threshold in compressed chest CT images: lung versus mediastinum and chest wall.** *Eur J Radiol* 2009, **69**:483–488.

24

Correlation of anterior segment optical coherence tomography measurements with graft trephine diameter following descemet stripping automated endothelial keratoplasty

Gavin S Tan[1,2], Mingguang He[3], Donald T Tan[1,2,4] and Jodhbir S Mehta[1,2,4,5*]

Abstract

Background: To assess repeatability of the Zhongshan Assessment Program (ZAP) software measurement of Anterior Segment Optical Coherence Tomography (ASOCT) images and correlate with graft trephine diameter following Descemet Stripping Automated Endothelial Keratoplasty (DSAEK)

Methods: Retrospectively evaluated interventional case series. 121 consecutive eyes undergoing DSAEK over a 26 month period underwent ASOCT imaging 1month after their surgery. ASOCT images were processed using ZAP software which measured the graft and cornea parameters including anterior and posterior graft arc length and cord length, posterior cornea arc length (PCAL) and anterior chamber width.

Results: The graft measurements showed good repeatability on ASOCT using ZAP with high intra class coefficient and small variation in the coefficient of variation. On ASOCT, the mean recipient PCAL was 12.99+/−0.69mm and the anterior chamber width was 11.16+/−0.57mm. The mean Graft anterior arc length was 9.69+/−0.66mm and the mean Graft anterior cord length was 8.92+/−2.94mm. The mean graft posterior arc length was 9.24+/−0.75mm and the mean graft posterior cord length was 8.15+/−0.57mm. Graft posterior arc length (rho=0.788, p< 0.001) correlated best with intra-operative graft trephine diameter. The mean ratio of posterior graft arc length to PCAL was 0.712 +/− 0.056.

Conclusions: We have validated the repeatability of the ZAP software for DSAEK graft measurements from ASOCT images and shown that the graft arc length parameters calculated from the ASOCT images correlate well with the intra-operative graft trephine diameter. This software may help surgeons determine the optimal DSAEK graft size based on pre-operative ASOCT measurements of the recipient eye.

Background

Descemet stripping automated endothelial keratoplasty (DSAEK), the main form of endothelial keratoplasty in which a posterior lamellar graft is attached to the posterior corneal surface is rapidly becoming the surgical alternative to penetrating keratoplasty (PK) for patients with corneal endothelial failure [1,2]. The size of the graft diameter in DSAEK usually exceeds that of conventional PK, and a 9.0mm graft, which is often possible in DSAEK, [1] will transfer 26% more surface area of healthy donor endothelial cells than a standard 8.0mm graft more commonly used in PK [3-5]. Although larger grafts offer the inherent advantage of transplanting more healthy donor endothelial cells, a larger diameter graft in DSAEK is technically more difficult to insert with an increased the risk of surgical graft trauma, and may crowd the chamber angle resulting in peripheral anterior synechiae (PAS) in eyes with shallow anterior chambers. Graft diameter has also been reported to have a small but statistically significant correlation with hyperopic shift post operatively [6,7].

Anterior segment optical coherence tomography (ASOCT) is a non-contact imaging technique that obtains high-resolution cross-sectional images of the cornea and

* Correspondence: jodmehta@gmail.com
[1]Singapore National Eye Centre (SNEC), 11 Third Hospital Avenue, Singapore 168751, Singapore
[2]Singapore Eye Research Institute (SERI), 11 Third Hospital Ave, Singapore 168751, Singapore
Full list of author information is available at the end of the article

anterior chamber. The ability of anterior segment OCT to render tissue planes with high axial resolution is potentially useful in evaluating the cornea after corneal lamellar procedures [8]. ASOCT has been used after DSAEK for assessing corneal deturgescence [9], predicting primary graft failure [10] and for quantitative imaging of the donor lamella and its anatomic effects within the anterior chamber [8].

The aim of this study was to (i) assess the reproducibility of post DSAEK graft measurements using the modified ZAP (Zhongshan Assessment Program) software (ii) to validate the measurements obtained from the ZAP readings and correlate this with intra-operative graft trephine measurements; (iii) to retrospectively analyze the graft sizing in our first 121 DSAEK cases to assess the size of the DSAEK graft in relation to the posterior corneal arc length (PCAL).

Methods

Approval for the study was granted by the Singapore National Eye Centre and Singapore Eye Research Institute institutional review board. The study was conducted in accordance with the Declaration of Helsinki. Written informed consent was obtained from all subjects before enrollment. One hundred and twenty one consecutive eyes undergoing DSAEK at the Singapore National Eye centre over a 26 month period, performed by a single corneal surgeon (DT), had ASOCT imaging performed one month after their surgery.

DSAEK surgical technique

DSAEK was performed using a similar technique, as described by Price [11], with the exception of the method of donor insertion. The taco folding technique was used in the first 20 eyes [12], followed by our previously described Sheets Glide technique in all subsequent 101 cases [13]. Microkeratome dissection of the donor was performed using an automated lamellar therapeutic keratoplasty unit (Carrazio-Barraquermicrokeratome, Moria). The diameter of the donor buttons ranged from 7.0 to 9.5mm with an increment of 0.25mm, and the trephine diameter was estimated at approximately 2mm less than the white-to-white measurement of the recipient corneal diameter, as measured by standard surgical calipers intra operatively. Graft thickness was determined by ultrasound pachymetry, after microkeratome dissection, prior to trephination.

Anterior segment optical coherence tomography

Anterior Segment images were scanned with the Zeiss Visante ASOCT (Carl Zeiss Meditec, Dublin, CA) within the first month post operation, with informed consent obtained from all participants, as part of our IRB approved study on DSAEK. The details of ASOCT imaging technology have been described previously [14-16]. To correct for errors caused by the different refractive indices of the cornea and aqueous, the software integral to the Visante ASOCT, initially de-warps the image at the air–tear interface and at the corneal–aqueous interface. Images were taken directly from the machine's output function as 816 x 636 pixel JPEG (lossless compression) files. All selected images were temporal/nasal i.e. horizontal scans, to maximize visibility of anatomical location and repeatability [17,18].

Image processing

All ASOCT images were assessed by one ophthalmologist (GT). For each image, the image file was opened using the Zhongshan Assessment Program and first, the two scleral spurs were identified, defined as the anatomical junction between the inner wall of the trabecular meshwork and the sclera (Figure 1) [19-21]. It is marked by a prominent inner extension of the sclera at its thickest part, and in this study it was defined as a change in curvature of the inner surface of the angle wall, often appearing as an inward protrusion of the sclera. Following this, the anterior and posterior lateral most edges of the DSAEK graft were marked, the software then calculated all parameters and the information was recorded (Figure 1).

The Zhongshan Assessment Program (ZAP, Guangzhou, China) is a proprietary non-commercially available anterior segment image processing software developed at the Zhongshan Ophthalmic centre, Guangzhou, China. This software may be requested free from the authors. The software automatically extracted the 300 x 600 8-bit greyscale (intensities from 0 to 255) image portion of the output file and performed noise and contrast conditioning [17]. A binary copy of the image was then produced where pixels were either 1 s (tissue) or 0 s (open space) depending on whether they were brighter or darker than a calculated threshold value. Algorithms defined the borders of the corneal epithelium and endothelium, and the anterior surface of the iris [17,22]. The anterior graft cord length and the posterior graft cord length were measured, defined as the straight line distance between the anterior edges and the posterior edges of the graft respectively. The anterior and posterior graft arc length were measured which represented the linear measurement of arc length of the anterior and posterior surfaces of the cornea. The posterior cornea arc length from scleral spur to sclera spur and the anterior chamber width using the scleral spurs as the landmarks were also measured. (Figure 1) Repeat measurements with the ZAP software were done for 20 randomly selected ASOCT images one month after the initial measurements were completed, with the observer masked to the results of the initial analysis to assess the intra-observer repeatability of the measurements.

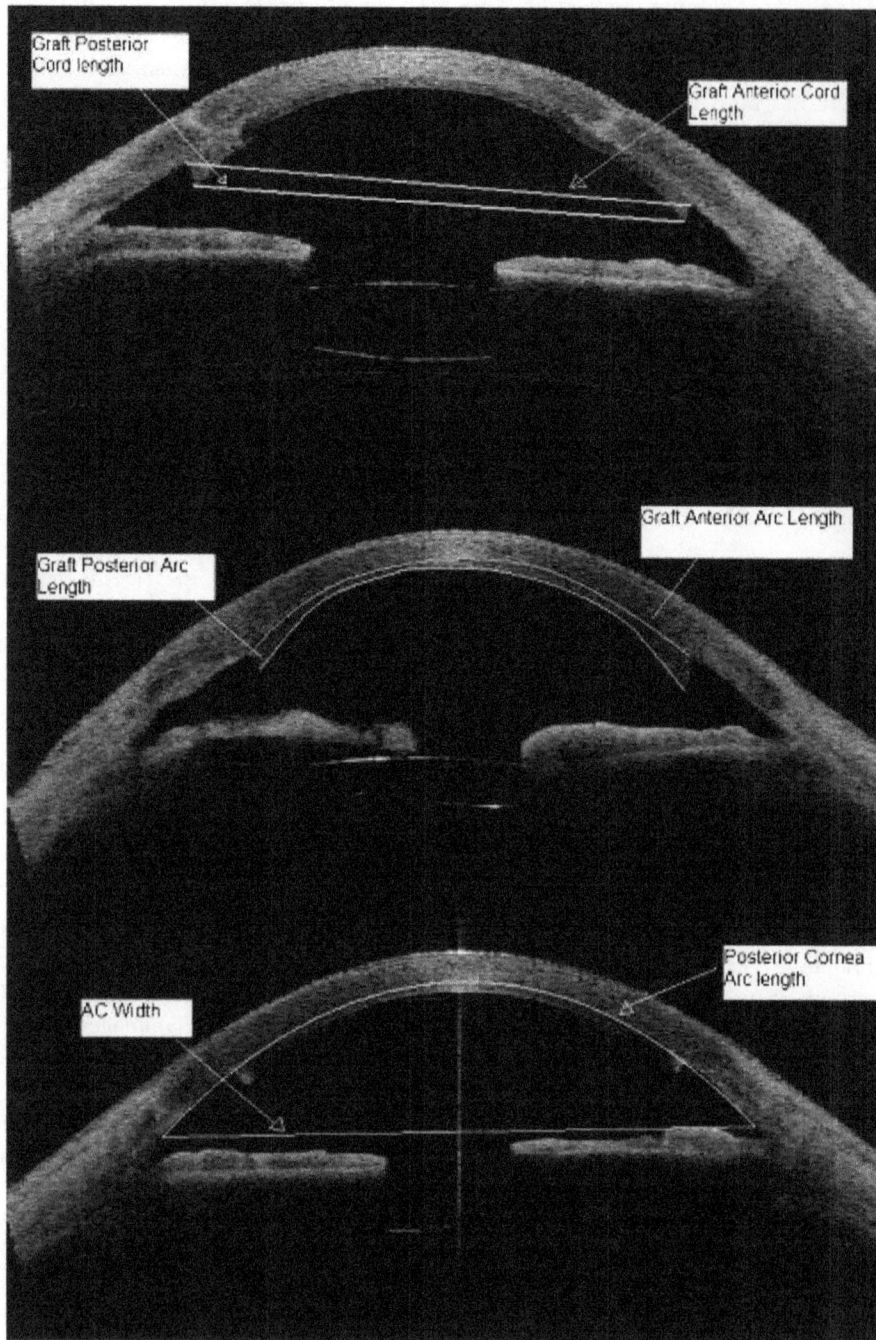

Figure 1 ASOCT image with markings and measurements.

Statistical methods

Parametric and non-parametric tests were used to compare continuous variables according to data distribution. Spearman's Rho correlation, linear regression and logistic regression analyses were used to assess factors relating to the posterior corneal arc length. $P < 0.05$ was considered statistically significant. Bland-Altman analysis was performed to analyze intra-observer agreement. Analysis of repeat measurements was done looking at limits of agreement, coefficient of variation and intraclass coefficient. Statistical analysis was performed by SPSS and microsoft® Excel software.

Results

Patient characteristics

A total of 121 eyes underwent DSAEK and had ASOCT done. 12 (9.9%) eyes were excluded because the ASOCT image was of insufficient quality to identify the sclera spur or to process the image with ZAP software. The remaining 109 eyes (56 right and 53 left) of 104 patients were included in this study. The mean age was 66.17+/−11.58 years and 53.2% were male (58 male patients & 46 female patients). The Sheets Glide insertion technique was used in 93 patients (85.3%) with acceptable ASOCT images. Mean pre-operative donor endothelial cell count was 2881.54 +/− 240.78 and the mean graft thickness was 194.50 +/− 43.10 um (Table 1). The graft trephine size used ranged from 7.0 to 9.5mm with a median and mode of 9.0mm (Figure 2).

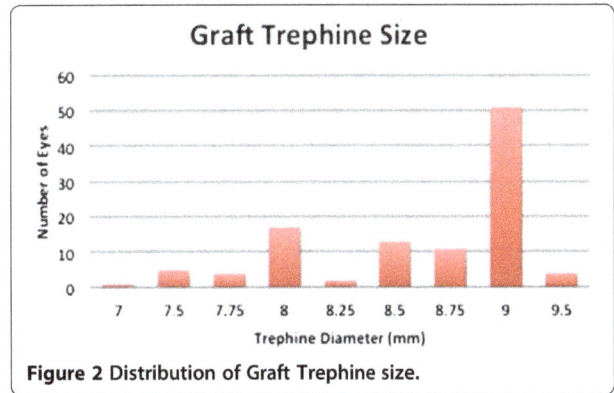

Figure 2 Distribution of Graft Trephine size.

ASOCT analysis

Intra-observer repeatability of graft parameters

We have previously shown good repeatability for the measurement of recipient posterior cornea arc length [22] but not graft measurements. On repeated measurements of the graft parameters on ASOCT, there was no significant difference in the intra-observer measurements. There was high intra class coefficient amongst all parameters, corneal recipient arc length, anterior chamber width, anterior graft arc length, anterior graft cord length, posterior graft arc length and posterior graft cord

Table 1 Demographics and graft parameters

	N=109 (Mean +/− SD)
Age (Years)	66.17 +/−11.58
Sex (Male)	58 (53.2%)
Side (OD)	56 (51.4%)
Glide Insertion technique	93 (85.3%)
Graft size (mm)	8.63 +/− 0.53
Endothelial Cell Count	2881.54 +/− 240.78
Graft thickness (um)	194.50 +/− 43.10
Posterior Cornea Arc length (mm)	12.99 +/− 0.69
Cornea Posterior Curvature (mm)	5.80 +/− 0.85
Posterior graft arc length (mm)	9.24 +/− 0.72
Posterior graft cord length (mm)	8.15 +/− 0.57
Anterior graft arc length (mm)	9.69 +/− 0.66
Anterior graft cord length (mm)	8.65 +/− 0.48
Ratio of posterior graft arc length to posterior Cornea arc length	0.712 +/− 0.516
Ratio of Anterior graft arc length to posterior Cornea arc length	0.745 +/−0.051
Ratio of posterior graft arc length to Posterior graft cord length	1.134 +/− 0.036
Ratio of anterior graft arc length to anterior graft cord length	1.122+/−0.048
Ratio of anterior graft arc length to posterior graft arc length	1.048 +/−0.048
Ratio of anterior graft Cord length to posterior graft cord length	1.096+/−0.339

length ranging from (0.900 to 0.989), which suggests a high level of agreement between repeated measurements. The coefficients of variation amongst all the graft parameters were small (1.24 to 3.71%) (Table 2). The Band Altman plots demonstrate that the mean difference between repeated measures are small and the limits of agreement are within an acceptable range (Figure 3).

Endothelial keratoplasty analysis

On ASOCT, the mean recipient posterior cornea arc length was 12.99 +/− 0.69mm and the mean anterior chamber width was 11.16 +/− 0.57mm. The mean Graft anterior arc length was 9.69 +/− 0.66mm and the mean Graft anterior cord length was 8.92 +/− 2.94mm. The mean graft posterior arc length was 9.24 +/− 0.75mm and the mean graft posterior cord length was 8.15 +/− 0.57mm. The mean ratio of posterior graft arc length to posterior cornea arc length was 0.712 +/− 0.056 (range 0.514 to 0.849) and the mean ratio of anterior graft arc length to posterior cornea arc length was 0.745 +/−0.051 (range 0.618 to 0.859).

Bivariate correlation showed that intraoperative graft trephine diameter correlated with graft anterior arc length, graft anterior cord length, graft posterior arc length and graft posterior cord length (all p< 0.001) (Table 3). The intraoperative graft trephine diameter correlated best with graft posterior arc length (Figure 4). Multivariate linear regression analysis was performed with graft posterior arc length as the dependent parameter in order to analyse the relationship with trephine diameter (Table 4). Models were analyzed using all the parameters significant on bivariate correlation together with age and sex. After performing forward and backward selection multivariate models, we found the model including cornea posterior curvature, AC width and trephine diameter had the greatest adjusted R^2 (0.697) for determining posterior graft arc length.

Examining the trend of graft size, we found that the posterior graft arc length increased with posterior cornea arc length. However, we noted that in our series, eyes

Table 2 Repeatability of ASOCT graft measurements

Parameter	Mean (SD) Observer 1	Mean (SD) Observer 2	P*	Mean difference (95%CI)	Limits of Agreement	Coefficient of variation (95% CI)	Intraclass Coefficient (95% CI)+
Posterior Cornea Arc length (mm)	13.08 (±0.61)	13.06 (±0.59)	0.634	0.02 (−0.06 to 0.10)	−0.32; 0.35	2.56% (1.50, 3.63)	0.959 (0.899 to 0.983)
Anterior chamber Width (mm)	11.24 (±0.50)	11.24 (±0.45)	0.942	0.00 (−0.10 to 0.10)	−0.42; 0.41	3.71% (0.25, 5.25)	0.900 (0.765 to 0.959)
Ant Graft Arc length (mm)	9.77 (±0.51)	9.783 (±0.53)	0.317	−0.02 (−0.06 to 0.02)	−0.18; 0.14	1.61% (0.94, 2.28)	0.988 (0.970 to 0.995)
Ant Graft Cord length (mm)	8.70 (±0.33)	8.73 (±0.34)	0.075	−0.02 (−0.05 to 0.00)	−0.14; 0.09	1.28% (0.75, 1.81)	0.985 (0.963 to 0.994)
Post Graft Arc length (mm)	9.43 (±0.52)	9.45 (±0.51)	0.240	−0.02 (−0.06 to 0.02)	−0.17; 0.13	1.55% (0.91, 2.19)	0.989 (0.973 to 0.996)
Post Graft Cord length (mm)	8.24 (±0.32)	8.26 (±0.34)	0.088	−0.02 (−0.05 to 0.00)	−0.12; 0.08	1.24% (0.73, 1.76)	0.988 (0.969 to 0.995)

*(2-sided).
+ all p< 0.001.

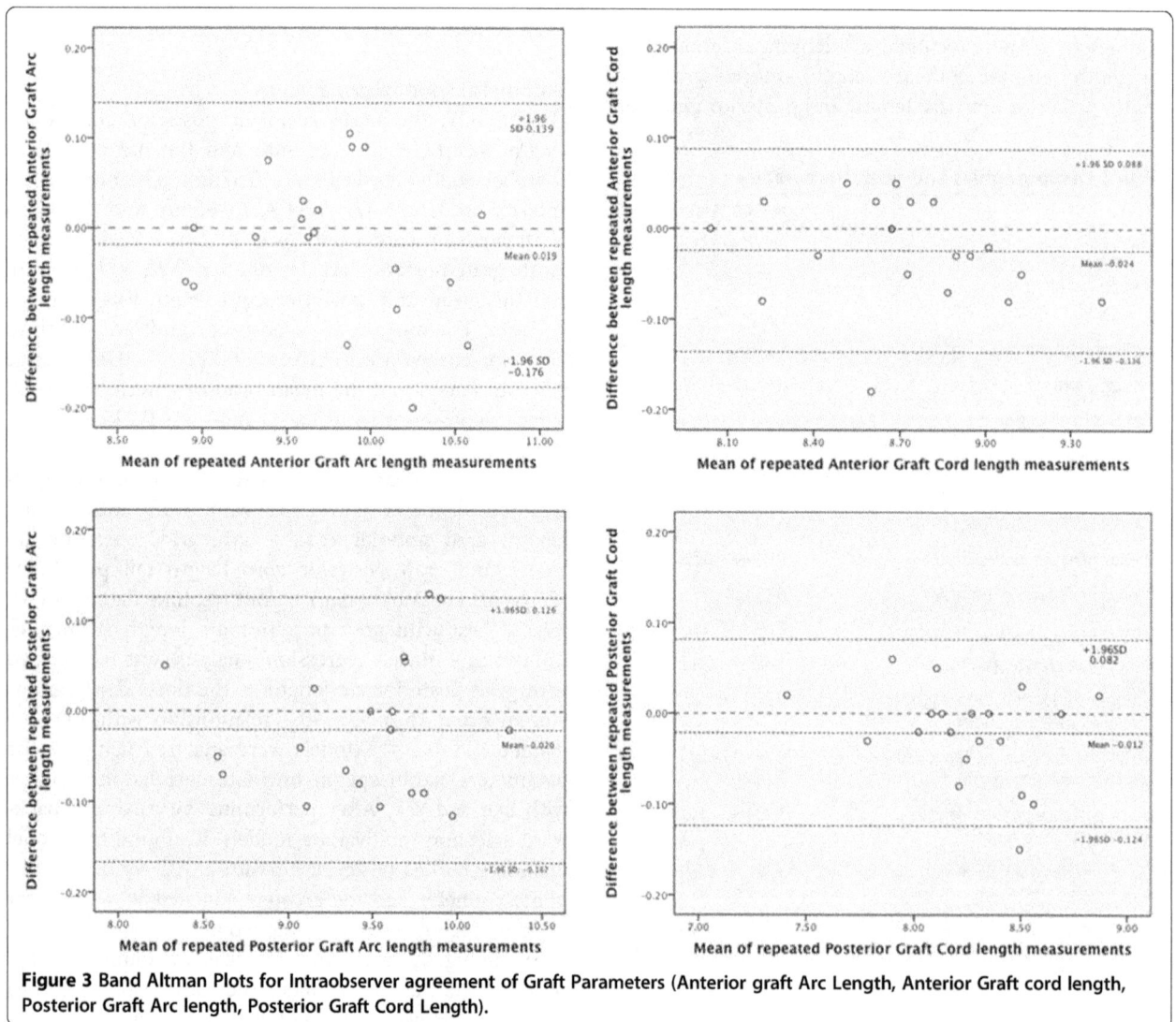

Figure 3 Band Altman Plots for Intraobserver agreement of Graft Parameters (Anterior graft Arc Length, Anterior Graft cord length, Posterior Graft Arc length, Posterior Graft Cord Length).

Table 3 Correlation between graft trephine diameter and ASOCT parameters measured

ASOCT Parameter	Spearman's Rho	p
Posterior Cornea Arc Length	0.298	<0.001
Cornea posterior curvature	0.011	0.909
Anterior Chamber Width	0.162	0.094
Graft Anterior Arc length	0.681	<0.001
Graft Anterior Cord Length	0.643	<0.001
Graft Posterior Arc length	0.788	<0.001
Graft Posterior Cord Length	0.636	<0.001
Graft Thickness	−0.167	0.088

with larger posterior cornea arc length, the ratio of graft posterior arc length to posterior cornea arc length was less than eyes with smaller posterior cornea arc length. (Figure 5).

Discussion

We have previously shown the utility of the ZAP software in providing reproducible measurements of posterior cornea arc lengths from ASOCT images [22]. In this study, ZAP was used to measure the graft parameters in ASOCT images of post-DSAEK eyes. We performed blinded intra-observer repeated measurements with the ZAP software on ASOCT images of endothelial keratoplasty in order to ascertain the repeatability of graft measurements which found that ZAP was able to provide reproducible measurements of DSAEK graft parameters from ASOCT images.

Although useful in providing anatomical detail of anterior segment structures, ASOCT does have its limitations. Images need to be dewarped with software algorithms to correct for index transitions [23], and calculations of anterior segment dimensions are also

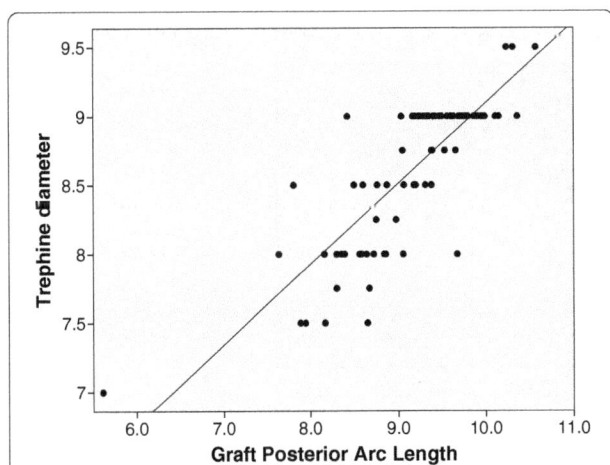

Figure 4 Correlation between trephine diameter and graft posterior arc length.

dependent on assumptions of cornea refractive index [24]. The time-domain ASOCT scans at 2000 axial lines per second and patient movement will affect the quality of the image and the accuracy of the dimensions measured from ASOCT scan. Therefore quantitative imaging on ASOCT may not always correlate with the actual tissue measurements. Our study compared an ex-vivo tissue measurement (the trephine diameter of the DSAEK graft), with the arc length of the graft measured post operatively on ASOCT. We found that among the in-vivo ASOCT graft measurements taken, the graft posterior arc length correlated best with graft trephine diameter. This may be expected since it would be less affected by the recipient cornea posterior curvature or the thickness of the graft, and the donor trephinations were all performed from the endothelial surface downwards.

Most of the grafts in this series were performed in eyes with pseudophakic bullous keratopathy where larger grafts with greater replacement of functional cornea endothelial cells were desirable. In our series, the mean ratio of posterior graft arc length to recipient posterior cornea arc length was 0.712 +/− 0.056 (Range 0.504 to 0.852). There was a small negative trend between the ratio of posterior graft arc length to posterior cornea arc length and the posterior cornea arc length, which suggested that we could have used larger grafts in eyes with larger posterior corneal arc lengths (Figure 5). For eyes in our series where the posterior cornea arc length was larger than the 75th percentile (13.52mm), the ratio of graft posterior arc length to posterior cornea arc length was less than the mean (0.712) in 70.4% of these eyes. This suggests that 70.4% of grafts in patients with PCAL> 13.5mm were undersized.

We feel that sizing of the DSAEK graft is not a "one size fits all" procedure. It is known that cornea dimensions can vary with ethnicity and adult stature [25]. Intra-operative graft sizing based on visual assessment of the horizontal white to white diameter does not take into account the cornea curvature, and may also be an underestimate in eyes with significant arcus or pannus. The main advantage of using the ZAP software is that it allows the surgeon to quantitatively assess the size of the recipient posterior corneal surface as opposed to the anterior surface. Using the anterior surface of the cornea may be appropriate for sizing for penetrating keratoplasty but it is inappropriate for EK surgery not only due to the position of the EK graft but also because the EK surgeon can potentially transplant a larger graft since there is no concern regarding the limbal vasculature. There is no published information as to the optimal graft size for endothelial keratoplasty and hence also the optimal ratio of graft posterior arc length to posterior cornea arc length, although it has been suggested that a larger graft with the same endothelial cell density would

Table 4 Multivariate regression between Graft Arc Length and Trephine diameter

Independent variables in regression model	B coefficient* (95%CI)	P value	Adjusted R²
Recipent age, sex, posterior cornea arc length	1.112 (0.935, 1.289)	<0.001	0.677
Recipent age, sex, posterior cornea arc length, AC width	1.134 (0.958, 1.310)	<0.001	0.686
Recipent age, sex, posterior cornea arc length, AC width, thickness	1.134 (0.955, 1.312)	<0.001	0.683
Recipent age, sex, Cornea posterior curvature	1.162 (0.999, 1.324)	<0.001	0.682
Cornea Posterior curvature	1.154 (0.998, 1.310)	<0.001	0.685
AC width	1.117 (0.959, 1.276)	<0.001	0.691
Recipent age, sex, Cornea posterior curvature, posterior cornea arc length, AC width	1.122 (0.951, 1.292)	<0.001	0.694
Cornea Posterior curvature, AC width**	1.112 (0.954, 1.269)	<0.001	0.697

*B coefficient for trephine diameter.
**Final model using backward selection.
All variables in the models were tested for colinearity with acceptable tolerence.

provide a greater total number of functioning endothelial cells to the recipient and may support greater long term endothelial cell survival [26,27]. Although one retrospective study demonstrated no significant difference in the loss of endothelial cell density comparing 8mm grafts and grafts larger than 8mm [28], this study only included patients with Fuch's endothelial dystrophy where the endothelial dysfunction is mainly in the central cornea and larger grafts may provide less of an advantage. Comparative studies between DSAEK and PK have shown that although DSAEK has a greater initial endothelial cell loss [29,30], the subsequent cell loss is at a slower rate in comparison to PK [26]. This may be related to the larger grafts with greater number of cells inserted during DSAEK. A large graft is not always an advantage, as an oversized graft may be more difficult to insert, and is also less tolerant to decentration, with a higher risk of crowding of the anterior chamber angle, contact with the peripheral iris leading to the development of peripheral anterior synechiae, and hence the potential for a higher risk of both angle-associated secondary glaucoma, and allograft rejection. The importance of DSAEK graft sizing may be of greater significance in our population of Asian eyes where the incidence of narrow angles and angle closure glaucoma is much higher than in Western and European populations [31]. Studies have also found that DSAEK grafts induce an initial hyperopic shift that decreases somewhat over time [32]. This hyperopic shift is reported to be correlated with central graft thickness, graft trephine

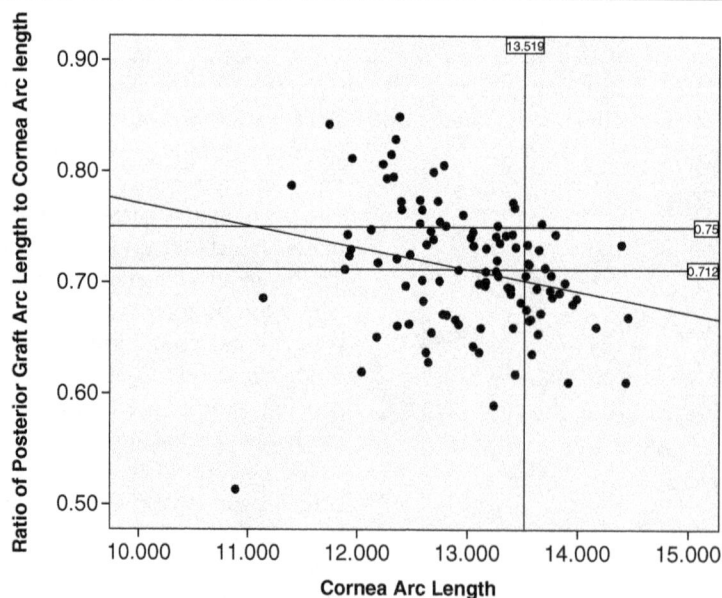

Figure 5 Graph of Ratio of posterior graft arc length to posterior cornea arc length vs cornea arc length. Vertical line represents the 75th percentile of posterior cornea arc length (13.52mm). Horizontal line represents the mean ratio of graft posterior arc length to posterior cornea arc length (0.71).

diameter as well as the thickness gradient between the centre and periphery of the graft [6,7,33]. Examining the relationship between the posterior and anterior graft arc length, in addition to the graft thickness and diameter, with the final refractive outcome, will allow us to better predict this hyperopic shift with the ZAP software.

In future, we aim to perform further studies to prospectively analyze the effect of graft size and the ratio of graft diameter to posterior cornea arc length, on postoperative outcomes including endothelial cell count and refractive outcome. Once we establish an optimal graft size ratio, we can estimate the appropriate graft trephine diameter based on the cornea posterior arc length from the pre-operative ASOCT image. Our multiple regression analysis showed that, a model using posterior cornea arc length and AC width measured on ASOCT would allow us to reasonably estimate the graft arc length based on the trephine diameter chosen (Table 4).

The use of ASOCT imaging and ZAP software in our study does have some limitations. It has previously been shown that there can be difficulty in detecting the sclera spurs on some ASOCT scans [34]. In some images, the internal surface of the sclera formed a smooth continuous line with no inward protrusion or change in curvature which made it impossible to detect the sclera spur. In addition, some ASOCT images were of suboptimal quality, which also affects the ability to accurately identify the sclera spur. Some of these poor quality images could not be processed by the ZAP software even if the sclera spur could be identified; this figure was 9.9% in our study. The study was also limited in that measurements were performed on horizontal (nasal/temporal) ASOCT scans only. We chose to use only horizontal scans since these scans have been shown to be the most consistent with respect to obtaining high quality images for ZAP software analysis, and also recognizing that most surgeons measure the horizontal rather than vertical white-to-white diameter [19]. In addition, ASOCT imaging of vertical scans can be limited by eyelid anatomy especially in our population of Asian eyes with small palpebral apertures. A further limitation to the software is that it can only be used on time domain scans that image the whole length of the anterior segment. The next generation of Fourier domain ASOCT scanners whilst providing better quality images have the disadvantage of not being able to scan the whole anterior segment in one scan.

Conclusion
In summary we have successfully validated the repeatability of the ZAP software measurements of ASOCT images from patients who have undergone DSAEK surgery. We have also shown that the graft arc length parameters calculated from the software correlate well with the intra operative graft trephine diameter. There will be much value in analyzing the correlation between graft parameters measured on ASOCT and DSAEK outcomes, which may enable us to optimize graft trephine diameter chosen for DSAEK surgery. The use of high resolution ASOCT scans in the future will also provide greater detail with more quantitative measurements that may be useful in studying outcomes and optimizing surgical decisions. The ability to accurately select the ideal donor diameter, to maximize endothelial cell transfer while reducing the risks of anterior chamber crowding and peripheral anterior synechiae, and predict the final refractive outcome, could help to improve graft survival, and visual outcomes, as well as reduce complications in DSAEK surgery.

Competing interests
The authors declare they have no competing interests.

Author details
[1]Singapore National Eye Centre (SNEC), 11 Third Hospital Avenue, Singapore 168751, Singapore. [2]Singapore Eye Research Institute (SERI), 11 Third Hospital Ave, Singapore 168751, Singapore. [3]Zhongshan Ophthalmic Centre, Guangzhou, China. [4]Yong Loo Lin School of Medicine, National University of Singapore, 1E Kent Ridge Road, Singapore, Singapore. [5]Department of Clinical Sciences, Duke-NUS Graduate Medical School, 8 College Rd, Singapore 169857, Singapore.

Authors' contributions
GT participated in the design of the study, performed the measurements on the ASOCT images, performed the statistical analysis and drafted the manuscript. MH advised on the design of the study, developed the software used for image measurements and advised on drafting the manuscript. DT performed the surgery on all patients in the study, advised on the design of the study and advised on the drafting of the manuscript. JM conceived of the study and participated in the design and coordination of the study as well as the drafting of the manuscript. All authors read and approved the final version of the manuscript.

Financial disclosure
National Research Foundation-Funded Translational & Clinical Research (TCR) Program Grant [NMRC/TCR/002 - SERI/2008 - TCR 621/41/2008].

References
1. Price MO, Price FW Jr: **Descemet's stripping with endothelial keratoplasty: comparative outcomes withmicrokeratome-dissected andmanually dissected donor tissue.** *Ophthalmology* 2006, 113:1936–1942.
2. Price FW Jr, Price MO: **Descemet's stripping with endothelial keratoplasty in 50 eyes: a refractive neutral corneal transplant.** *J Refract Surg* 2005, 21:339–345.
3. Thompson RW Jr, Price MO, Bowers PJ, Price FW Jr: **Long-term graft survival after penetrating keratoplasty.** *Ophthalmology* 2003, 110:1396–1402.
4. Tan DT, Janardhanan P, Zhou H, Chan YH, Htoon HM, Ang LP, Lim LS: **Penetrating keratoplasty in Asian eyes: the Singapore Corneal Transplant Study.** *Ophthalmology* 2008, 115:975–982 e971.
5. Bertelmann E, Pleyer U, Rieck P: **Risk factors for endothelial cell loss post-keratoplasty.** *Acta Ophthalmol Scand* 2006, 84:766–770.
6. Lombardo M, Terry MA, Lombardo G, Boozer DD, Serrao S, Ducoli P: **Analysis of posterior donor corneal parameters 1 year after Descemet stripping automated endothelial keratoplasty (DSAEK) triple procedure.** *Graefes Arch Clin Exp Ophthalmol* 2010, 248:421–427.

7.   Jun B, Kuo AN, Afshari NA, Carlson AN, Kim T: **Refractive change after descemet stripping automated endothelial keratoplasty surgery and its correlation with graft thickness and diameter.** *Cornea* 2009, **28**:19–23.

8.   Lim LS, Aung HT, Aung T, Tan DT: **Corneal imaging with anterior segment optical coherence tomography for lamellar keratoplasty procedures.** *Am J Ophthalmol* 2008, **145**:81–90.

9.   Di Pascualem A, Prasher P, Schlecte C, Arey M, Bowman RW, Cavanagh HD, McCulley JP, Mootha W: **Corneal deturgescence after Descemet stripping automated endothelial keratoplasty evaluated by Visante anterior segment optical coherence tomography.** *Am J Ophthalmol* 2009, **148**:32–37 e31.

10. Shih CY, Ritterband DC, Palmiero PM, Seedor JA, Papachristou G, Harizman N, Liebmann JM, Ritch R: **The use of postoperative slit-lamp optical coherence tomography to predict primary failure in descemet stripping automated endothelial keratoplasty.** *Am J Ophthalmol* 2009, **147**:796–800–800 e791.

11. Price FW Jr, Price MO: **Descemet's stripping with endothelial keratoplasty in 200 eyes: Early challenges and techniques to enhance donor adherence.** *J Cataract Refract Surg* 2006, **32**:411–418.

12. Melles GR, Lander F, Nieuwendaal C: **Sutureless, posterior lamellar keratoplasty: a case report of amodified technique.** *Cornea* 2002, **21**:325–327.

13. Mehta JS, Por YM, Beuerman RW, Tan DT: **Glide insertion technique for donor cornea lenticule during Descemet's stripping automated endothelial keratoplasty.** *J Cataract Refract Surg* 2007, **33**:1846–1850.

14. Su DH, Friedman DS, See JL, Chew PT, Chan YH, Nolan WP, Smith SD, Huang D, Zheng C, Li Y, *et al*: **Degree of angle closure and extent of peripheral anterior synechiae: an anterior segment OCT study.** *Br J Ophthalmol* 2008, **92**:103–107.

15. Radhakrishnan S, Huang D, Smith SD: **Optical coherence tomography imaging of the anterior chamber angle.** *Ophthalmol Clin North Am* 2005, **18**:375–381. vi.

16. Radhakrishnan S, Rollins AM, Roth JE, Yazdanfar S, Westphal V, Bardenstein DS, Izatt JA: **Real-time optical coherence tomography of the anterior segment at 1310 nm.** *Arch Ophthalmol* 2001, **119**:1179–1185.

17. Console JW, Sakata LM, Aung T, Friedman DS, He M: **Quantitative analysis of anterior segment optical coherence tomography images: the Zhongshan Angle Assessment Program.** *Br J Ophthalmol* 2008, **92**:1612–1616.

18. Lavanya R, Teo L, Friedman DS, Aung HT, Baskaran M, Gao H, Alfred T, Seah SK, Kashiwagi K, Foster PJ, Aung T: **Comparison of anterior chamber depthmeasurements using the IOLMaster, scanning peripheral anterior chamber depth analyser, and anterior segment optical coherence tomography.** *Br J Ophthalmol* 2007, **91**:1023–1026.

19. Sakata LM, Lavanya R, Friedman DS, Aung HT, Seah SK, Foster PJ, Aung T: **Assessment of the scleral spur in anterior segment optical coherence tomography images.** *Arch Ophthalmol* 2008, **126**:181–185.

20. Pavlin CJ: **Practical application of ultrasound biomicroscopy.** *Can J Ophthalmol* 1995, **30**:225–229.

21. Pavlin CJ, Harasiewicz K, Foster FS: **Ultrasound biomicroscopy of anterior segment structures in normal and glaucomatous eyes.** *Am J Ophthalmol* 1992, **113**:381–389.

22. Yuen L, He M, Aung T, Htoon HM, Tan DT, Mehta JS: **Biometry of the Cornea and Anterior Chamber in Chinese Eyes: an Anterior Segment Optical Coherence Tomography Study.** *Invest Ophthalmol Vis Sci* 2010, **51**:3433–3440.

23. Westphal V, Rollins A, Radhakrishnan S, Izatt J: **Correction of geometric and refractive image distortions in optical coherence tomography applying Fermat's principle.** *Opt Express* 2002, **10**:397–404.

24. Lin RC, Shure MA, Rollins AM, Izatt JA, Huang D: **Group index of the human cornea at 1.3-microm wavelength obtained in vitro by optical coherence domain reflectometry.** *Opt Lett* 2004, **29**:83–85.

25. Wong TY, Foster PJ, Johnson GJ, Klein BE, Seah SK: **The relationship between ocular dimensions and refraction with adult stature: the Tanjong Pagar Survey.** *Invest Ophthalmol Vis Sci* 2001, **42**:1237–1242.

26. Price FW Jr, Price MO: **Does endothelial cell survival differ between DSEK and standard PK?** *Ophthalmology* 2009, **116**:367–368.

27. Amann J, Holley GP, Lee SB, Edelhauser HF: **Increased endothelial cell density in the paracentral and peripheral regions of the human cornea.** *Am J Ophthalmol* 2003, **135**:584–590.

28. Terry MA, Li J, Goshe J, Davis-Boozer D: **Endothelial keratoplasty: the relationship between donor tissue size and donor endothelial survival.** *Ophthalmology* 2011, **118**:1944–1949.

29. Price MO, Gorovoy M, Benetz BA, Price FW Jr, Menegay HJ, Debanne SM, Lass JH: **Descemet's stripping automated endothelial keratoplasty outcomes compared with penetrating keratoplasty from the Cornea Donor Study.** *Ophthalmology*, **117**:438–444.

30. Price MO, Price FW Jr: **Endothelial cell loss after descemet stripping with endothelial keratoplasty influencing factors and 2-year trend.** *Ophthalmology* 2008, **115**:857–865.

31. Foster PJ, Oen FT, Machin D, Ng TP, Devereux JG, Johnson GJ, Khaw PT, Seah SK: **The prevalence of glaucoma in Chinese residents of Singapore: a cross-sectional population survey of the Tanjong Pagar district.** *Arch Ophthalmol* 2000, **118**:1105–1111.

32. Holz HA, Meyer JJ, Espandar L, Tabin GC, Mifflin MD, Moshirfar M: **Corneal profile analysis after Descemet stripping endothelial keratoplasty and its relationship to postoperative hyperopic shift.** *J Cataract Refract Surg* 2008, **34**:211–214.

33. Dupps WJ Jr, Qian Y, Meisler DM: **Multivariatemodel of refractive shift in Descemet-stripping automated endothelial keratoplasty.** *J Cataract Refract Surg* 2008, **34**:578–584.

34. Dorairaj S, Liebmann JM, Ritch R: **Quantitative evaluation of anterior segment parameters in the era of imaging.** *Trans Am Ophthalmol Soc* 2007, **105**:99–108. discussion 108–110.

25

Segmentation of corpus callosum using diffusion tensor imaging: validation in patients with glioblastoma

Mohammad-Reza Nazem-Zadeh[1,2,3], Sona Saksena[4], Abbas Babajani-Fermi[4,5], Quan Jiang[3], Hamid Soltanian-Zadeh[1,4,6*], Mark Rosenblum[5], Tom Mikkelsen[7] and Rajan Jain[4,7]

Abstract

Background: This paper presents a three-dimensional (3D) method for segmenting corpus callosum in normal subjects and brain cancer patients with glioblastoma.

Methods: Nineteen patients with histologically confirmed treatment naïve glioblastoma and eleven normal control subjects underwent DTI on a 3T scanner. Based on the information inherent in diffusion tensors, a similarity measure was proposed and used in the proposed algorithm. In this algorithm, diffusion pattern of corpus callosum was used as prior information. Subsequently, corpus callosum was automatically divided into Witelson subdivisions. We simulated the potential rotation of corpus callosum under tumor pressure and studied the reproducibility of the proposed segmentation method in such cases.

Results: Dice coefficients, estimated to compare automatic and manual segmentation results for Witelson subdivisions, ranged from 94% to 98% for control subjects and from 81% to 95% for tumor patients, illustrating closeness of automatic and manual segmentations. Studying the effect of corpus callosum rotation by different Euler angles showed that although segmentation results were more sensitive to azimuth and elevation than skew, rotations caused by brain tumors do not have major effects on the segmentation results.

Conclusions: The proposed method and similarity measure segment corpus callosum by propagating a hypersurface inside the structure (resulting in high sensitivity), without penetrating into neighboring fiber bundles (resulting in high specificity).

Keywords: Corpus callosum, Fiber bundle segmentation, Level-set, Glioblastoma, Diffusion tensor imaging

Background

Corpus callosum is the largest inter-hemispheric fiber bundle in the human brain [1,2]. Most of the fibers interconnect homologue cortical areas in roughly mirror image sites but a large number of the fibers have heterotypic connections ending in asymmetrical areas [3]. Previous studies have mainly investigated effects of various pathologies on the corpus callosum [4-7]. However, a fully automated, fast, and accurate method for segmenting corpus callosum without penetrating into irrelevant neighboring

structures, using data acquired in routine clinical protocols, is still lacking.

Previously, image processing methods have been proposed for segmenting corpus callosum in anatomical magnetic resonance images (MRI) [8-10]. These methods rely on intensity information of two-dimensional images and their results may need pruning. Recently, attention has been oriented towards diffusion tensor imaging (DTI) to segment white matter tracts of the brain [11,12]. Although the tensor model fails to describe higher order anisotropies in heterogeneous areas where more than one fiber population exists, it is practically useful for extracting major white matter tracts, particularly the ones with predominant diffusivity pattern such as corpus callosum. When using DTI data, the fiber bundles can be

* Correspondence: hamids@rad.hfh.edu
[1]Control and Intelligent Processing Center of Excellence, School of Electrical and Computer Engineering, University of Tehran, Tehran 14399, Iran
Full list of author information is available at the end of the article

extracted by: a) clustering of fibers resulting from tractography into fiber bundles [13-19]; or b) segmenting fiber bundles via hyper-surface propagation based on local properties of diffusion tensor, diffusion signal, or orientation distribution function (ODF) [20-27]. Since clustering methods rely on the tractography results, they do not work properly if the tractography results are inaccurate. On the other hand, segmentation methods based on hyper-surface propagation do not use the tractography results and are thus more robust to noise.

In a region-based segmentation framework, a similarity measure between successive tensors is typically used. Some of the hyper-surface propagating methods in the literature concentrated on scalar quantities derived from the tensor data which do not reflect complete tensor information [20]. Other methods benefit from the entire information contained in the DTI data [21-30]. Wang and Vemuri [22] proposed a statistical level-set segmentation method. However, the tensors derived in this framework are not necessarily positive semi-definite, leading to inappropriate results especially when consecutive tensors are much different. Metrics like Kullback-Leibler divergence and J-divergence [23,24] have also been proposed. One of the most promising methods is introduced by Jonasson et al. [25]. They defined a new similarity measure called normalized tensor scalar product (NTSP). Comparing NTSP with other similarity measures, they demonstrated superiority of their proposed measure. To segment brain structures like thalamic nuclei, they modified their framework to favor the propagation of multiple hyper surfaces without overlapping [26]. Lenglet et al. [27] defined a dissimilarity measure and statistics between tensors based on the Riemannian distances. Although improving the segmentation results, this approach is computationally expensive. Defining a Log-Euclidean distance, another metric was defined by Arsigny et al. [28] which has lower computational burden. Weldeselassie and Hamarneh [29] used their proposed similarity measure in an energy minimization framework. Awate et al. [30] used the similarity measure in a Markov random field framework.

In terms of quantitative evaluation of diffusion parameters, previous studies have compared DTI-based indices in normal appearing white matter and corpus callosum in multiple sclerosis [4], stroke [5], schizophrenia [6], and Huntington's [7] and also studied the DTI methods to assess corpus callosum regions across the human lifespan [31]. For segmenting corpus callosum and its subdivisions in these studies, however, two-dimensional (2D) methods were applied and DTI-based indices compared in the mid-sagittal plane. However, without recruiting a three dimensional (3D) method to segment the whole corpus callosum and its subdivisions, the extracted quantities may be inaccurate.

Since the tensor model is not capable of describing heterogeneous diffusion behavior in the crossing fiber bundles, some studies used High Angular Resolution Diffusion Imaging (HARDI) data to segment specific bundles [32-38]. However, the HARDI data is not widely acquired in clinical centers and hence, the tensor-based methods are still of more practical use in clinical research.

In this manuscript, we present a 3D method to segment corpus callosum. Based on tensor and anisotropy values of neighboring voxels, a similarity measure is proposed and used as a speed function in the proposed level-set method. In this method, the principal diffusion direction (PDD) and prior information about the diffusivity pattern in corpus callosum are used to avoid inclusion of neighboring fiber bundles. Then, the Witelson subdivisions of corpus callosum are automatically identified [39]. The idea of using diffusivity pattern in corpus callosum has been used by Lee et al. [40]. However, they performed a 2D segmentation on the mid-sagittal plane. Moreover, since their method uses the left-right component of PDD to delineate corpus callosum boundaries, it is not applicable in more lateral sagittal planes, where corpus callosum connects to minor and major forceps and considerable anterior-posterior component of PDD exists.

The proposed segmentation method can be identically used for segmenting corpus callosum of control subjects as well as patients with glioblastoma. However, since we use the geometric information of the diffusivity pattern in corpus callosum and the glioblastoma tumor may change the original shape and diffusivity pattern of corpus callosum, we validate the reproducibility of the proposed method through realistic simulations of corpus callosum rotations under glioblastoma tumor pressure. We study the effects of rotation by different Euler angles (azimuth, elevation and skew) quantitatively and demonstrate that even in extreme cases with large rotations, brain tumors do not have major effects on the segmentation results generated by our proposed method. We apply the method to the DTI data of normal subjects and brain cancer patients with glioblastoma and show its superiority to some of the previously published methods in the literature.

Methods
Patient population
This study is approved by the institutional review board and is compliant with the Health Insurance Portability and Accountability Act (HIPAA). Between February 2006 and December 2008, 19 patients (8 males, 11 females; mean age 60.7 years) with treatment naïve glioblastoma underwent MRI with DTI using a 3 T scanner at our institution. Based on anatomical MRI findings, the patients were divided into two groups: Group 1

including patients with tumors not infiltrating corpus callosum (n = 12); and Group 2 including patients with tumors infiltrating corpus callosum (n = 7). For the control group, 11 patients (5 males, 6 females; mean age 48 years) who underwent brain MRI for nonspecific headache or single idiopathic seizure with normal MRI were included.

Magnetic resonance imaging protocol
All the patients underwent both conventional MRI and DTI on a 3 T scanner (Excite HD, GE Medical Systems, Milwaukee, WI) using an 8-channel head coil. Diffusion weighted images (DWIs) were acquired in 25 diffusion gradient directions. The reconstructed DWIs have intra-slice resolution of 256 × 256 with voxel size of 0.98 × 0.98 × 2.5 mm. To have the same step size in each direction for the front propagation in the level-set method and to avoid extensive computation, we interpolated the data into 128 × 128 grid with cubical, 1.9 × 1.9 × 1.9 mm voxels.

Level-set approach
We use a level-set method that takes into account several properties when formulating the segmentation problem [41,42]. The method smoothes the propagating hyper-surface automatically and leads to a regularized segmentation. Among the advantages of the method, its property of generalizing from 2D to 3D and higher dimensions and automatic splitting and merging of the surfaces are notable. In addition, it simplifies calculation of geometric quantities needed in the proposed method such as normal to surface and curvature.

For bundle segmentation in areas with high level of similarity in diffusion, the hyper-surface needs to grow in the direction normal to the surface. Moreover, the resulting fiber bundles must be smooth. Consequently, we use a level-set whose growing hyper-surface is the zero level-set of the following function which is a reduced form of the Hamilton-Jacobi partial differential equation:

$$D_t\varphi(r,t) + F(r,t)||\nabla\varphi(r,t)|| - \kappa(r,t)||\nabla\varphi(r,t)|| = 0 \quad (1)$$

where r ∈ $\Re^n$ is the state space, ϕ: $\Re^n \times \Re \to \Re$ is the level set function, $D_t\phi$ is the partial derivative of ϕ with respect to the time variable t, $\nabla\phi = D_r\phi$ is the gradient of ϕ with respect to the state space variables, and F(r, t) is the speed in the direction normal to the surface, extracted from the spherical harmonic coefficients of the neighboring voxels. The sign $||\cdot||$ stands for the magnitude operator. The curvature $\kappa(r, t)$ is used to fulfill the smoothness constraint. To calculate the first order spatial partial derivative $\nabla\phi(r, t)$, we use the 5th order of the upwind method [41].

Corpus callosum segmentation
Corpus callosum is a commissural fiber bundle with a specific diffusion pattern which can be coded as prior knowledge in the segmentation framework. Using this information, we prevent the hyper-surface from propagating into adjacent white matter structures such as cingulum, tapetum, minor and major forceps, and tracts of the corona radiata. Although dissimilarity among tensors helps in this case, smooth and gradual transition in shape and direction of the DTI tensors from corpus callosum to minor and major forceps makes the segmentation difficult.

We define a similarity measure between every voxel on the propagating hyper-surface and its neighbors in the propagation direction, based on tensor and anisotropy values. This similarity measure is used as the speed term F(r, t) in Equation (1). The hyper-surface propagation in each step depends only on the speed function of the boundary voxels. This speed function term moves the hyper-surface to fill the whole fiber bundle, while the regularizing curvature term in Equation (1) is in charge of smoothing corpus callosum without changing its real structure.

Using the fact that the diffusivity in corpus callosum is perpendicular to the mid-sagittal plane of the brain, we consider a threshold (PDD_x Threshold) for the x-component (left-right component) of the PDD ($PDD_x(r)$) for propagating the front only inside the corpus callosum. The x-component of the PDD is large throughout the structure body. However, corpus callosum fibers project to the cortical area at its genu and splenium, where the x-component of PDD is not large anymore. Fortunately, these fibers are considered as different fiber tracts of minor and major forceps, and most of studies investigating the different diffusion indices within the corpus callosum, exclude the minor and major forceps from that.

In the proposed algorithm, we consider two more thresholds on collinearity of the PDD vectors (Collinearity_Threshold) and similarity of fractional anisotropy (FA) values (FA_Threshold) in the neighboring voxels.

The proposed segmentation steps are as follows:

1. Select the initial seeds in corpus callosum in mid-sagittal plane manually.
2. Initiate the hyper-surface as the congregation of small spheres around the seed points.
3. Do until convergence
   - For each point r on the hyper-surface at step t:
     a) Calculate the normal direction to the surface.
     b) Calculate the 26-neighborhood and keep the neighbors n_r for r, which are collinear with the normal, with respect to the r.

c) If $PDD(r). PDD(n_r) >Collinearity\_Thres$-$hold$ & $FA\ (n_r) >FA\_Threshold$ & $PDD_x\ (r) >PDD_x\_Threshold$

Then $\quad F(r, t) = \sum_{n_r} FA(r).FA(n_r). \dfrac{tr\left[D(r)^*D(n_r)\right]}{tr\left[D(r)\right]^* tr\left[D(n_r)\right]}$ (2)

- Threshold $F(r, t)$ with $F\_Threshold$ to diminish the effect of negligible speeds.
- Use the resultant speed in the level-set framework.

4. Extract the zero level-set as the segmented corpus callosum.

In Equation (2), $tr(.)$ is the matrix trace and $D(r)$ is the tensor at point r.

After segmenting corpus callosum, Witelson subdivisions of corpus callosum are automatically extracted [39]. First, the critical point between genu and rostrum of corpus callosum is calculated, where the curvature of the structure boundary in mid-sagittal plane changes. Then, the segmented corpus callosum is automatically subdivided into Witelson subdivisions in the mid-sagittal plane: rostrum, genu, rostral body, anterior mid-body, posterior mid-body, isthmus and splenium [39]. Moreover, the user can visualize and confirm the calculated mid-sagittal plane and the critical joining point between genu and rostrum. The critical point can be selected manually if close supervision is preferred or needed.

Results

Segmentation using proposed method

We implemented the proposed algorithm in MATLB R2008a using a PC with Intel® Core™ 2Duo CPU (E8400@ 3.00 GHz, 3.00 GHz) and 4 GByte RAM and 64 bit VISTA operating system.

To evaluate quality of the segmentation results, the dice correctness measure [43] is calculated using the following relation:

$$Correctness = \frac{N(S_a \cap S_y)}{[N(S_a) + N(S_y)]/2} \quad (3)$$

where S_a and S_r are the automatic and manual (reference) segmentation results, respectively, and N is the number of voxels in each bundle. Here, $N(S_a \cap S_y)$ is the number of the True-Positives. The Dice correctness measure is appropriately bounded, normalized, well-understood, and applied widely in evaluating segmentation methods. Two of the co-authors (a clinical expert and a technical expert) sat down together and carried out the manual segmentation which is considered as the reference segmentation results.

We tested sensitivity of corpus callosum Witelson segments to $PDD_x\_Threshold$ for a normal subject. Figures 1 and 2 show the number of True-Positives, the number of False-Positives, and the Dice correctness measure over a range of $PDD_x\_Threshold$ for the Witelson segments of the Corpus Callosum of a normal subject and a tumor patient, respectively. As shown in these figures, for $PDD_x\_Threshold$ values within a specific range (here 0.5 to 0.6), the Dice correctness measure is maximized. For a higher $PDD_x\_Threshold$, both the number of True-Positives and False-Positives start to decrease, however, the number of False-Positives tend to saturate by increasing the $PDD_x\_Threshold$. This occurs conversely for $PDD_x\_Threshold$ values lower than a specific range, i.e., both the number of True-Positives and False-Positives start to increase, however, the number of True-Positives tends to saturate by decreasing $PDD_x\_Threshold$. As seen, there is a small difference between the optimal selection of $PDD_x\_Threshold$ for the normal subject and the tumor case, suggesting that we can apply the same $PDD_x\_Threshold$ for all datasets.

Figure 3 shows the number of True-Positives, the number of False-Positives, and the Dice correctness measure over a range of $Collinearity\_Threshold$ for the Witelson segments of the Corpus Callosum of a normal subject. It is shown that when $Collinearity\_Threshold$ values are in a specific range (here 0.65 to 0.75), the Dice correctness measure is maximized. However, the sensitivity of the segmentation method to $Collinearity\_Threshold$ is less than its sensitivity to $PDDx\_Threshold$. We found the following set of parameters optimal for segmenting corpus callosum: $PDD_x\_Threshold$ = 0.55, $Collinearity\_Threshold$ = 0.7, $FA\_Threshold$ = 0.1, and $F\_Threshold$ = 0.05.

The tensor-based method proposed by Jonasson et al. [32] with NTPP similarity measure is quite sensitive to the speed threshold. If the speed threshold is selected high enough to prevent the front from propagating into the neighboring structures, corpus callosum is not segmented entirely (low sensitivity). However, if the speed threshold is chosen low enough to segment the entire corpus callosum, the front propagates into irrelevant fiber structures such as superior longitudinal fasciculus, cingulum, minor forceps, and tracts of corona-radiata (low specificity). Figure 4a shows the results of our implementation of their method. In this figure, we tuned the speed threshold so that the whole structure is segmented. Figure 4b demonstrates high sensitivity (segmenting almost the whole structure) and high specificity (without major penetration into the neighbouring structures) of our proposed method compared to the Jonasson's method.

We have also compared the results of the proposed method with those of the Jonasson's method

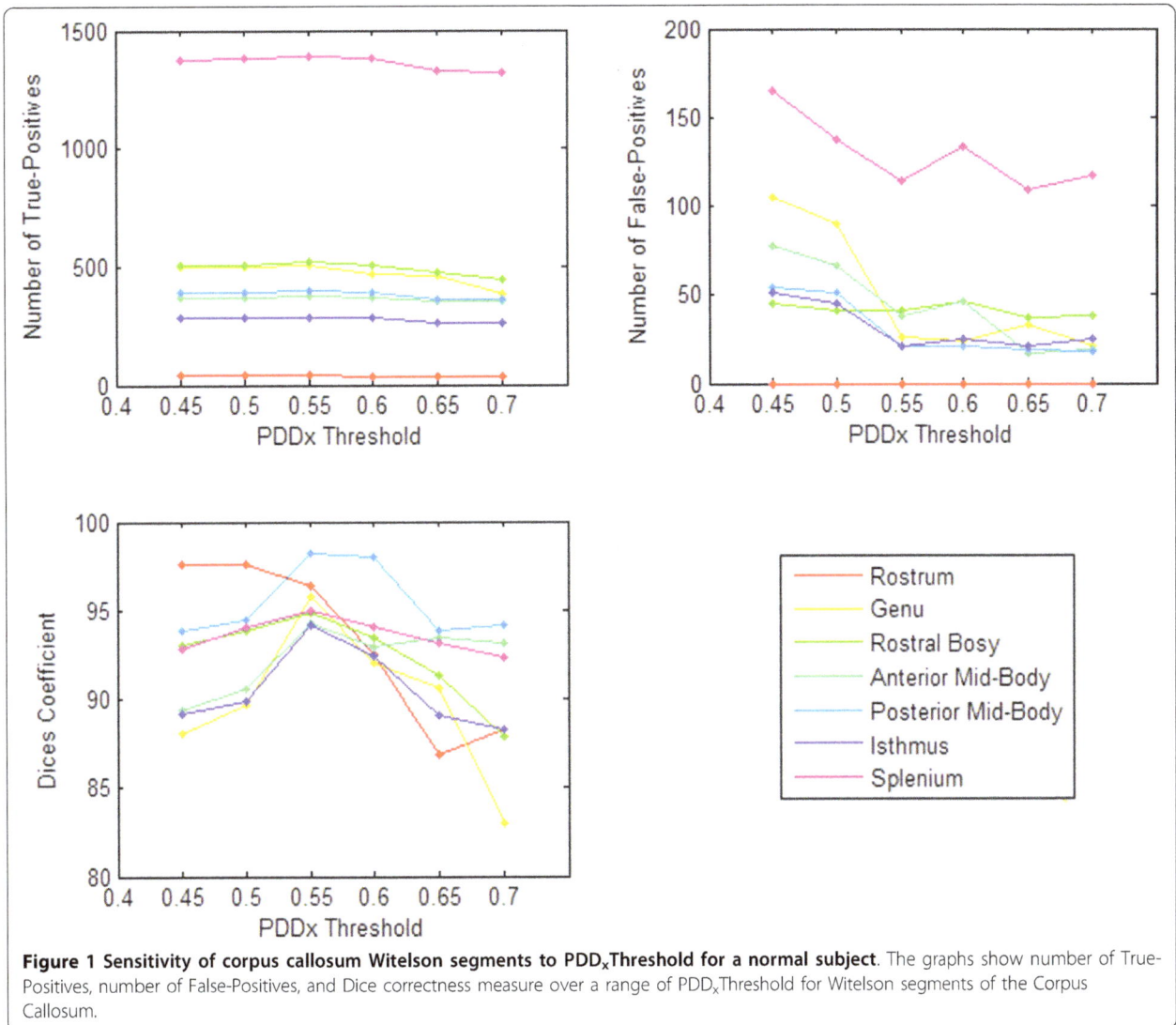

Figure 1 Sensitivity of corpus callosum Witelson segments to PDD$_x$Threshold for a normal subject. The graphs show number of True-Positives, number of False-Positives, and Dice correctness measure over a range of PDD$_x$Threshold for Witelson segments of the Corpus Callosum.

quantitatively. Table 1 shows the average Dice measures for different Witelson subdivisions of corpus callosum for the control subjects. Note that the best performance is obtained in the genu area with least penetration inside adjacent fiber bundles and the worst performance is obtained in the posterior mid-body subdivision with penetration mainly inside cingulum and tracts of corona-radiata. For the tumor patients, the performance of the Jonasson's method was poor and thus we do not present them.

Table 2 shows the average Dice measure for different Witelson subdivisions of corpus callosum in the control subjects, Group 1 patients (tumor not infiltrating corpus callosum), and Group 2 patients (tumor infiltrating corpus callosum). Dice measures ranging from 90% to 98% indicate that the automatic segmentation results generated for the control subjects and the Group 1 patients are in excellent agreement with the manual segmentation

results. For Group 2 patients where the tumors infiltrated corpus callosum, the Dice measures ranging from 81% to 92% indicate good agreements of the automatic and manual segmentation results.

Performance of the proposed method can be ascertained by visualizing the segmentation results (Figures 5, 6, 7). Figure 5 shows the segmentation results of the proposed method for 11 control subjects. Figure 6 shows the results for 12 Group 1 patients where the glioblastoma tumor does not infiltrate corpus callosum. These 12 patients were selected based on the severity of the effect of tumor on the rotation of corpus callosum. Note that although these cases include major geometric deviations from the normal state, the proposed method has successfully segmented corpus callosum and its subdivisions. Figure 7 shows the segmentation results for 7 Group 2 patients where the glioblastoma tumor has infiltrated corpus callosum. This figure illustrates that

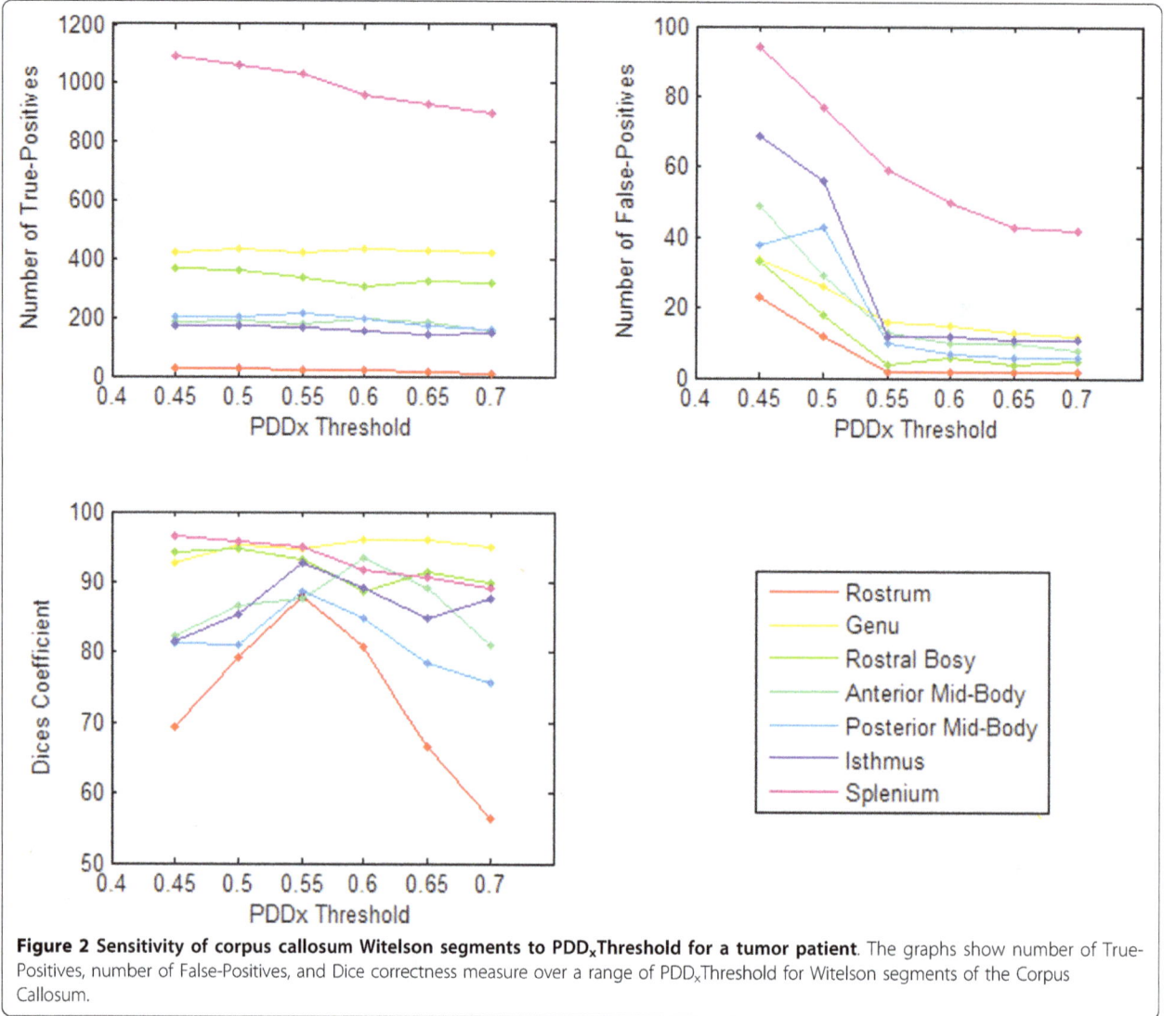

Figure 2 Sensitivity of corpus callosum Witelson segments to PDD$_x$Threshold for a tumor patient. The graphs show number of True-Positives, number of False-Positives, and Dice correctness measure over a range of PDD$_x$Threshold for Witelson segments of the Corpus Callosum.

the proposed method has successfully segmented corpus callosum and its subdivisions in these extreme cases. Note that in all cases, the segmented corpus callosum does not penetrate into the adjacent fiber bundles such as cingulum, tapetum, minor and major forceps, superior longitudinal fasciculus, or tracts of corona radiata.

Rotational effect of tumor on proposed method
We have used the geometric information of the diffusivity pattern in corpus callosum to prevent the front from penetrating into the neighboring structures. However, a tumor may change the shape and diffusivity pattern of corpus callosum from its original shape and diffusivity pattern.

To study the rotational effect of a tumor on the segmentation process, we rotate the segmented corpus callosum and its neighbors up to 5 voxels in different Euler angles (*azimuth-elevation-skew*), the tensor (T),

and the principal diffusion direction (PDD) of each voxel for all control subjects.

$$R(\varphi, \theta, \psi) = R_x(\varphi)R_y(\theta)R_z(\psi) \tag{4}$$

where R(ϕ,θ,ψ) is the rotation matrix with respect to the spherical Euler angles of ϕ,θ and ψ respectively. $R_x(\phi)$, $R_y(\theta)$, and $R_z(\psi)$ are rotational matrices for rotations around x, y, and z axes, respectively. Then,

$$(x', y', z') = R(\varphi, \theta, \psi)*(x, y, z) \tag{5}$$

where (x, y, z) is the coordinates for a voxel within a 5-voxel neighborhood of corpus callosum, while (x', y'z') is the rotated voxel coordinates.

For each of the rotated coordinates, we calculate the tensor (T) and the principal diffusion direction (PDD) by:

$$T(x', y', z') = R^t(\phi,\theta,\psi)*T(x,y,z)*R(\phi,\theta,\psi) \tag{6}$$

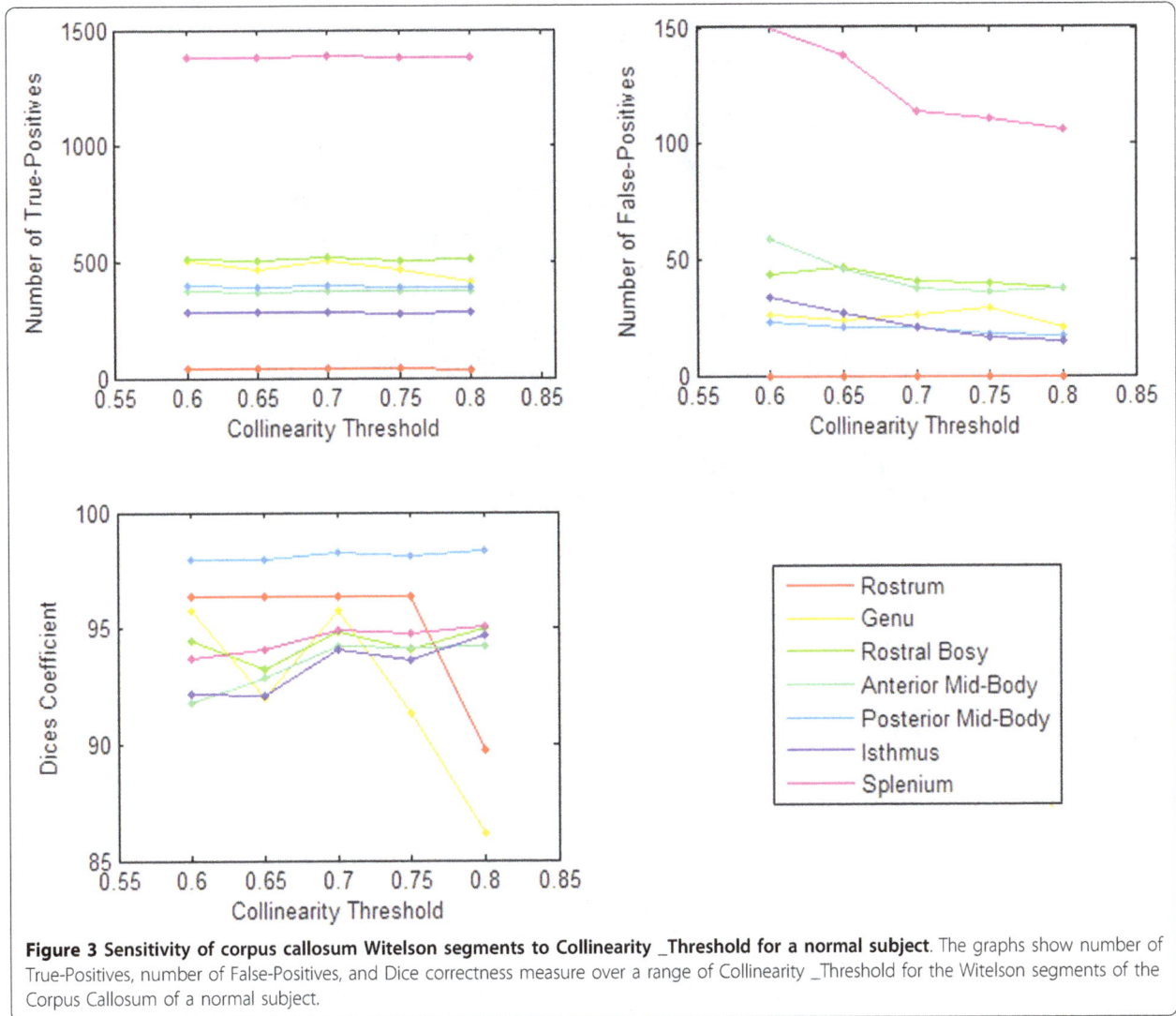

Figure 3 Sensitivity of corpus callosum Witelson segments to Collinearity _Threshold for a normal subject. The graphs show number of True-Positives, number of False-Positives, and Dice correctness measure over a range of Collinearity _Threshold for the Witelson segments of the Corpus Callosum of a normal subject.

$$PDD(x', y', z') = R(\phi, \theta, \psi) * PDD(x, y, z) \qquad (7)$$

The means and standard deviations of the Dice measures for the subdivisions of the corpus callosum rotated in different Euler angles (5, 10, 15, 20, 25, and 30 degrees) in 11 control subjects are shown in Table 3. The top, middle, and bottom rows represent the segmentation results of the rotated corpus callosum and its neighbors under different azimuth angles (around x axis), elevation angles (around y axis), and skew angles (around z axis), respectively. As can be seen from the Tables 2 and 3, the rotation of corpus callosum does not have a major effect on the segmentation results. It means that although the segmentation algorithm relies on the geometric information of corpus callosum and its diffusion pattern, it segments a corpus callosum deformed under the potential tumor pressure.

We used the Wilcoxon two sample tests to compare sensitivity of the outer subdivisions (rostrum, genu, and splenium) and the inner subdivisions (rostral body, anterior and posterior mid-body, and isthmus) of corpus callosum with respect to the rotation. For two arrays A and B, the Wilcoxon test performs a paired two-sided signed rank test of the null hypothesis that data in the vector A-B come from a symmetric distribution with zero median. P-values less than 0.01 are considered statistically significant. From the p-values in Table 4, it can be inferred that the outer subdivisions have significantly lower average Dice measures than the inner subdivision for all azimuth and elevation rotation angles (p-values less than 0.0004). For skew angles, however, the outer subdivisions do not show significantly lower average Dice measures than the inner subdivision (5 out of 6 p-values are more than 0.01). Considering the overall diffusivity inside corpus

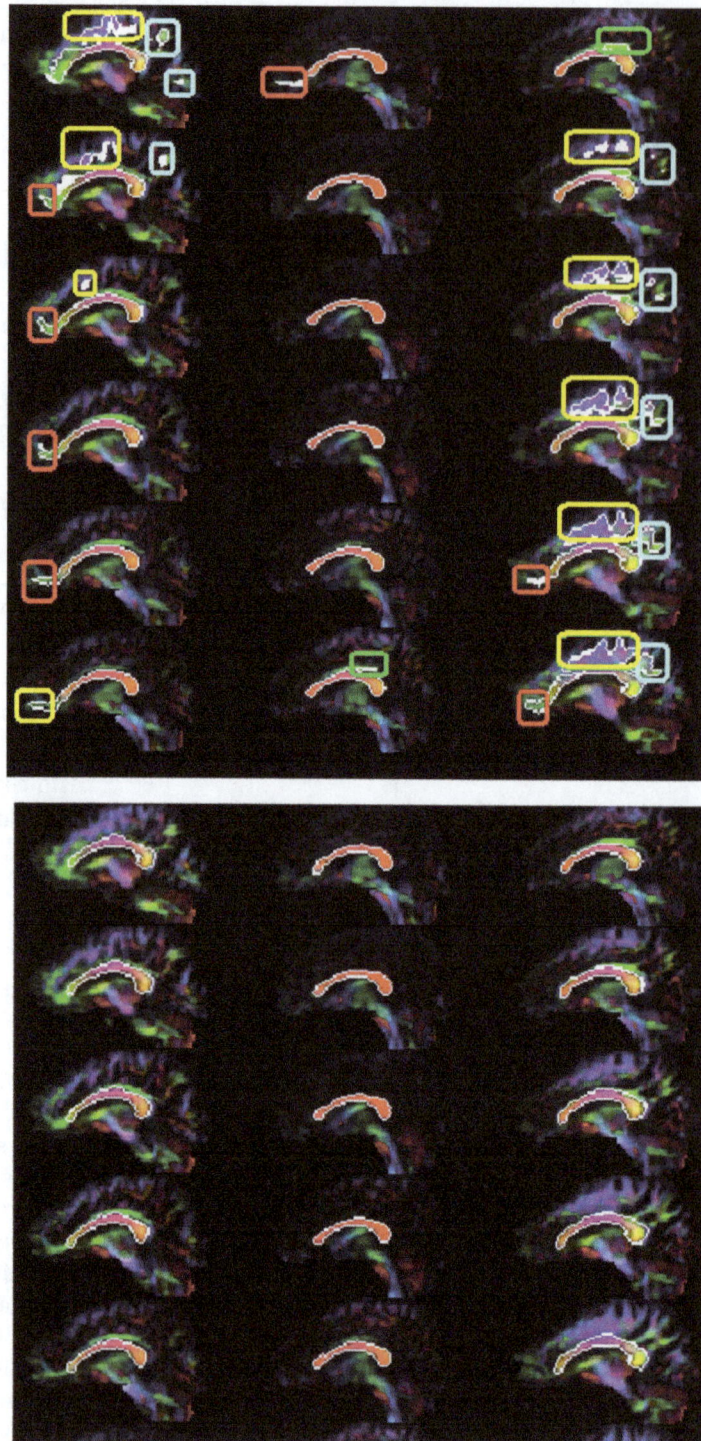

Figure 4 Comparing of corpus callosum segmentations by the proposed method and the Jonasson's method [25]. In (**a**) for the Jonasson's method, the speed threshold was chosen low enough to capture the corpus callosum structure. However, the segmentation front propagates inside irrelevant fiber structures such as superior longitudinal fasciculus (cyan rounded rectangles), cingulum (green rounded rectangles), minor forceps (red rounded rectangles), and tracts of corona-radiata (yellow rounded rectangles). In (**b**), our method segments the corpus callosum structure with high sensitivity (segmenting the whole structure) and high specificity (without major leakage into the neighboring structures).

Table 1 Comparison of the proposed method with the Jonasson's method

Witelson Subdivisions	Proposed Method	Jonasson's Method
Rostrum	94.41	75.15
Genu	98.25	91.24
Rostral Body	97.27	83.10
Anterior Mid-Body	95.44	79.33
Posterior Mid-Body	96.07	71.54
Isthmus	94.24	81.46
Splenium	97.29	80.25

The average Dice measures for different Witelson subdivisions of the corpus callosum for the control subjects. Note that the best performance is obtained in the genu area with least penetration inside adjacent fiber bundles, and the worst performance is obtained in the posterior mid-body subdivision with penetration mainly inside cingulum and tracts of corona-radiata.

callosum perpendicular to its main axis, the overall diffusivity pattern changes more dramatically around the x and y axes (azimuth and elevation) than around the z axis (skew). Therefore, the segmentation results are more sensitive to rotations in the azimuth and elevation directions. Figures 8, 9 and 10 show the segmentation results of the proposed method for the corpus callosum and its neighbors rotated 30° in the azimuth, elevation, and skew directions, respectively.

Discussion

Novel aspects of proposed method

1. New similarity measure based on local diffusion characteristics

The proposed method is more accurate than the tensor-based method that uses the NTSP similarity measure [25]. Comparing with the manual segmentation by experts, we demonstrated accuracy of our proposed method even when the tumor infiltrates corpus callosum.

Table 2 Average Dice measures for different Witelson subdivisions of the corpus callosum

Witelson Subdivisions	Control Subjects	Group 1 Patients	Group 2 Patients
Rostrum	94.41	94.04	90.72
Genu	98.25	94.99	92.61
Rostral Body	97.27	94.05	84.73
Anterior Mid-Body	95.44	91.45	81.58
Posterior Mid-Body	96.07	94.1	83.29
Isthmus	94.24	94.57	85.09
Splenium	97.29	90.16	89.56

The subjects are classified to control subjects, Group 1 patients with tumors not infiltrating the corpus callosum, and Group 2 patients with tumors infiltrating the corpus callosum. Note that the high quality of the results for the control subjects as well as the tumor patients.

2. 3D segmentation of the entire corpus callosum

The proposed method works in 3D. Extraction of diffusion indices such as mean diffusivity and fractional anisotropy over the entire corpus callosum generates a reliable quantification of the structure that cannot be achieved by an analysis of the mid-sagittal plane only [4-7].

3. Preventing from penetrating inside neighboring fiber bundles

An optimal set of parameters is chosen to segment the entire corpus callosum (with high sensitivity) without penetrating into adjacent fiber structures (with high specificity). We have used *Collinearity_Threshold* to prevent the front from penetrating into cingulum. The threshold for the x-component of the principal diffusion direction ($PDD_x\_Threshold$) is used to prevent the front from propagating into major and minor forceps. *FA_Threshold* is also important to prevent from penetrating inside tapetum (as in general, it has diffusivity patterns similar to corpus callosum in crossing areas with lower FA values). To segment the entire corpus callosum in patients with low FA values, one should choose *FA_Threshold* and *F_Threshold* quite small. However, one should be cautious that in this case, the front may propagate outside of white matter in some areas.

4. Automatically extracting Witelson subdivisions of corpus callosum

The proposed method defines Witelson subdivisions of corpus callosum automatically.

5. Applicability to glioblastoma tumor patients as well as normal subjects using the same set of parameters

The proposed method has successfully segmented corpus callosum and its subdivisions in diffusions MRI data of normal subjects and brain tumor patients.

6. Evaluating potential effects of tumor on segmentation of corpus callosum

Depending on size, shape, type and proximity to the corpus callosum, the glioblastoma tumor may cause rotation, shrinkage or more severe disruptions like tearing of the corpus callosum fibers. Amongst the mentioned effects, we evaluated the linear rotational effect of tumor on corpus callosum. With this simplification and without loss of generality, we showed that the change in diffusivity pattern due to a tumor does not change the segmentation accuracy dramatically. However, if the effect of tumor infiltration inside the corpus callosum is sever and changes the structure dramatically, it may be impossible to segment the structure entirely and accurately.

Selection of initial seeds

The proposed segmentation method is seed-based and needs the initial seed points for hyper-surface to propagate. This requires the operators to define the seeds

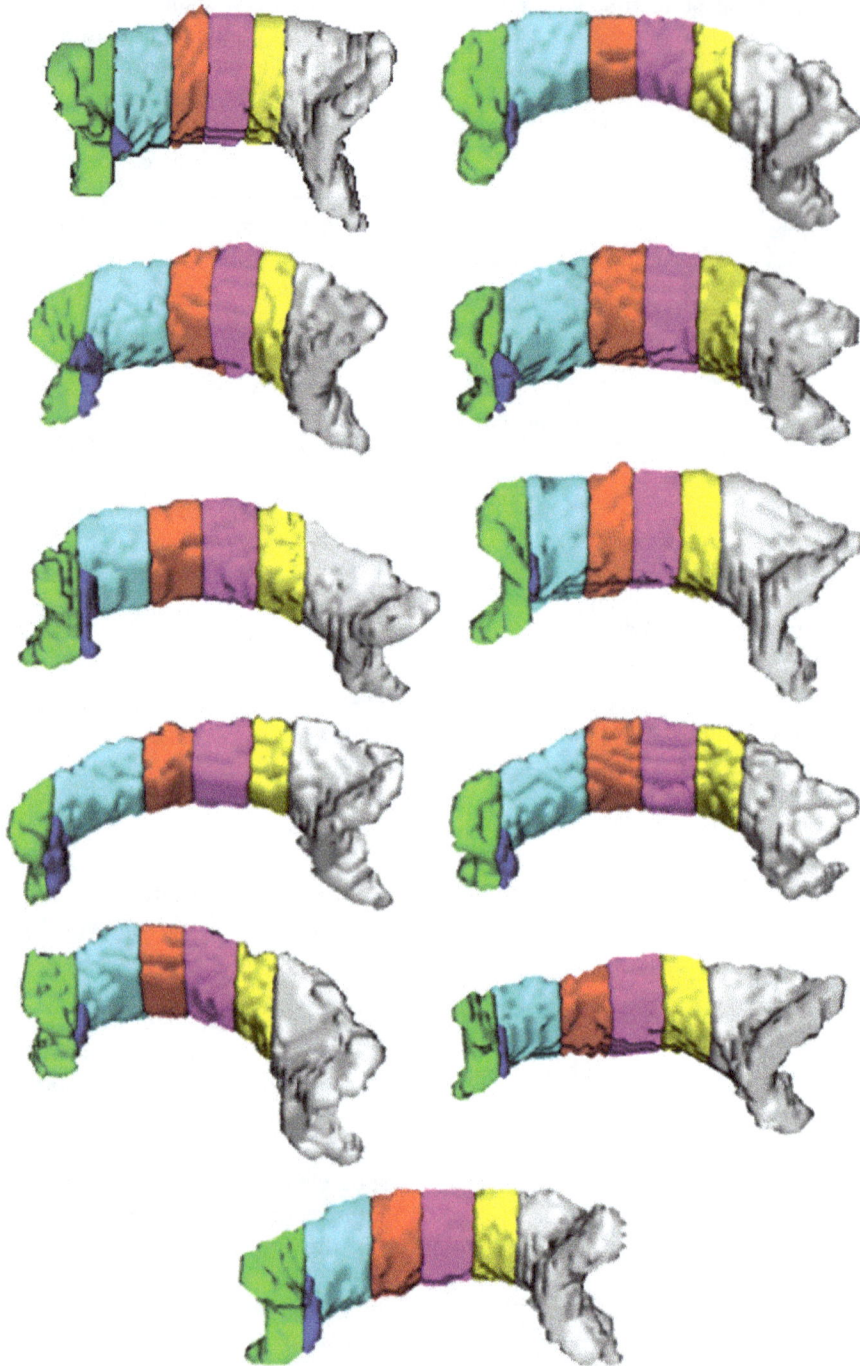

Figure 5 Segmented corpus callosum by the proposed method for 11 control subjects. The colors show the Witelson subdivisions results for the corpus callosum. Rostrum: blue, Genu: green, Rostral Body: cyan, Anterior Mid-body: red, Posterior Mid-body: turquoise, Isthmus: yellow, Splenium: gray.

manually using anatomical landmarks. To automate the process, the initial seeds may be obtained from fiber atlases of control subjects [34,44]. However, when segmenting fiber bundles of pathological cases, abnormalities like tumors may change the fiber bundles and thus conventional atlas registration methods may not be

applicable. To solve this problem, Zacharaki et al. [45] proposed a method for transferring structural and functional information from neuro-anatomical brain atlases into individual patient's data. Application of such methods in our case of segmenting corpus callosum in patients with tumors would be still in question.

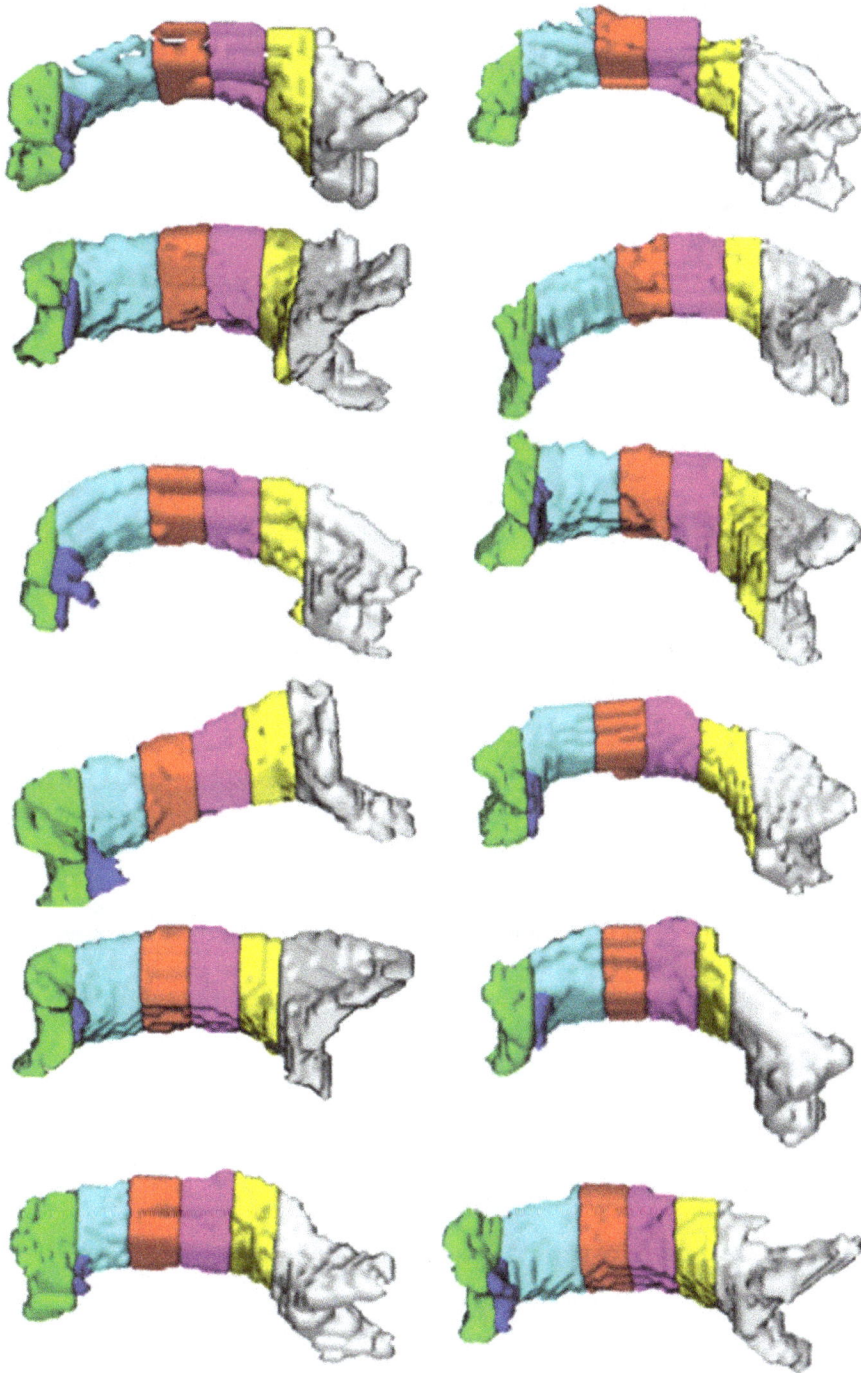

Figure 6 Segmented corpus callosum by the proposed method for 12 glioblastoma patients with non-infiltrating tumors. The colors show the Witelson subdivisions results for the corpus callosum. Rostrum: blue, Genu: green, Rostral Body: cyan, Anterior Mid-body: red, Posterior Mid-body: turquoise, Isthmus: yellow, Splenium: gray.

Segmentation of fiber structures in HARDI

Since the tensor model is not capable of describing heterogeneous diffusion behavior in crossing fiber bundles, some studies segmented the desired fiber bundles using HARDI data. Generalizing the level-set method presented in [22] to the HARDI data, Descoteaux and Deriche [35] applied a region-based statistical surface evolution to the image of the ODFs to find coherent white matter fiber bundles. This is equivalent to the maximization of a posteriori probability which obtains

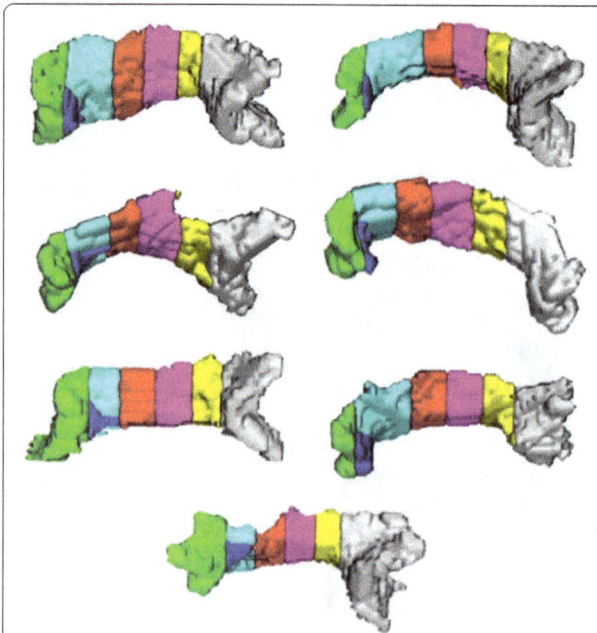

Figure 7 Segmented corpus callosum by the proposed method for 7 glioblastoma patients with infiltrating tumors. The colors show the Witelson subdivisions results for the corpus callosum. Rostrum: blue, Genu: green, Rostral Body: cyan, Anterior Mid-body: red, Posterior Mid-body: turquoise, Isthmus: yellow, Splenium: gray.

Table 4 The *p*-value of Wilcoxon two-sample tests between outer (rostrum, genu, and splenium) and inner (rostral body, anterior and posterior mid-body, and isthmus) subdivisions of corpus callosum

	Azimuth Rotation Angle					
	5	10	15	20	25	30
P-value	8.2E-05	8.1E-05	8.1E-05	7.1E-03	8.2E-05	8.2E-05
	Elevation Rotation Angle					
	5	10	15	20	25	30
P-value	8.2E-05	3.9E-04	1.4E-04	8.2E-05	8.0E-05	8.2E-05
	Skew Rotation Angle					
	5	10	15	20	25	30
P-value	7.6E-02	8.2E-02	9.2E-01	2.4E-04	5.8E-03	3.6E-02

The outer subdivisions have significantly lower average Dice measures than the inner subdivision for all azimuth and elevation rotation angles (p-values less than 0.0004). For skew angles, however, the outer subdivisions do not show significantly lower average Dice measures than the inner subdivision (5 out of 6 p-values are more than 0.01). See Table 3 for the means and standard deviations of the 11 subjects.

the desired segmentation for the observed ODFs and presumes Gaussian distributions in different partitions of the Q-ball images. Although their method appropriately propagates through the regions of fiber crossings, it propagates the hyper-surface inside all of the crossing fiber bundles and segments them as a whole, not individually. They applied their method to extract corpus callosum and tracts of corona-radiata. However, their

Table 3 Means and standard deviations of the Dice measures in 11 normal subjects where corpus callosum subdivisions are rotated under different Euler angles

Witelson Subdivisions of Corpus Callosum		Rostrum	Genu	Rostral Body	Anterior Mid-Body	Posterior Mid-Body	Isthmus	Splenium
Azimuth Rotation Angle	5	94.51 ± 1.15	96.46 ± 1.43	99.07 ± 0.84	98.48 ± 0.77	99.28 ± 0.56	96.84 ± 0.91	96.23 ± 0.93
	10	91.44 ± 0.99	95.48 ± 0.98	95.02 ± 1.13	95.45 ± 0.99	97.36 ± 1.03	96.27 ± 0.93	94.11 ± 1.01
	15	91.00 ± 1.47	90.77 ± 1.15	94.17 ± 0.95	94.47 ± 0.96	94.97 ± 0.70	92.84 ± 1.01	90.55 ± 0.97
	20	88.29 ± 1.24	89.33 ± 1.07	89.65 ± 0.75	90.61 ± 1.23	88.86 ± 0.86	89.18 ± 1.23	88.40 ± 1.06
	25	84.24 ± 1.03	88.47 ± 1.12	89.16 ± 0.86	87.32 ± 1.03	88.83 ± 1.06	89.01 ± 1.49	84.69 ± 1.20
	30	80.16 ± 1.70	82.96 ± 1.23	85.09 ± 1.21	85.45 ± 1.13	85.36 ± 0.98	83.07 ± 1.11	81.23 ± 0.97
Elevation Rotation Angle	5	93.64 ± 0.92	96.29 ± 1.28	97.75 ± 0.97	96.91 ± 1.02	98.65 ± 1.16	96.29 ± 0.72	95.83 ± 1.09
	10	91.27 ± 0.88	96.24 ± 1.08	97.74 ± 1.00	95.46 ± 1.06	94.14 ± 1.09	91.56 ± 1.17	91.96 ± 1.41
	15	87.75 ± 0.86	95.28 ± 1.15	93.86 ± 0.89	93.81 ± 0.97	94.95 ± 0.83	89.30 ± 0.91	91.08 ± 1.14
	20	85.37 ± 1.01	92.58 ± 0.77	90.59 ± 0.89	89.98 ± 1.29	92.51 ± 1.05	87.36 ± 1.32	86.29 ± 0.88
	25	83.47 ± 0.90	86.67 ± 0.77	86.25 ± 1.32	89.27 ± 1.17	87.66 ± 0.99	84.88 ± 1.27	84.48 ± 1.10
	30	79.39 ± 1.29	81.60 ± 1.10	85.00 ± 1.10	84.35 ± 1.01	85.22 ± 1.03	83.41 ± 0.88	81.58 ± 0.89
Skew Rotation Angle	5	97.96 ± 1.09	98.75 ± 0.63	99.09 ± 0.68	98.00 ± 1.07	98.73 ± 1.00	96.62 ± 0.73	98.85 ± 0.59
	10	95.29 ± 1.12	96.38 ± 0.80	94.72 ± 1.04	94.46 ± 1.45	94.80 ± 1.28	94.98 ± 1.00	94.21 ± 0.88
	15	91.88 ± 1.04	95.00 ± 1.34	92.56 ± 1.16	94.22 ± 0.97	92.73 ± 1.31	94.72 ± 1.44	93.66 ± 1.01
	20	89.79 ± 0.83	87.92 ± 1.18	85.83 ± 1.29	88.35 ± 1.16	86.99 ± 1.27	87.85 ± 0.98	89.28 ± 1.16
	25	87.55 ± 1.22	86.11 ± 1.21	85.73 ± 1.08	86.34 ± 1.28	86.22 ± 1.08	85.55 ± 1.27	87.35 ± 0.87
	30	84.61 ± 1.17	83.39 ± 0.89	84.58 ± 1.13	84.09 ± 1.03	85.26 ± 1.12	86.43 ± 1.16	85.00 ± 1.00

It can be inferred that the rotation of corpus callosum does not have a major effect on the segmentation results.

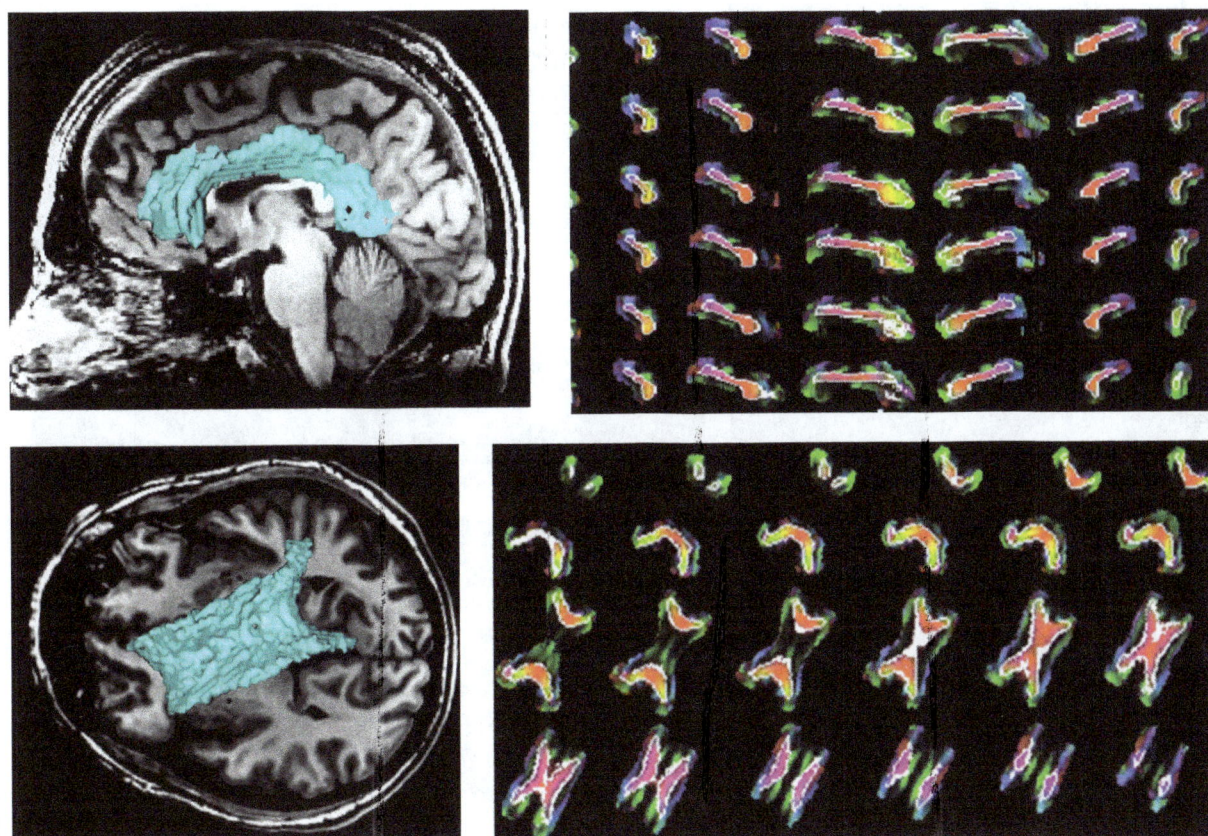

Figure 8 Segmentation results by the proposed method for a normal corpus callosum and its neighbors rotated 30° under the azimuth angle. (**a**), (**b**): Segmented corpus callosum in green overlaid on the T1 sagittal and axial images, respectively. (**c**), (**d**): Boundaries of the corpus callosum delineated in white in the sagittal and axial slices, respectively, overlaid on the color coding of the principal diffusion direction in each pixel.

method is sensitive to initial seeds and suffers from limited anatomical knowledge of the operator who defines the seeds. In another study, a k-means algorithm has been employed to find the clusters using Euclidean distance as dissimilarity measure [36].

In a different study, a Position-Orientation Space (POS) is introduced by combining the geometric space with the spherical ODF space from the HARDI data, where two crossing fiber populations with different orientations in the spatial domain are resolved by applying a front propagation method in the level-set framework in a five-dimensional space [32]. Hagmann et al. [36] performed fiber bundle segmentation in POS based on the Markov Random Fields (MRF). In a similar study, McGraw et al. [37] proposed a mixture of von Mises-Fisher distributions to model the ODF again in MRF. Assuming that the spatial relationships are modeled by the MRF, this method estimates a hidden random field of fiber bundles from the observed ODF profiles using a Maximum a Posteriori (MAP) formulation. However, dimensional reinforcement of the

problem causes disadvantages such as increasing the computational cost.

Using Spherical Harmonic Coefficients (SHC) as features of functions on the sphere [38], a method has been proposed for fiber bundle segmentation [33]. However, without masking the speed term with a measure of anisotropy (such as FA) that has low values in the crossing areas, the growing hyper-surface may penetrate into irrelevant fiber bundles that have common areas with the bundle of interest. In another work [34], the authors proposed an atlas-based method introducing a novel similarity based on PDD's and spherical harmonic coefficients. Integrating PDD's into the framework, along with a proper PDD-selection algorithm, leads to the segmentation of most of important fiber bundles in the brain without penetration into irrelevant fiber bundles that have common areas with the bundle of interest. Using an atlas [44] to find the initial seeds for the fiber bundles, the proposed method overcomes limitations of the semi-automatic methods that suffer from limited anatomical knowledge and subjectivity of the operator

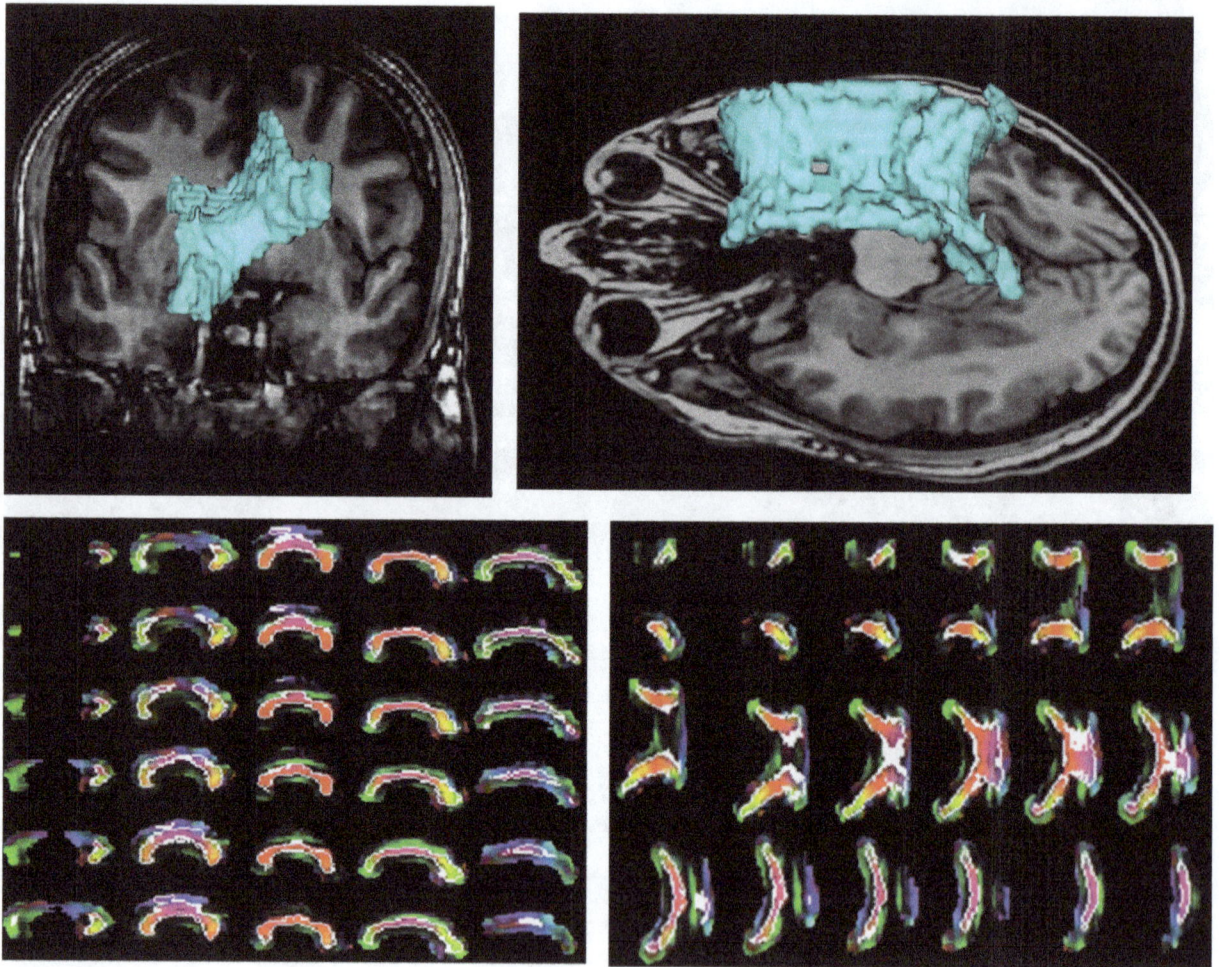

Figure 9 Segmentation results by the proposed method for a normal corpus callosum and its neighbors rotated 30° under the elevation angle. (a), (b): Segmented corpus callosum in green overlaid on the T1 sagittal and axial images, respectively. (c), (d): Boundaries of the corpus callosum delineated in white in the sagittal and axial slices, respectively, overlaid on the color coding of the principal diffusion direction in each pixel.

who defines the seed voxels. Note that since the number of diffusion measurements in the tensor data is not adequate for fitting SHC and estimating more than one PDD, we used the same methods originally applied on the HARDI data.

Although the success of recent studies in segmenting fiber bundles in the HARDI data is promising, such protocol in not being widely used in clinical centers. On the other hand, diffusion tensor imaging is clinically feasible and thus the tensor-based methods are of more interest.

Conclusion

In this paper, we have proposed a 3D method based on a new DTI similarity measure to segment corpus callosum and determine its subdivisions. The method propagates a hyper-surface within corpus callosum without

penetration into the neighboring fiber bundles. Segmentation of corpus callosum, the largest commissural fiber bundle in the brain, makes it possible to quantify various diffusion characteristics in its subdivisions, opening new perspectives for monitoring disease evolution or prognosis.

Ethics statement

MRI and other data of the tumor patients originally acquired for patient care are retrospectively and anonymously used in this research to train, test, and evaluate the proposed methods. This usage was reviewed and approved by the Institutional Review Board (IRB) committee of Henry Ford Hospital, Detroit, Michigan, USA. Details of the data and results are described in the manuscript.

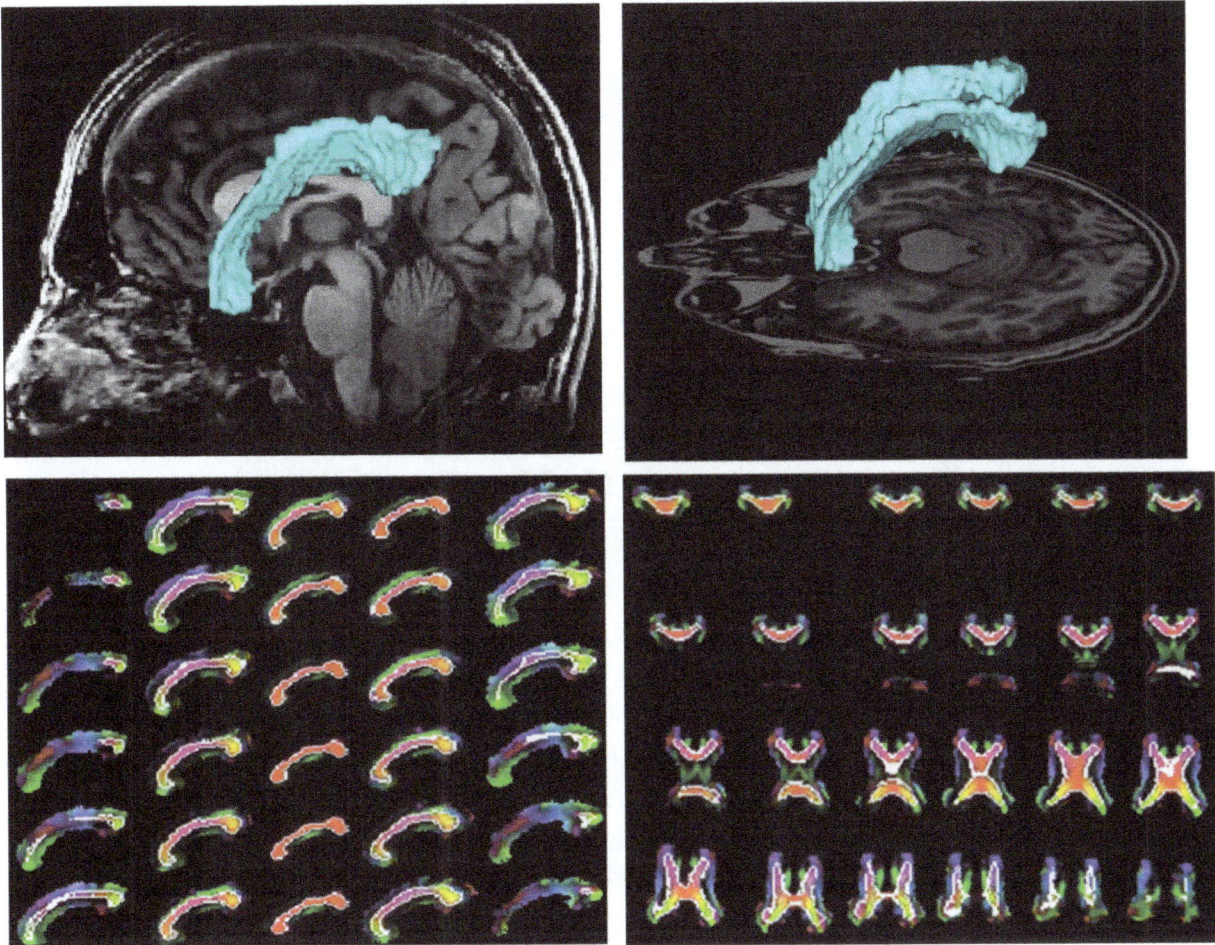

Figure 10 Segmentation results by the proposed method for a normal corpus callosum and its neighbors rotated 30° under the skew angle. (**a**), (**b**): Segmented corpus callosum in green overlaid on the T1 sagittal and axial images, respectively. (**c**), (**d**): Boundaries of the corpus callosum delineated in white in the sagittal and axial slices, respectively, overlaid on the color coding of the principal diffusion direction in each pixel.

Author details
[1]Control and Intelligent Processing Center of Excellence, School of Electrical and Computer Engineering, University of Tehran, Tehran 14399, Iran. [2]Department of Radiation Oncology and Radiology, University of Michigan, Ann Arbor, MI 48109-0010, USA. [3]Department of Neurology, Henry Ford Health System, Detroit, MI 48202, USA. [4]Department of Radiology, Henry Ford Health System, Detroit MI 48202, USA. [5]Washington University School of Medicine, Mallinckrodt Institute of Radiology, St. Louis MO 63110, USA. [6]Department of Radiology, Wayne State University, Detroit, MI 48202, USA. [7]Department of Neurosurgery, Henry Ford Health System, Detroit, MI 48202, USA.

Authors' contributions
MN implemented the algorithms presented in the manuscript, tested the algorithms, and prepared the first draft of the manuscript. RJ participated in the design and coordination of the study, helped with the testing and evaluation of the proposed method, and revised the manuscript. SS contributed to the manual segmentation, revision of the manuscript, and final evaluation of the results. AB performed the statistics on the segmentation results. HS contributed to the revision of the manuscript and analysis of the results. MR, QJ, TM contributed to the image acquisition,

selection of the cases, and classifying them into different groups. All authors read and approved the final manuscript.

Competing interests
The authors declare that they have no competing interests.

References
1. de Lacoste MC, Kirkpatrick JB, Ross ED: **Topography of the human corpus callosum.** *J Neuropathol Exp Neurol* 1985, **44**:578-591.
2. Clarke S, Miklossy J: **Occipital cortex in man: organization of callosal connections, related myelo- and cytoarchitecture, and putative boundaries of functional visual areas.** *J Comp Neurol* 1990, **298**:188-214.
3. Dorion A, Chantôme M, Hasboun D, *et al*: **Hemispheric asymmetry and corpus callosum morphometry: a magnetic resonance imaging study.** *Neuroscience Research* 2000, **36**:9-13.
4. Hasan K, Gupta R, Santos R, Wolinsky J, Narayana P: **Diffusion tensor fractional anisotropy of the normal-appearing seven segments of the corpus callosum in healthy adults and relapsing-remitting multiple sclerosis patients.** *Journal of Magnetic Resonance Imaging* 2005, **21**:735-743.
5. Gupta R, Saksena S, Hasan K, *et al*: **Focal Wallerian degeneration of the corpus callosum in large middle cerebral artery stroke: serial diffusion tensor imaging.** *Journal of Magnetic Resonance Imaging* 2006, **24**:549-555.

6. Kubicki M, Styner M, Bouix S, *et al*: **Reduced interhemispheric connectivity in schizophrenia-tractography based segmentation of the corpus callosum.** *Schizophrenia research* 2008, **106**:125-131.

7. Rosas HD, Lee SY, Bender AC, Zaleta AK, Vangel M, Yu P, Fischl B, Pappu V, Onorato C, Cha JH, Salat DH, Hersch SM: **Altered white matter microstructure in the corpus callosum in Huntington's disease: Implications for cortical.** *Neuroimage* 2010, **49**:2995-3004.

8. Lundervold A, Duta N: *Taxt T.* Jain A: **Model-guided segmentation of corpus callosum in MR images.** *Citeseer* 1999, 231-237.

9. Lee C, Huh S, Ketter T, Unser M: **Automated segmentation of the corpus callosum in midsagittal brain magnetic resonance images.** *Optical Engineering* 2000, **39**:924-935.

10. Brejl M, Sonka M: **Object localization and border detection criteria design in edge-based image segmentation: automated learning from examples.** *IEEE Transactions on Medical Imaging* 2000, **19**:973-985.

11. Basser P, Mattiello J, Le Bihan D: **MR diffusion tensor spectroscopy and imaging.** *Biophys* 1994, **66**:259-267.

12. Basser P, Mattiello J, Le Bihan D: **Estimation of the effective self-diffusion tensor from the NMR spin echo.** *J Magn Reson* 1994, **103**:247-254.

13. Brun A, Knutsson H, Park H, Shenton M, Westin C: **Clustering fiber traces using normalized cuts.** *MICCAI LNCS* 2004, **3216**:368-375.

14. Maddah M, Grimson W, Warfield S, Wells W: **A unified framework for clustering quantitative analysis of white matter fiber tracts.** *Med Imag Analysis* 2008, **12**:191-202.

15. Xu Q, Anderson A, Gore J, Ding Z: **Unified Bundling and Registration of Brain White Matter Fibers.** *IEEE Transactions on Medical Imaging* 2009, **28**(9):1399-1411.

16. Voineskos A, Rajji T, Lobaugh N, *et al*: **Age-related decline in white matter tract integrity and cognitive performance: A DTI tractography and structural equation modeling study.** *Neurobiology of Aging* 2010, doi:10.1016/j.neurobiolaging.2010.02.009.

17. Wassermann D, Bloy L, Kanterakis E, Verma R, Deriche R: **Unsupervised white matter fiber clustering and tract probability map generation: Applications of a Gaussian process framework for white matter fibers.** *Neuroimage* 2010, **51**(1):228-241.

18. Li H, Xue Z, Guo L, Liu T, Hunter J, Wong S: **A hybrid approach to automatic clustering of white matter fibers.** *Neuroimage* 2010, **49**:1249-1258.

19. Eckstein I, Shattuck D, Stein J, *et al*: **Active fibers: Matching deformable tract templates to diffusion tensor images.** *Neuroimage* 2009, **47**:82-89.

20. Zhukov L, Museth K, Breen D, Whitaker R, Barr A: **Level set modeling and segmentation of DT-MRI brain data.** *J Electron Imag* 2003, **12**:125-133.

21. Vemuri B, Chen Y, McGraw T, Wang Z, Mareci T: **Fiber tract mapping from diffusion tensor MRI.** *Proc IEEE Workshop on Variational and Level Set Methods in Computer Vision* 2001, 81-88.

22. Wang Z, Vemuri B: **Tensor field segmentation using region based active contour model.** *ECCV LNCS* 2004, **3024**:304-315.

23. Rousson M, Lenglet C, Deriche R: **Level set and region based surface propagation for diffusion tensor MRI segmentation.** *Computer vision and mathematical methods in medical and biomedical image analysis* 2004, 123-134.

24. Feddern C, Weickert J, Burgeth B: *Level set methods for tensor valued images* 2003, 65-72, Geometric and Level Set Methods in Computer Vision: In Proceedings of the Second IEEE Workshop on Variational.

25. Jonasson L, Bresson X, Hagmann P, Cuisenaire O, Meuli R, Thiran J: **White matter fiber tract segmentation in DT-MRI using geometric flows.** *Med Imag Analysis* 2005, **3**:223-236.

26. Jonasson L, Hagmann P, Pollo C, Bresson X, Wilson C, Meuli R, Thiran J: **A level set method for segmentation of the thalamus and its nuclei in DT-MRI.** *Signal Processing* 2007, **87**:309-321.

27. Lenglet C, Rousson M, Deriche R: **A statistical framework for DTI segmentation.** *IEEE Trans Med Imag* 2006, **25**:675-700.

28. Arsigny V, Fillard P, Pennec X, Ayache N: **Log-Euclidean metrics for fast and simple calculus on diffusion tensors.** *Magnetic Resonance in Medicine* 2006, **56**:411-421.

29. Weldeselassie Y, Hamarneh G: **DT-MRI segmentation using graph cuts.** *Citeseer: 65121 K-65121* .

30. Awate S, Hui Z, Gee J: **A fuzzy, nonparametric segmentation framework for DTI and MRI analysis: With applications to DTI-tract extraction.** *IEEE Transactions on Medical Imaging* 2007, **26**:1525-1536.

31. Hasan K, Ewing-Cobbs L, Kramer L, Fletcher J, Narayana P: **Diffusion tensor quantification of the macrostructure and microstructure of human midsagittal corpus callosum across the lifespan.** *NMR in Biomedicine* 2008, **21**:1094-1101.

32. Jonasson L, Bresson X, Thiran J, Wedeen V, Hagmann P: **Representing diffusion MRI in 5-D simplifies regularization and segmentation of white matter tracts.** *IEEE Trans On Med Imaging* 2007, **26**:1547-1554.

33. Nazem-Zadeh M, Davoodi-Bojd E, Soltanian-Zadeh H: **Level set fiber bundle segmentation using spherical harmonic coefficients.** *Computerized Medical Imaging and Graphics* 2010, **34**:192-202.

34. Nazem-Zadeh M, Davoodi-Bojd E, Soltanian-Zadeh H: **Atlas-Based Fiber Bundle Segmentation Using Principal Diffusion Directions and Spherical Harmonic Coefficients.** *NeuroImage* 2011, **54**:246-164, Supplement 1.

35. Descoteaux M, Deriche R: **High angular resolution diffusion MRI segmentation using region-based statistical surface evolution.** *Journal of Mathematical Imaging and Vision* 2008, **33**(2):239-252.

36. Hagmann P, Jonasson L, Deffieux T, Meuli R, Thiran J, Wedeen V: **Fibertract segmentation in position orientation space from high angular resolution diffusion MRI.** *Neuroimage* 2006, **32**:665-675.

37. McGraw T, Vemuri B, Yezierski R, Mareci T: **Segmentation of High Angular Resolution Diffusion MRI modeled as a field of von mises-fisher mixtures.** *Proc European Conf on Computer Vision* 2006, 463-475.

38. Hess C, Mukherjee P, Han E, Xu D, Vigneron D: **Q-ball reconstruction of multimodal fiber orientations using the spherical harmonic basis.** *Magn Reson Med* 2006, **56**:104-117.

39. Witelson S: **Hand and sex differences in the isthmus and genu of the human corpus callosum: a postmortem morphological study.** *Brain* 1989, **112**:799.

40. Lee S, Cheng J, Chen C, Tseng W: **An automatic segmentation approach for boundary delineation of corpus callosum based on cell competition.** *Proc Engineering in Medicine and Biology Society Conf of the IEEE* 2008, 5514-5517.

41. Osher S, Sethian J: **Fronts propagating with curvature dependent speed: algorithms based on Hamilton-Jacobi formulations.** *J Comput Phys* 1988, **79**:12-49.

42. Osher S, Paragios N: **Chapter: Level set methods. Geometric level set methods in imaging, vision, and graphics.** *Springer-Verlag New York Inc* 2003, 3-20.

43. Dice LR: **Measures of the amount of ecologic association between species.** *Ecology* 1945, **26**:297-302.

44. Wakana S, Caprihan A, Panzenboeck M, *et al*: **Reproducibility of quantitative tractography methods applied to cerebral white matter.** *Neuroimage* 2007, **36**:630-644.

45. Zacharaki E, Hogea C, Shen D, Biros G, Davatzikos C: **Non-diffeomorphic registration of brain tumor images by simulating tissue loss and tumor growth.** *Neuroimage* 2009, **46**:762-774.

Permissions

List of Contributors

Elin Trägårdh, David Jakobsson and Lars Edenbrandt
Clinical Physiology and Nuclear Medicine Unit, Skåne University Hospital, Lund University, Malmö, Sweden

Karl Sjöstrand
Informatics and Mathematical Modeling, Technical University of Denmark, Copenhagen, Denmark

Tomoyuki Minezawa, Takuya Okamura, Sayako Morikawa, Teppei Yamaguchi, Yoshikazu Niwa, Tomoko Takeyama, Yuki Mieno, Tami Hoshino, Sakurako Uozu, Yasuhiro Goto, Masamichi Hayashi, Sumito Isogai, Toru Nakanishi and Kazuyoshi Imaizumi
Division of Respiratory Medicine and Clinical Allergy, Department of Internal Medicine, Fujita Health University, 1-98 Dengakugakubo, Kutsukake-cho, Toyoake, Aichi 470-1192, Japan

Hiroshi Yatsuya
Department of Public Health, Fujita Health University, Toyoake, Aichi, Japan

Naoki Yamamoto
Laboratory of Molecular Biology & Histochemistry, Fujita Health University, Toyoake, Aichi, Japan

Naozumi Hashimoto and Mariko Morishita
Department of Respiratory Medicine, Nagoya University Graduate School of Medicine, Nagoya, Japan

Masaki Matsuo
Department of Respiratory Medicine, Chubu Rosai Hospital, Nagoya, Japan.

Mitsushi Okazawa
Department of Respiratory Medicine, Daiyu-kai Hospital, Ichinomiya, Aichi, Japan

Jan Erik Otterstad
Department of Cardiology, Vestfold Hospital Trust, 3103 Tønsberg, Norway

Ingvild Billehaug Norum and Vidar Ruddox
University of Oslo, Faculty of Medicine, Pb 1078 Blindern, 0316 Oslo, Norway

Department of Cardiology, Vestfold Hospital Trust, 3103 Tønsberg, Norway

Thor Edvardsen
Department of Cardiology, Oslo University Hospital, Rikshospitalet, Nydalen, 0424 Oslo, Norway
University of Oslo, Faculty of Medicine, Pb 1078 Blindern, 0316 Oslo, Norway

Örjan Smedby
Department of Medical and Health Sciences (IMH), Linköping University, Linköping, Sweden

S. Ehsan Saffari
Sabzevar University of Medical Sciences, Sabzevar, Iran
Department of Medical and Health Sciences (IMH), Linköping University, Linköping, Sweden

Áskell Löve
Department of Diagnostic Radiology, Lund University, Clinical Sciences, Lund, Sweden
Department of Radiology, Landspitali University Hospital, Reykjavik and Faculty of Medicine, University of Iceland, Reykjavik, Iceland

Mats Fredrikson
Department of Clinical and Experimental Medicine, Linköping University, Linköping, Sweden

Örjan Smedby
KTH Royal Institute of Technology, School of Technology and Health, Alfred Nobels allé 10, SE-141 52 Huddinge, Stockholm, Sweden

Jing-xin Zhao
Department of Orthopedics, Chinese PLA 82nd Hospital, No.100 East Jiankang Road, Qinghe District, Huai'an, Jiangsu Province 223001, People's Republic of China

Pei-fu Tang, Li-hai Zhang, Hai-long Du, Li-ning Zhang and Li-cheng Zhang
Department of Orthopedics, Chinese PLA General Hospital, No.28 Fuxing Road, Beijing, Haidian District 100853, People's Republic of China

Zhe Zhao
Department of Orthopedics, Beijing Tsinghua Chang Gung Hospital, No.1 Block Tiantongyuan North, Beijing 102218, People's Republic of China
Department of Orthopedics, Chinese PLA General Hospital, No.28 Fuxing Road, Beijing, Haidian District 100853, People's Republic of China

Xiu-yun Su
Department of Orthopedics, Affiliated Hospital of the Academy of Military Medical Sciences, No.8 Dongdajie Road, Beijing 100071, People's Republic of China
Department of Orthopedics, Chinese PLA General Hospital, No.28 Fuxing Road, Beijing, Haidian District 100853, People's Republic of China

Malin Andersson and Karl Jägervall
Center for Medical Image Science and Visualization (CMIV), Linköping University, Linköping, Sweden
Department of Radiology and Department of Medical and Health Sciences, Linköping University, Linköping, Sweden

Per Eriksson and Anders Persson
Department of Nephrology and Department of Medical and Health Sciences, Linköping University, Linköping, Sweden

Göran Granerus
Department of Clinical Physiology and Department of Medical and Health Sciences, Linköping University, Linköping, Sweden

Chunliang Wang and Örjan Smedby
School of Technology and Health (STH), KTH Royal Institute of Technology, Stockholm, Sweden
Center for Medical Image Science and Visualization (CMIV), Linköping University, Linköping, Sweden
Department of Radiology and Department of Medical and Health Sciences, Linköping University, Linköping, Sweden

Tarique Hussain, Sarah A. Peel, Israel Valverde, Markus Henningsson, Rene M. Botnar, John Simpson and Gerald F. Greil
Division of Imaging Sciences, King's College London, NIHR Biomedical Research Centre at Guy's & St Thomas' NHS Foundation Trust, London, UK

Karolina Bilska, John Simpson, Israel Valverde and Sujeev Mathur
Department of Paediatric Cardiology, Evelina London Children's Hospital, Guy's & St Thomas' NHS Foundation Trust, Westminster Bridge Road, London, UK

Gerald F. Greil and Tarique Hussain
Department of Pediatrics, UT Southwestern Medical Center, Children's Medical Center, 1935 Medical District Drive, Dallas, TX, USA
Department of Paediatric Cardiology, Evelina London Children's Hospital, Guy's & St Thomas' NHS Foundation Trust, Westminster Bridge Road, London, UK

Zhi-gang Chu, Meng-qi Liu, Fa-jin Lv and Yu Ouyang
Department of Radiology, The First Affiliated Hospital of Chongqing Medical University, 1# Youyi street, Chongqing 400016, China

Zhi-yu Zhu
Department of Stomatology, The First Affiliated Hospital of Chongqing Medical University, 1# Youyi street, Chongqing 400016, China

Thomas Westermaier, Thomas Linsenmann, Mario Loehr, Christian Stetter, Nadine Willner and Ralf-Ingo Ernestus
Department of Neurosurgery, University of Wuerzburg, Josef-Schneider-Str. 11, 97080 Wuerzburg, Germany

Laszlo Solymosi and György A. Homola
Department of Neuroradiology, University of Wuerzburg, Josef-Schneider-Str. 11, 97080 Wuerzburg, Germany

Giles H. Vince
Abteilung für Neurochirurgie, Klinikum Klagenfurt, Feschnigstraße 11, 9020 Klagenfurt am Woerthersee, Austria

Sakon Noriki
Division of Tumor Pathology, Department of Pathological Sciences, School of Medical Sciences, University of Fukui, 23-3 Shimoaizuki, Matsuoka Eiheiji-cho, Yoshida-gun, 910-1193 Fukui, Japan
Autopsy Imaging Center, School of Medical Sciences, University of Fukui, Fukui, Japan

Toyohiko Sakai, Hirohiko Kimura and Kazuyuki Kinoshita
Division of Radiology, Department of Radiology and Laboratory Medicine, School of Medical Sciences, University of Fukui, 23-3 Shimoaizuki, Matsuoka Eiheiji-cho, Yoshida-gun, 910-1193 Fukui, Japan
Autopsy Imaging Center, School of Medical Sciences, University of Fukui, Fukui, Japan

Hironobu Naiki and Kunihiro Inai
Division of Molecular Pathology, Department of Pathological Sciences, School of Medical Sciences, University of Fukui, Fukui, Japan
Autopsy Imaging Center, School of Medical Sciences, University of Fukui, Fukui, Japan

Takahiro Yamauchi
Division of Hematology and Oncology, Faculty of Medical Sciences, University of Fukui, 23-3 Shimoaizuki, Matsuoka Eiheiji-cho, Yoshida-gun, 910-1193 Fukui, Japan

Masayuki Iwano
Division of Nephrology, Department of General Medicine, University of Fukui, 23-3 Shimoaizuki, Matsuoka Eiheiji-cho, Yoshida-gun, 910-1193 Fukui, Japan

H. M. M. T. B. Herath, S. P. Pahalagamage and Sunethra Senanayake
National hospital, Colombo, Sri Lanka

Jamshid Sadiqi, Najibullah Rasouly and Hidayatullah Hamidi
Radiology Department of French Medical Institute for Mothers and Children (FMIC), Kabul, Afghanistan

Salahuddin Siraj
Orthopedic Department of French Medical Institute for Mothers and Children (FMIC), Kabul, Afghanistan

Jamshid Sadiqi
Radiology Department, French Medical Institute for Mothers & Children (FMIC), behind Kabul Medical University Aliabad, Kabul, Afghanistan

Kyu-Chong Lee, Jongmee Lee, Kyeong Ah Kim and Cheol Min Park
Department of Radiology, Korea University Guro Hospital, Korea University College of Medicine, 80 Guro-dong, Guro-gu, Seoul 152-703, South Korea

Baek Hui Kim
Department of Pathology, Korea University Guro Hospital, Korea University College of Medicine, Seoul, South Korea

Yasutoshi Ishihara
School of Science and Technology, Meiji University, Higashimita Tama, Kawasaki, Kanagawa, Japan

Takumi Honma
Graduate School of Science and Technology, Meiji University, Higashimita, Tama, Kawasaki, Kanagawa, Japan

Satoshi Nohara and Yoshio Ito
The Nagoya Research Laboratory, Meito Sangyo Co., Ltd, Kaechi Nishibiwajima, Kiyosu, Aichi, Japan

Margaret M O'Keeffe and Kerry Siminoski
Department of Radiology and Diagnostic Imaging, University of Alberta, and Medical Imaging Consultants, 11010-101 Street, Edmonton, AB T5H 4B9, Canada

Todd M Davis
Intelerad, Montreal, QC, Canada
3295 Midpark Way SE, Suite 380, Calgary, AB T2X 2A8, Canada

Stephen HJ Andrews
Department of Biomedical Engineering, Schulich School of Engineering, University of Calgary, Human Performance Lab, 2500 University Drive NW, Calgary, AB T2N 1N4, Canada

Nigel G Shrive and Janet L Ronsky
Mechanical and Manufacturing Engineering, Schulich School of Engineering, Faculty of Kinesiology, University of Calgary, Calgary, Canada
McCaig Institute for Bone and Joint Health, University of Calgary, Calgary, Canada

Jerome B Rattner and Heather A Jamniczky
Department of Cell Biology and Anatomy, The McCaig Institute for Bone and Joint Health, Faculty of Medicine, University of Calgary, Calgary, Canada

Yingwei Wu, Weiwen Shen and Yushan Du
Radiology Department, East Hospital, Tongji University, school of Medicine, Shanghai 200120, China

Ying Yuan and Xiaofeng Tao
Radiology Department, Shanghai People's Ninth Hospital, Shanghai Jiaotong University, School of Medicine, Shanghai 200011, China

Xiuhui Yue
Radiology Department, Shanghai Changzheng Hospital, Shanghai, China

Cheuk Ying Tang
Radiology Department, Mount Sinai School of Medicine, New York 10029, USA

Christian von Falck, Bernhard Meyer, Frank Wacker and Thomas Rodt
Department of Radiology, Hannover Medical School, Hannover 30625, Germany

Christine Fegbeutel
Department of Cardiothoracic, Transplant and Vascular Surgery, Hannover Medical School, Hannover, Germany

Florian Länger
Institute of Pathology, Hannover Medical School, Hannover, Germany

Frank Bengel
Department of Nuclear Medicine, Hannover Medical School, Hannover, Germany

Ajediran I Bello and Oluwasegun J Alabi
Department of Physiotherapy, School of Allied Health Sciences, College of Health Sciences, University of Ghana, Accra, Ghana

Eric K Ofori
Department of Radiography, School of Allied Health Sciences, College of Health Sciences, University of Ghana, Accra, Ghana

David N Adjei
Department of Medical Laboratory Sciences, School of Allied Health Sciences, College of Health Sciences, University of Ghana, Accra, Ghan

Goran Djuričić, Tijana Radović, Nataša Milčanović and Predrag Djukić
Department of Radiology, University Children's Hospital, Belgrade, School of Medicine, University of Belgrade, Tiršova 10, 11000 Belgrade, Republic of Serbia

Marko Radulovic and Zorica Milošević
Institute of Oncology and Radiology of Serbia, School of Medicine, University of Belgrade, Pasterova 14, 11000 Belgrade, Republic of Serbia

Jelena Sopta
Institute of Pathology, School of Medicine, University of Belgrade, Dr Subotica 1, 11000 Belgrade, Republic of Serbia

Elin Trägårdh, Sven Valind and Lars Edenbrandt
Clinical Physiology and Nuclear Medicine Unit, Skåne University Hospital, Lund University, Entrance 44, 205 05 Malmö, Sweden

Sumeyra U Demir, Roya Hakimzadeh and Eric V Myer
Signal Processing Technologies LLC, Richmond, VA, USA

Rosalyn Hobson Hargraves
Department of Electrical Engineering, Virginia Commonwealth University, Richmond, VA, USA
Signal Processing Technologies LLC, Richmond, VA, USA

Kayvan Najarian
Department of Emergency Medicine, Virginia Commonwealth University, Richmond, VA, USA
Signal Processing Technologies LLC, Richmond, VA, USA
Virginia Commonwealth University Reanimation Engineering Science (VCURES), Richmond, VA, USA
Department of Computer Science, Virginia Commonwealth University, Richmond, VA, USA

Kevin R Ward
Department of Computer Science, Virginia Commonwealth University, Richmond, VA, USA
Department of Emergency Medicine, Michigan Center for Integrative Research in Critical Care, University of Michigan, Ann Arbor, MI, USA
Signal Processing Technologies LLC, Richmond, VA, USA

Alexander C Flint
Interconnect Medical, LLC, Menlo Park, CA 94025, USA

Gavin S Tan
Singapore National Eye Centre (SNEC), 11 Third Hospital Avenue, Singapore 168751, Singapore
Singapore Eye Research Institute (SERI), 11 Third Hospital Ave, Singapore 168751, Singapore

Donald T Tan
Singapore National Eye Centre (SNEC), 11 Third Hospital Avenue, Singapore 168751, Singapore
Singapore Eye Research Institute (SERI), 11 Third Hospital Ave, Singapore 168751, Singapore
Yong Loo Lin School of Medicine, National University of Singapore, 1E Kent Ridge Road, Singapore, Singapore

Jodhbir S Mehta
Singapore National Eye Centre (SNEC), 11 Third Hospital Avenue, Singapore 168751, Singapore
Singapore Eye Research Institute (SERI), 11 Third Hospital Ave, Singapore 168751, Singapore
Yong Loo Lin School of Medicine, National University of Singapore, 1E Kent Ridge Road, Singapore, Singapore
Department of Clinical Sciences, Duke-NUS Graduate Medical School, 8 College Rd, Singapore 169857, Singapore

Mingguang He
Zhongshan Ophthalmic Centre, Guangzhou, China

Mohammad-Reza Nazem-Zadeh
Department of Radiation Oncology and Radiology, University of Michigan, Ann Arbor, MI 48109-0010, USA
Control and Intelligent Processing Center of Excellence, School of Electrical and Computer Engineering, University of Tehran, Tehran 14399, Iran
Department of Neurology, Henry Ford Health System, Detroit, MI 48202, USA

Quan Jiang
Department of Neurology, Henry Ford Health System, Detroit, MI 48202, USA

Sona Saksena
Department of Radiology, Henry Ford Health System, Detroit MI 48202, USA

Mark Rosenblum
Washington University School of Medicine, Mallinckrodt Institute of Radiology, St. Louis MO 63110, USA
Department of Radiology, Henry Ford Health System, Detroit MI 48202, USA

Abbas Babajani-Fermi
Washington University School of Medicine, Mallinckrodt Institute of Radiology, St. Louis MO 63110, USA

Hamid Soltanian-Zadeh
Department of Radiology, Wayne State University, Detroit, MI 48202, USA
Department of Radiology, Henry Ford Health System, Detroit MI 48202, USA
Control and Intelligent Processing Center of Excellence, School of Electrical and Computer Engineering, University of Tehran, Tehran 14399, Iran

Tom Mikkelsen
Department of Neurosurgery, Henry Ford Health System, Detroit, MI 48202, USA

Rajan Jain
Department of Neurosurgery, Henry Ford Health System, Detroit, MI 48202, USA
Control and Intelligent Processing Center of Excellence, School of Electrical and Computer Engineering, University of Tehran, Tehran 14399, Iran
Department of Radiology, Henry Ford Health System, Detroit MI 48202, USA

Index

www.ingramcontent.com/pod-product-compliance
Lightning Source LLC
Chambersburg PA
CBHW08203519032B
41458CB00010B/3375